Food Biofortification Technologies

Contemporary Food Engineering

Series Editor

Professor Da-Wen Sun, Director

Food Refrigeration & Computerized Food Technology

National University of Ireland, Dublin

(University College Dublin) Dublin, Ireland http://www.ucd.ie/sun/

Food Biofortification Technologies, *edited by Agnieszka Agnieszka* (2017)

Trends in Fish Processing Technologies, *edited by Daniela Borda, Anca I. Nicolau, and Peter Raspor* (2017)

High Pressure Processing of Fruit and Vegetable Juices, *edited by Milan Houška and Filipa Vinagre Marques da Silva* (2017)

Advances in Meat Processing Technology, by *Alaa El-Din A. Bekhit* (2017)

Advances in Postharvest Fruit and Vegetable Technology, *edited by Ron B.H. Wills and John Golding* (2017)

Food Nanotechnology: Principles and Applications, *edited by C. Anandharamakrishnan and S. Parthasarathi* (2017)

Engineering Aspects of Food Emulsification and Homogenization, *edited by Marilyn Rayner and Petr Dejmek* (2017)

Engineering Aspects of Food Biotechnology, *edited by Jose A. Teixeira and Antonio A. Vicente* (2017)

Edible Oils: Extraction, Processing, and Applications, *edited by Smain Chemat* (2017)

Engineering Aspects of Membrane Separation and Application in Food Processing, *edited by Robert W. Field, Erika Bekassy-Molnar, Frank Lipnizki, and Gyula Vatai* (2017)

Advances in Fruit Processing Technologies, *edited by Sueli Rodrigues and Fabiano Andre Narciso Fernandes* (2016)

Thermal Food Processing: New Technologies and Quality Issues, Second Edition, *edited by Da-Wen Sun* (2016)

Enhancing Extraction Processes in the Food Industry, *edited by Nikolai Lebovka, Eugene Vorobiev, and Farid Chemat* (2016)

Engineering Aspects of Cereal and Cereal-Based Products, *edited by Raquel de Pinho Ferreira Guine, and Paula Maria dos Reis Correia* (2016)

Fermentation Processes Engineering in the Food Industry, *edited by Carlos Ricardo Soccol, Ashok Pandey, and Christian Larroche* (2016)

Physical Properties of Foods: Novel Measurement Techniques and Applications, *edited by Ignacio Arana* (2016)

Juice Processing: Quality, Safety and Value-Added Opportunities, *edited by Victor Falguera and Albert Ibarz* (2016)

Modified Atmosphere and Active Packaging Technologies, *edited by Ioannis Arvanitoyannis* (2016)

Advances in Food Extrusion Technology, *edited by Medeni Maskan and Aylin Altan* (2016)

Operations in Food Refrigeration, *edited by Rodolfo H. Mascheroni* (2016)

Emerging Technologies for Food Quality and Food Safety Evaluation, *edited by Yong-Jin Cho and Sukwon Kang* (2016)

Advances in Technologies for Producing Food-relevant Polyphenols, *edited by Jose Cuevas Valenzuela, Jose Rodrigo Vergara-Salinas, and Jose Ricardo Perez-Correa* (2016)

Advances in Heat Transfer Unit Operations: Baking and Freezing in Bread Making, *edited by Georgina Calderón-Domínguez, Gustavo F. Gutiérrez-López, and Keshavan Niranjan* (2016)

Innovative Processing Technologies for Foods with Bioactive Compounds, *edited by Jorge J. Moreno* (2016)

Light Scattering Technology for Food Property, Quality and Safety Assessment, *edited by Renfu Lu* (2016)

Edible Food Packaging: Materials and Processing Technologies, *edited by Miquel Angelo Parente Ribeiro Cerqueira, Ricardo Nuno Correia Pereira, Oscar Leandro da Silva Ramos, Jose Antonio Couto Teixeira, and Antonio Augusto Vicente* (2016)

Handbook of Food Processing: Food Preservation, *edited by Theodoros Varzakas and Constantina Tzia* (2015)

Handbook of Food Processing: Food Safety, Quality, and Manufacturing Processes, *edited by Theodoros Varzakas and Constantina Tzia* (2015)

Advances in Postharvest Fruit and Vegetable Technology, *edited by Ron B. H. Wills and John Golding* (2015)

Engineering Aspects of Food Emulsification and Homogenization, *edited by Marilyn Rayner and Petr Dejmek* (2015)

Handbook of Food Processing and Engineering, Volume II: Food Process Engineering, *edited by Theodoros Varzakas and Constantina Tzia* (2014)

Handbook of Food Processing and Engineering, Volume I: Food Engineering Fundamentals, *edited by Theodoros Varzakas and Constantina Tzia* (2014)

Juice Processing: Quality, Safety and Value-Added Opportunities, *edited by Víctor Falguera and Albert Ibarz* (2014)

Engineering Aspects of Food Biotechnology, *edited by José A. Teixeiraand António A. Vicente* (2013)

Engineering Aspects of Cereal and Cereal-Based Products, *edited by Raquel de Pinho Ferreira Guiné and Paula Maria dos Reis Correia* (2013)

Fermentation Processes Engineering in the Food Industry, *edited by Carlos Ricardo Soccol, Ashok Pandey, and Christian Larroche* (2013)

Modified Atmosphere and Active Packaging Technologies, *edited by Ioannis Arvanitoyannis* (2012)

Advances in Fruit Processing Technologies, *edited by Sueli Rodrigues and Fabiano Andre Narciso Fernandes* (2012)

Biopolymer Engineering in Food Processing, *edited by Vânia Regina Nicoletti Telis* (2012)

Operations in Food Refrigeration, *edited by Rodolfo H. Mascheroni* (2012)

Thermal Food Processing: New Technologies and Quality Issues, Second Edition, *edited by Da-Wen Sun* (2012)

Physical Properties of Foods: Novel Measurement Techniques and Applications, *edited by Ignacio Arana* (2012)

Handbook of Frozen Food Processing and Packaging, Second Edition, *edited by Da-Wen Sun* (2011)

Advances in Food Extrusion Technology, *edited by Medeni Maskan and Aylin Altan* (2011)

Enhancing Extraction Processes in the Food Industry, *edited by Nikolai Lebovka, Eugene Vorobiev, and Farid Chemat* (2011)

Emerging Technologies for Food Quality and Food Safety Evaluation, *edited by Yong-Jin Cho and Sukwon Kang* (2011)

Food Process Engineering Operations, *edited by George D. Saravacos and Zacharias B. Maroulis* (2011)

Biosensors in Food Processing, Safety, and Quality Control, *edited by Mehmet Mutlu* (2011)

Physicochemical Aspects of Food Engineering and Processing, *edited by Sakamon Devahastin* (2010)

Infrared Heating for Food and Agricultural Processing, *edited by Zhongli Pan and Griffiths Gregory Atungulu* (2010)

Mathematical Modeling of Food Processing, *edited by Mohammed M. Farid* (2009)

Engineering Aspects of Milk and Dairy Products, *edited by Jane Sélia dos Reis Coimbra and José A. Teixeira* (2009)

Innovation in Food Engineering: New Techniques and Products, *edited by Maria Laura Passos and Claudio P. Ribeiro* (2009)

Processing Effects on Safety and Quality of Foods, *edited by Enrique Ortega-Rivas* (2009)

Engineering Aspects of Thermal Food Processing, *edited by Ricardo Simpson* (2009)

Ultraviolet Light in Food Technology: Principles and Applications, *Tatiana N. Koutchma, Larry J. Forney, and Carmen I. Moraru* (2009)

Advances in Deep-Fat Frying of Foods, *edited by Serpil Sahin and Servet Gülüm Sumnu* (2009)

Extracting Bioactive Compounds for Food Products: Theory and Applications, *edited by M. Angela A. Meireles* (2009)

Advances in Food Dehydration, *edited by Cristina Ratti* (2009)

Optimization in Food Engineering, *edited by Ferruh Erdoˇgdu* (2009)

Optical Monitoring of Fresh and Processed Agricultural Crops, *edited by Manuela Zude* (2009)

Food Engineering Aspects of Baking Sweet Goods, *edited by Servet Gülüm Sumnu and Serpil Sahin* (2008)

Computational Fluid Dynamics in Food Processing, *edited by Da-Wen Sun* (2007)

Food Biofortification Technologies

Edited by
Agnieszka Saeid
Department of Chemistry
Department of Advanced Materials Technologies
Wrocław University of Science and Technology
Poland

CRC Press
Taylor & Francis Group
Boca Raton London New York

CRC Press is an imprint of the
Taylor & Francis Group, an **informa** business

CRC Press
Taylor & Francis Group
6000 Broken Sound Parkway NW, Suite 300
Boca Raton, FL 33487-2742

Printed on acid-free paper
International Standard Book Number-13: 978-1-4987-5659-4 (Hardback)

Visit the Taylor & Francis Web site at
http://www.taylorandfrancis.com

and the CRC Press Web site at
http://www.crcpress.com

Contents

Series Preface

Contemporary Food Engineering

Food engineering is the multidisciplinary field of applied physical sciences combined with the knowledge of product properties. Food engineers provide the technological knowledge transfer essential to the cost-effective production and commercialization of food products and services. In particular, food engineers develop and design processes and equipment to convert raw agricultural materials and ingredients into safe, convenient, and nutritious consumer food products. However, food engineering topics are continuously undergoing changes to meet diverse consumer demands, and the subject is developing rapidly to reflect market needs.

One of the many challenges in the development of food engineering is to employ modern tools and knowledge, such as computational materials science and nanotechnology, to develop new products and processes. Simultaneously, improving food quality, safety, and security continue to be critical issues in food engineering studies. New packaging materials and techniques are being developed to provide more protection to foods, and novel preservation technologies are emerging to enhance food security and defense. In addition, process control and automation regularly appear among the top priorities identified in food engineering. Advanced monitoring and control systems are developed to facilitate automation and flexible food manufacturing processes. Furthermore, energy-saving and minimization of environmental problems continue to be important food engineering issues, and significant progress is being made in waste management, efficient utilization of energy, and reduction of effluents and emissions in food production.

The *Contemporary Food Engineering* series, consisting of edited books, attempts to address some of the recent developments in food engineering. The series covers advances in classical unit operations in engineering applied to food manufacturing as well as topics such as progress in the transport and storage of liquid and solid foods; heating, chilling, and freezing of foods; mass transfer in foods; chemical and biochemical aspects of food engineering and the use of kinetic analysis; dehydration, thermal processing, non-thermal processing, extrusion, liquid food concentration, membrane processes, and applications of membranes in food processing; shelf-life and electronic indicators in inventory management; sustainable technologies in food processing; and packaging, cleaning, and sanitation. These books are aimed at professional food scientists, academics researching food engineering problems, and graduate-level students.

The editors of these books are leading engineers and scientists from different parts of the world. All the editors were asked to present their books to address the market's needs and pinpoint cutting-edge technologies in food engineering.

All contributions are written by internationally renowned experts who have both academic and professional credentials. All authors have attempted to provide critical, comprehensive, and readily accessible information on the art and science of a relevant topic in each chapter, with reference lists for further information.

Therefore, each book can serve as an essential reference source to students and researchers in universities and research institutions.

Da-Wen Sun
Series Editor

Preface

Malnutrition or *hidden hunger* can be a symptom of too low an intake of nutrients, which is a common phenomenon in developed countries even if the amount of digested food and delivered calories is more than required. Some reports suggest that approximately 50% of the world's population are afflicted with micronutrient deficiency of iron, zinc, calcium, iodine, and selenium. A proper balance of micronutrients is crucial to the proper growth and development of crops, animals, and humans. The intensity of agricultural production coupled with improper fertilization is causing ever greater soil impoverishment with every vegetation season.

There are three ways to alleviate malnutrition resulting from the lack of micronutrients:

1. Direct nutrient supplementation
2. Dietary modification and diversification
3. Indirect interventions, such as biofortification

For many decades, agricultural production has been facing the problem of low-quality plant and animal produce. Adding exogenous nutrients to foodstuffs can increase the latter's nutrient content, but such practices are restricted due to the limited stability of additives and their negative impact on food quality.

Dietary modification and diversification can barely be implemented in developing countries and does not always bring the desired results. Biofortification, which can be defined as the process of increasing the content/density of essential nutrients and/or its bioavailability of food with valuable compounds, is a promising means of increasing nutrient intakes. The *designer food* with higher content of nutrients can be obtained as a result of genetic modification, the classical breeding with modified fodder, and by the agronomic pathway. Genetic biofortification involves either genetic engineering or classical plant breeding. Modern plant breeding has been oriented toward achieving high agricultural yields rather than nutritional quality; additionally, this approach to overcoming micronutrient deficiencies is related to certain ethical problems and hence negative social attitudes.

The production of biofortified foodstuffs can be ensured through the proper supplementation of nutrients in the animal diet as well as the application of the designed fertilization in agriculture. The fastest and simplest solution seems to be the combined fertilization strategy that will ensure the proper level of phytoavailability of mineral micronutrients in the soil. Products obtained with an increased amount of nutrients applied in animal feeding will result in a higher density of microelements in the animal products such as milk, meat, and eggs. Developing a new generation of feed additives with balanced fertilization could help in the elaboration of new designer food products that will support the treatment of such disorders as anemia or other nutrient deficiencies. This approach allows for the production of food components (e.g., animal food products, such as farmed fish, beef, pork, lamb, chicken, eggs, and milk fortified with microelements, vitamins, or fatty acids, as well as plant products, such as maize) that are rich in nutrients.

This book deals with fortification methods and agricultural treatments that can improve the quality of food products or other agricultural compounds, providing them with a higher density of valuable nutrients. The utilization of novel products, such as feed additives and fertilizers, can avert nutrient depletion in food products. We describe new and conventional methods of introducing valuable compounds into food components and present the application of biosorption, bioaccumulation, and utilization of fertilizers in obtaining designer food. Attention is paid to the use of biomass as a carrier of nutrients, such as microelements, into the food components. The chapters are dedicated to specific food products and their nutrient components. The first chapter discusses the agronomic biofortification with micronutrients where the fertilization strategies are pointed out as a key to plant/cereal fortification. Other chapters present the fortification of animal foodstuffs such as meat, fish, milk, and eggs, in addition to the fortification of plant foodstuffs such as vegetables, fruits, and cereals. We also explore advances in food fortification with vitamins and co-vitamins, essential minerals, essential fatty and amino acids, phytonutrients, and enzymes.

Agnieszka Saeid
Wrocław University of Technology
Wrocław, Poland

Series Editor

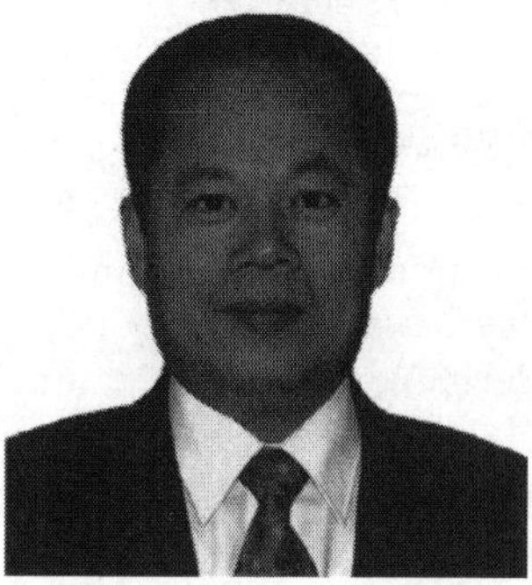

Prof. Da-Wen Sun, born in southern China, is a global authority in food engineering research and education; he is a member of the Royal Irish Academy (RIA), which is the highest academic honor in Ireland; he is also a member of Academia Europaea (The Academy of Europe) and a fellow of the International Academy of Food Science and Technology. He has contributed significantly to the field of food engineering as a researcher, academic authority, and educator.

His main research activities include cooling, drying, and refrigeration processes and systems, quality and safety of food products, bioprocess simulation and optimization, and computer vision/image processing and hyperspectral imaging technologies. His many scholarly works have become standard reference materials for researchers, especially in the areas of computer vision, computational fluid dynamics modeling, vacuum cooling, and related subjects. Results of his work have been published in over 800 papers, including more than 390 peer-reviewed journal-papers (Web of Science h-index = 62). He has also edited 14 authoritative books. According to Thomson Scientific's *Essential Science Indicators* SM, based on data derived over a period of 10 years from Web of Science, there are about 4,500 scientists who are among the top 1% of the most cited scientists in the category of agriculture sciences; for many years, Professor Sun has consistently been ranked among the top 50 scientists in the world (he was at 25th position in March 2015, and at 1st position if ranking is based on "Hot Papers," and in 2nd position if ranking is based on "Top Papers" or "Highly Cited Papers").

He received a first class BSc honors and MSc in mechanical engineering, and a PhD in chemical engineering in China before working in various universities in Europe. He became the first Chinese national to be permanently employed in an Irish university when he was appointed college lecturer at the National University of Ireland, Dublin (University

College Dublin, UCD), in 1995, and was then progressively promoted in the shortest possible time to senior lecturer, associate professor, and full professor. Dr. Sun is now a professor of food and biosystems engineering and the director of the UCD Food Refrigeration and Computerized Food Technology Research Group.

As a leading educator in food engineering, Professor Sun has trained many PhD students, who have made their own contributions to the industry and academia. He has also frequently delivered lectures on advances in food engineering at academic institutions worldwide, and delivered keynote speeches at international conferences. As a recognized authority in food engineering, he has been conferred adjunct/visiting/consulting professorships from 10 top universities in China, including Zhejiang University, Shanghai Jiaotong University, Harbin Institute of Technology, China Agricultural University, South China University of Technology, and Jiangnan University. In recognition of his significant contribution to food engineering worldwide and for his outstanding leadership in the field, the International Commission of Agricultural and Biosystems Engineering (CIGR) awarded him the "CIGR Merit Award" in 2000, and again in 2006, the Institution of Mechanical Engineers based in the United Kingdom named him "Food Engineer of the Year 2004." In 2008, he was awarded the "CIGR Recognition Award" in honor of his distinguished achievements as one of the top 1% among agricultural engineering scientists in the world. In 2007, he was presented with the only "AFST(I) Fellow Award" given in that year by the Association of Food Scientists and Technologists (India), and in 2010, he was presented with the "CIGR Fellow Award"; the title of Fellow is the highest honor at CIGR and is conferred to individuals who have made sustained, outstanding contributions worldwide. In March 2013, he was presented with the "You Bring Charm to the World" Award by Hong Kong-based Phoenix Satellite Television with other award recipients including the 2012 Nobel Laureate in Literature and the Chinese Astronaut Team for Shenzhou IX Spaceship. In July 2013, he received the "Frozen Food Foundation Freezing Research Award" from the International Association for Food Protection (IAFP) for his significant contributions to enhancing the field of food-freezing technologies. This is the first time that this prestigious award was presented to a scientist outside the United States.

He is a fellow of the Institution of Agricultural Engineers and a fellow of Engineers Ireland (the Institution of Engineers of Ireland). He is editor-in-chief of *Food and Bioprocess Technology—An International Journal* (2012 Impact Factor = 4.115), former editor of *Journal of Food Engineering* (Elsevier), and a member of the editorial boards for a number of international journals, including the *Journal of Food Process Engineering, Journal of Food Measurement and Characterization,* and *Polish Journal of Food and Nutritional Sciences.* He is also a chartered engineer.

On May 28, 2010, he was awarded membership in the RIA, which is the highest honor that can be attained by scholars and scientists working in Ireland. At the 51st CIGR General Assembly held during the CIGR World Congress in Quebec City, Canada, on June 13–17, 2010, he was elected incoming president of CIGR, became CIGR president in 2013–2014, and is now CIGR past president. On September 20, 2011, he was elected to Academia Europaea (The Academy of Europe), which is functioning as the European Academy of Humanities, Letters and Sciences, and is one of the most prestigious academies in the world; election to the Academia Europaea represents the highest academic distinction.

Contributors

Angel Antonio Carbonell Barrachina
Department Agro-food Technology
Universidad Miguel Hernandez de Elche
Elche, Alicante, Spain

Katarzyna Chojnacka
Department of Advanced Material Technologies
Faculty of Chemistry
Wrocław University of Science and Technology
Wrocław, Poland

Grażyna Czyżak-Runowska
Poznan University of Life Sciences
Poznan, Poland

Ankit Goyal
Mansinhbhai Institute of Dairy and Food Technology
Mehsana, Gujarat, India

Magdalena Jastrzębska
Department of Agroecosystems
Faculty of Environmental Management and Agriculture
University of Warmia and Mazury in Olsztyn
Olsztyn, Poland

Damian Konkol
Department of Environmental Hygiene and Animal Welfare
Wrocław University of Environmental and Life Sciences
Wrocław, Poland

Mariusz Korczyński
Department of Environmental Hygiene and Animal Welfare
Wrocław University of Environmental and Life Sciences
Wrocław, Poland

Malgorzata Korzeniowska
Department of Animal Products Technology and Quality Management
Wrocław University of Environmental and Life Sciences
Wrocław, Poland

Robert Kupczyński
Department of Environmental Hygiene and Animal Welfare
Wrocław University of Environmental and Life Sciences
Wrocław, Poland

Bogusława Łęska
Faculty of Chemistry
Adam Mickiewicz University in Poznan
Poznan, Poland

Izabela Michalak
Department of Advanced Material Technologies
Faculty of Chemistry
Wrocław University of Science and Technology
Wrocław, Poland

Sebastian Opaliński
Department of Environmental Hygiene and Animal Welfare
Wrocław University of Environmental and Life Sciences
Wrocław, Poland

Ami Patel
Mansinhbhai Institute of Dairy and Food Technology
Mehsana, Gujarat, India

Agnieszka Saeid
Department of Advanced Material Technologies
Faculty of Chemistry
Wrocław University of Science and Technology
Wrocław, Poland

Mateusz Samoraj
Department of Advanced Material Technologies
Faculty of Chemistry
Wrocław University of Science and Technology
Wrocław, Poland

Nihir Shah
Mansinhbhai Institute of Dairy and Food Technology
Mehsana, Gujarat, India

Manvesh Sihag
Mansinhbhai Institute of Dairy and Food Technology
Mehsana, Gujarat, India

D. Suresh Kumar
Cymbio Pharma Private Limited
Industrial Suburb
Yeshwanthpur, Bangalore, India

Marita Świniarska
Department of Environmental Hygiene and Animal Welfare
Wrocław University of Environmental and Life Sciences
Wrocław, Poland

Beenu Tanwar
Mansinhbhai Institute of Dairy and Food Technology
Mehsana, Gujarat, India

Łukasz Tuhy
Department of Advanced Material Technologies
Faculty of Chemistry
Wrocław University of Science and Technology
Wrocław, Poland

Aneta Wojdylo
Department of Fruit and Vegetables Technology and Plant Nutraceuticals
Wrocław University of Environmental and Life Sciences
Wrocław, Poland

chapter one

Agronomic biofortification as a key to plant/cereal fortification in micronutrients

Agnieszka Saeid and Magdalena Jastrzębska

Contents

1.1 Introduction

Agronomic biofortification through fertilization (its application to soils, seeds, and/or leaves) helps to increase plant nutrient content without changing the plant's genetic makeup (Figure 1.1) (Almendros et al., 2015). Agronomic biofortification provides an immediate and effective route to enhancing micronutrient concentrations in edible crop products, although genetic biofortification may be more cost effective in the long run (de Valença et al., 2017).

Soil deficiency is reflected in the poor nutrients composition of crops. This problem is aggravated by growing cereal crops on soils potentially deficient in nutrients. Nutrient deficiency in humans is seen mainly in regions where soils have this deficiency problem and cereals are a major source of daily calorie intake (Bilski et al., 2012). Agricultural intervention to improve production of micronutrient-rich foods is one of the priority areas for research and an effective strategy compared to supplementation and food diversification (Żuk-Gołaszewska et al., 2016; Pandey et al., 2016). The agronomic biofortification of cereal crops appears to be a rapid and simple solution to the deficiency of these elements in soils and plants. Care should be exercised not to overfertilize crops with micronutrients because of consequent toxicity and losses in quality and quantity of grain yield (Rengel et al., 1999). The potential of agronomic fortification is strongly related with micronutrient bioavailability at three stages: from soil to plant, form plant/crop to food, and from food to humans. The losses of micronutrients occur at many stages, for example as an effect of nutrient and other components interaction in soil as well as in the plant or human body (de Valença et al., 2017). Agronomic biofortification can increase both yields and the nutritional quality of staple crops. Micronutrient fertilization is most effective in combination with NPK, organic fertilizers, and improved crop varieties, highlighting the importance of integrated soil fertility management.

The soil-plant system is instrumental to human nutrition and forms the basis of the food chain in which there is micronutrient cycling, resulting in an ecologically sound and sustainable flow of micronutrients. Developing special micronutrient fertilizers and integrated nutrient management technologies for increasing both the density of the micronutrients in the edible parts of plants and their bioavailability to humans is crucial (Yang et al., 2007).

1.2 Forms of fertilizer

The simplest way to increase the density of mineral elements in edible crops is enhancement of the availability of nutrients delivered through fertilization, so that plants can uptake the nutrient from soil in a more

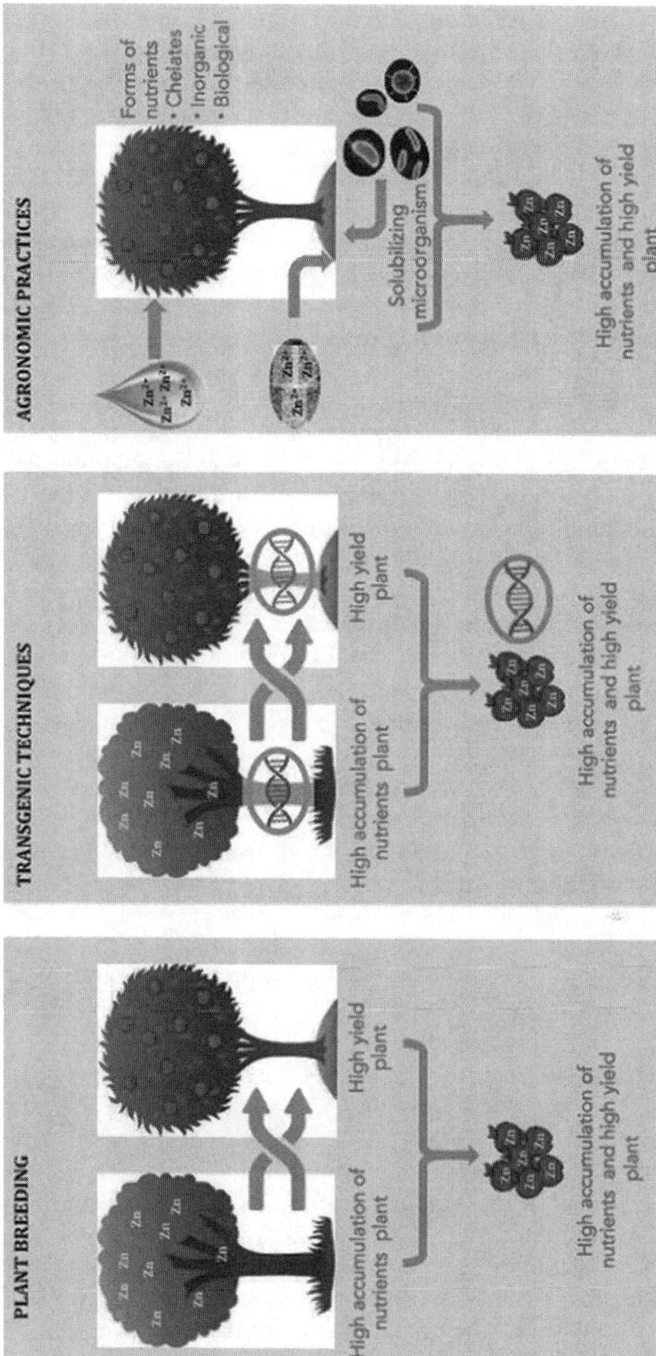

Figure 1.1 Three strategies for biofortification.

efficient way (Almendros et al., 2015). The kind of nutrients source and soil characteristics have a great influence on agronomic biofortification in plants and therefore also on the quality and plant biomass of the crop. Soils differ greatly in their mineral composition and nutrients' phytoavailability depends on several factors (Pinto and Ferreira, 2015) such as pH, water holding capacity, cation exchange capacity of soil, specific surface area, surface charge density, as well as cation-exchange capacity.

The bioavailability of micronutrients used in fertilization is mostly defined by the form of delivered macronutrient, as the form of the nutrients and interactions between them can have positive as well as neutral or even negative effects on yields and nutrient use efficiencies (Saha et al., 2015; Rietra et al., 2015).

By applying nutrients into the soil we can expect an increase of their content in the plant tissues, but the size of this increase depends on the fertilizers applied and their availability, which is essentially governed by the adsorption–desorption characteristics of soils (Dai et al., 2009). Several critical factors determine the availability of nutrients from fertilizers. A large number of diverse materials can serve as sources of plant nutrients. These can be natural, synthetic, recycled wastes, or a range of biological products including microbial inoculants. Figure 1.2 presents the four main groups of forms of nutrients that can be delivered into the soil during fertilization.

1.2.1 *Inorganic fertilizers*

With rising expectations toward agricultural production, the importance of micronutrient fertilization has increased over the years. Soil supplies that are insufficient to meet increased crop requirements are especially important for several microelements since they affect both crop yields and produce quality. Increasingly, micronutrients have become yield-limiting factors and are partly responsible for decreasing the efficiency of NPK fertilizers. Therefore, standard NPK-based fertilization must often be supplemented by the deficient micronutrients. Table 1.1 collects inorganic form of nutrients that are commonly used if micronutrient fertilization by adding to the NPK fertilizers.

Application of microelement fertilizers in the form of inorganic salts is the most common procedure within the agronomic biofortification practice. It brings good results that are strongly related to the kind of supplemented micronutrient and the chemical properties of fertilized soil. Zinc sulfate ($ZnSO_4{\cdot}7H_2O$) and copper sulfate ($CuSO_4{\cdot}5H_2O$) are the most tested fertilizers, since Zn and Fe are of mainly deficiency concerns (Rosado et al., 2009) among the others that are essential elements: Fe, Zn, Se, I, Cu, Ca, and Mg (Zhao and McGrath, 2009). Their application results

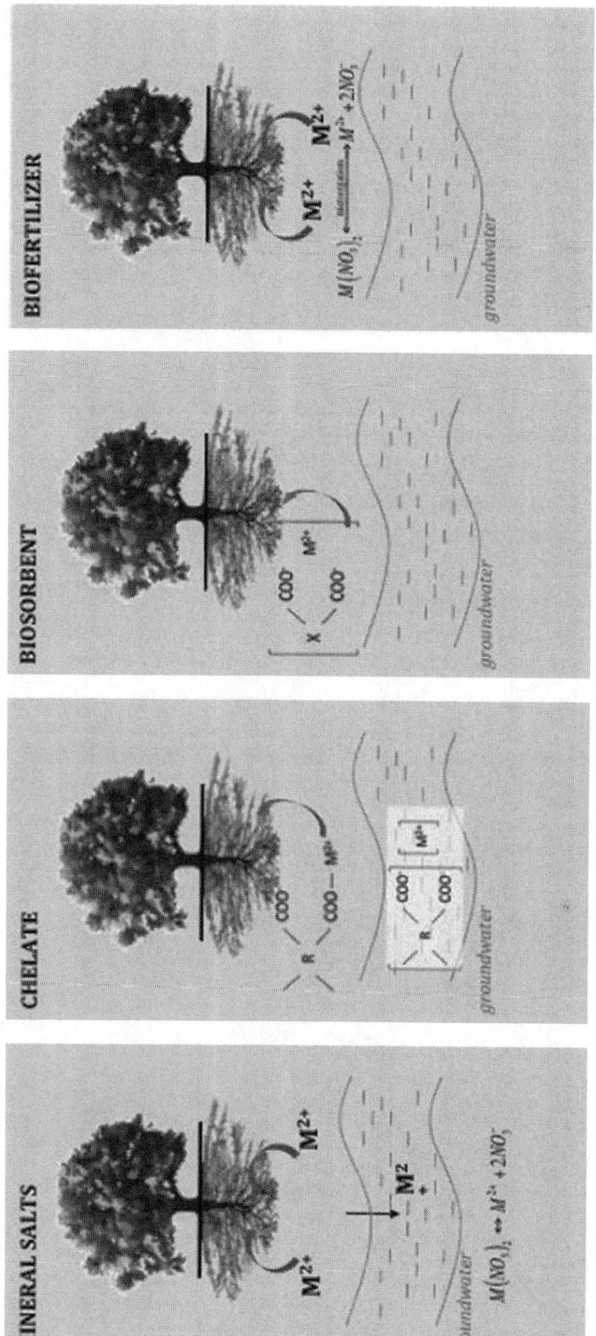

Figure 1.2 Mechanism of uptake of micronutrient ions from the soil by plants. (Modified from Tuhy, L. et al., *Open Chemistry*, 13, 1119–1126, 2012.)

Table 1.1 Inorganic form of nutrients used nowadays by adding to NPK fertilizers

No.	Nutrient	Salt	Form	Content %
1.	B	Sodium tetraborate or borax	$Na_2B_4O_7{\cdot}10H_2O$	10.5
		Boric acid	H_3BO_3	17
		Solubor	$Na_2B_4O_7{\cdot}5H_2O$ + $Na_2B_{10}O_{16}{\cdot}10H_2O$	19
		Boron frits		Variable B content
2.	Cl	Potassium chloride	KCl	47
		NP/NPK complexes in which KCl	KCl	
		Sodium chloride	NaCl	60
		Ammonium chloride	NH_4Cl	66
3.	Cu	Copper sulfate	$CuSO_4{\cdot}5H_2O$	24
		Copper sulfate	$CuSO_4{\cdot}H_2O$	35
		Copper oxychloride		
		Metallic oxide and silicate		
4.	Fe	Ferrous sulfate	$FeSO_4{\cdot}7H_2O$	19–21
		Ferrous ammonium sulfate	$(NH_4)_2SO_4{\cdot}FeSO_4{\cdot}6H_2O$	16
		Ferrous ammonium phosphate	$Fe(NH_4)PO_4{\cdot}H_2O$	29
		Ferric sulfate	$Fe(SO_4)_3{\cdot}4H_2O$	23
5.	Mn	Manganese sulfate	$MnSO_4{\cdot}H_2O$	30.5
		Manganese oxide	MnO	41–68
		Manganese frits		10–35
		Manganese oxides		Variable Mn content
		Manganese carbonate		
		Manganese phosphate		
6.	Mo	Sodium molybdate	$Na_2MoO_4{\cdot}2H_2O$	40
		Ammonium molybdate	$[(NH_4)_6Mo_7O_{24}{\cdot}4H_2O]$	54
		Molybdenum oxide	MoO_3	66
		Molybdenum frits		

(*Continued*)

Table 1.1 (Continued) Inorganic form of nutrients used nowadays by adding to NPK fertilizers

No.	Nutrient	Salt	Form	Content %
7.	Zn	Zinc sulfates	$ZnSO_4{\cdot}7H_2O$	21
			$ZnSO_4{\cdot}zH_2O$	33
		Chelate	Zn-EDTA	12
		Zinc oxide	ZnO	55
		Zinc frits		Variable Zn content
8.	Co	Cobalt sulfate	$CoSO_4$	21

Source: Jones, J. B., *Plant Nutrition Manual*, Boca Raton, CRC Press, 1997; Roy, R. N. et al., In: *Sources of Plant Nutrients and Soil Amendments. Ferilizer and Plant Nutrition Biuletin*, Italy, Food and Agriculture Organization of the United Nations, 2006.

in higher density in harvested plants but lower than in the case of chelates (Liu et al., 2015).

A modification that could improve the effectiveness of inorganic microelement fertilizers would be their simultaneous use in soil and foliar application. It was proven that Zn applied at 25.0 kg $ZnSO_4$; $7H_2O$/ha through soil and 2 foliar sprays of 0.5% solution of $ZnSO_4$; $7H_2O$ significantly increased Zn content in the harvested grains and straws/stalks (Saha et al., 2015). Similar findings were described also for field peas (Poblaciones and Rengel, 2016) and *B. oleracea* (Barrameda-Medina et al., 2017). It can be recognized that inorganic fertilizers yielded better results when foliar was applied or used in the fertigation (Smoleń and Sady, 2012) as compared to pre-sowing soil fertilization. The methods of application are described in detail in this chapter (see Section 3.1 Methods of Application). Another interesting approach for the biofortification is the use of inorganic salt to obtain a new formulation, as in the case of Se-enriched peat. The peat was enriched by thoroughly mixing it with a solution of sodium selenite and then applied during the pre-transplanting stage (Businelli et al., 2015).

1.2.2 Organic fertilizers

Organic fertilizers were the source of micronutrient for plants long before they began to be applied in their mineral form. In early agricultural societies, it was observed that crop yields could be increased by adding animal manure or plant debris to soil. A new study reveals that Neolithic farmers used livestock manure to enhance crop yields (Bogaard et al., 2013). We continue this practice today with regular additions of organic matter (from different sources), which is used mainly in organic and integrated farming systems (Kizos et al., 2010).

Organic fertilizers are materials whose basic ingredient is organic matter (Adegoke et al., 2016). They traditionally derived from animal excreta (livestock manure, slurry, poultry feces) and vegetable matter (compost, straw, green manures). Naturally occurring organic fertilizers include peat, seaweed, and guano (Hazra, 2016). Recently, municipal and industrial wastes were taken into account as organic renewable resources of plant nutrients (Schulz and Rornheld, 1997). The most important organic materials that accumulate in industrial countries and which could be used as secondary fertilizers are sewage sludge, and increasingly in the last few years bio-compost and by-products from the food and foodstuff industry. Organic waste from the food and luxury item industries (i.e., by-products from the processing of agricultural products) can also be utilized in agricultural production; for example, from breweries (yeast, brewer's grain, diatomaceous marl), from fruit and vegetable production, from potato processing and the starch production industry, from wine production (husk), and from slaughterhouses. In addition, organic waste from forestry and pulp and paper industries (bark mulch and sawdust) can also be used in agricultural production.

Organic matter is an important secondary source of micronutrients. Most micronutrients are held tightly in complex organic compounds and may not be readily available to plants (Das, 2014). However, they are slowly released into a form available to plants as organic matter decomposes (Hazra, 2016). In general, micronutrients are present in very small amounts in organic fertilizers and these products do not have a nutrient guarantee (Das, 2014). On the other hand, organic fertilizers perform soil-conditioning functions. The addition of organic matter also improves the physical, chemical, and biological properties of soils (El Sayed Hameda et al., 2012).

It is difficult for farmers to find precise information on the micronutrient content of organic fertilizers, because more attention has been given to determining the NPK content. This is unfortunate, because in our times, with the availability of purified commercial fertilizers, the micronutrients in organic residues may be more important than the major nutrients (Jones and Jacobsen, 2009). Owing to the small amounts of micronutrients present in organic materials, large fluctuations can exist. For example, the nutrient content of manure may vary depending on animal type and diet, type and amount of bedding, manure moisture content, and storage method (Eghball et al., 2002). Green manure elemental composition is mainly related to plant species and stage (Silva et al., 2008), and this of sewage sludge depends on the source from which it has been generated, such as industrial or residential facilities and the processes used in sewage treatment stations (da Silva et al., 2011). The values presented in Table 1.2 are useful only in showing the possible magnitude of the micronutrient content.

Table 1.2 Micronutrient contents of the selected organic fertilizers, mg/kg

Organic fertilizers	Fe	Cu	Mn	Mo	Zn	B	Se	I	Cd	Cr	Pb	Source
Cattle manure	1075	8.80	247		44							Uyanöz (2007)
Cattle manure		31	230		174		0.6			0.16		Hamnér and Kirchmann (2015)
Pig manure	1416	502	367		563				4.65			Li et al. (2009)
Pig manure	2158	156	355		286							Gondek et al. (2013)
Pig slurry		178	302	4.9	635		1.6			0.17		Hamnér and Kirchmann (2015)
Chicken manure	34[a]	3.8[a]	72[a]		41[a]							Shaban et al. (2009)
Sheep manure compost	1248.9	4.0	45.6		68.9				0.7	8.9	15.8	Wang et al. (2016)
Rice straw	225	3.73	467		49.6				0.97			Li et al. (2009)
Sewage sludge		390	280	6.7	550		1.3			1.3		Hamnér and Kirchmann (2015)
Sewage sludge	5391	80	112		950							Gondek et al. (2013)
Sewage sludge	2275–3322	7–11	100–287		68–177	3–5			1–2			Tennakoon and Bandara (2003)
Green manure red clover					45.6							Aghili et al. (2014)
Green manure sunflower					104.4							Aghili et al. (2014)
Green manure *Accacia*	870–994	7–9	78–92		54–61	46–49			0.5–1			Tennakoon and Bandara (2003)
Green manure *Pueraria*	117–280	4–6	82–120		64–70	20–24			0.5–1			Tennakoon and Bandara (2003)
Seaweed *Laminaria*								746–1862				Teas et al. (2004)

[a] DTPA extractable

As organic fertilizers release nutrients over a fairly long period, their potential drawback is that they may not release enough of their principal nutrient at a time to give the plant what it needs for best growth. Because organic fertilizers depend on soil organisms to mineralize, most of them are effective only when soil is moist and soil temperature is sufficiently warm for the soil organisms to be active (Jones and Jacobsen, 2009).

Much has been published which has considered the possibilities and limitations of fertilizing with biodegradable organic wastes (Schulz and Rornheld, 1997). There are various risks involved with the application of those materials to agricultural lands. These are related to environmental pollutants such as heavy metals and organic contaminants, over-application of fertilizer due to the high level of management difficulties relative to that of mineral fertilizers, hygienic aspects, contamination with extraneous materials, for example, glass, stones, plastic. (Schulz and Rornheld, 1997). However, application of manure from intensive livestock farms may also result in significant increase in the content of toxic pollutants in crops (Li et al., 2009).

The influence of organic soil fertilization on micronutrient content in crops has been studied by many authors and different results have been recorded.

Numerous reports have recommend organic fertilizer as a tool of crop biofortification in macronutrients. Application of farmyard manure in Egypt (El-Ghamry et al., 2009) gave a significant increase in Fe, Mn, and Zn concentration in wheat grain as compared with the control treatment. In the same country, substantial increases in rice plants concentrations of Fe, Mn, and Zn were noted under application of chicken manure (Shaban et al., 2009). Fe and Zn concentrations in barley grains increased through vermicompost application in Iran (Farahani et al., 2011). Application of animal manure has been also proposed as a method to increase crop Se content in deficient soils (e.g., Borowska and Koper, 2006; Borowska et al., 2012; Kabata-Pendias, 2010). Experiments conducted in Poland showed that Se content in potato tubers (Borowska and Koper, 2006) increased with increasing doses of cattle manure (up to 80 t/ha), but the highest Se concentrations in aboveground biomass of winter wheat were observed when plots were treated with the doses of 20 and 40 Mg/ha, which was about 70% higher in comparison with the control plant (Borowska et al., 2012). The application of manure in the dose of 80 Mg/ha resulted in a decrease in the selenium content in aboveground wheat biomass. By applying seaweed, which is known as an iodine-rich organic material (Mouritsen, 2013), to soils, crops are able to increase the absorption and accumulation of this trace element (Lawson et al., 2015). Aghili et al. (2014) proved that the addition of green manure of red clover and sunflower to a calcareous soil may increase grain Zn concentration in bread wheat.

Some studies have delivered less optimistic information. In the experiments carried out in China (Wang et al., 2016), using sheep manure compost increased the concentrations of Fe and Zn in wheat grain, but the Cu and Mn concentrations tended to decrease with the compost treatments compared with the corresponding control. In a similar study conducted in Poland (Rutkowska et al., 2014) farmyard manure treatment decreased the Fe and Zn concentrations in wheat. In the experiments in Turkey, cattle manure caused increase of Cu content in dry bean grain while not changing Fe, Mn, and Zn concentrations (Uyanöz, 2007) and did not have significant effect on Fe, Zn, Cu and Mn amount of onion bulbs (Yoldas et al., 2011). According to data from long-term field trials carried out in Sweden, trace metals (Cd, Cu, Mn, Mo, Se) concentrations in spring barley and winter wheat grains were not affected by regular additions of manure and sewage sludge when applied at rates being normal for Swedish agriculture (Hamnér and Kirchman, 2015).

In favor of organic fertilizers as a valuable source of micronutrients for plants, some research has shown that the content of these elements in crops is higher due to organic materials application than after fertilization with mineral NPK. It was confirmed, for example, in the cropping of rice (Shaban et al., 2009), barley (Farahani et al., 2011), and *Amaranthus spinosus* (Mofunanya et al., 2015), but there are also reports that document the lack of differences or even worse effects (Uyanöz, 2007).

Varied effects of organic fertilizers on the content of micronutrients in crops have not been precisely explained. Some authors claim that the application of organic amendments improve the soil nutrient content, but do not always increase the plant nutrient concentration (Roe, 1998; Warman, 2005). As mentioned earlier (see chapter 2), quite apart from genetic characteristics of the crop itself, not only the content of microelements in soil but also their bioavailability is crucial for plants (Gondek et al., 2013). It is observed that long-term organic fertilization influences the content of available microelement forms in soil as well as in the soil solution, but together with increasing contents of organic matter in soil, mobility of Cu, Fe, and Mn in the soil solution decreases (Rutkowska et al., 2014). In general, these elements show high affinity to organic matter and as a result they form stable bonds (Rutkowska et al., 2014). Changes in soil properties caused by organic fertilization can also be of greater importance for the phytoavailability of trace elements and crop uptake (Hamnér and Kirchman, 2015). For example, adding organic matter may influence soil pH, the essential factor for availability of the majority of micronutrients (Jayalath et al., 2016; McCauley et al., 2009). Higher microbial activity influenced by organic materials may be beneficial for crops; however, microorganisms can compete with plants for microelements as they rely on the same nutrients for growth (Coyne and Mikkelsen, 2015).

By changing soil physical condition organic matter can alter development of root systems and thus uptake of nutrients (Watson et al., 2012).

It must be taken into consideration that individual micronutrients have different properties and specific chemical behaviors. As Zn is an easily plant available metal in soil (Kabata-Pendias, 2010), the addition in organic fertilizers usually increases its concentration in crops (Hamnér and Kirchman, 2015). Cu is strongly bound to organic matter (Hwang et al., 2015). Even when organic matter decomposes and Cu is released, there are still a large number of binding sites available for Cu to rebind. The addition of organic fertilizers may therefore not significantly affect concentrations of Cu in crops (Hamnér and Kirchman, 2015). Mn is abundant in soils and plant availability is mainly controlled by soil pH and redox conditions, therefore fertilization with organic amendments do not significantly alter crop uptake unless pH and redox are affected (Hamnér and Kirchman, 2015). Crop availability of Mo is mainly affected by pH values in soil (Gupta and Lipsett, 1981). As addition of Mo to organic fertilizers is usually small, organic fertilizer may have no effect unless soil pH is affected (Hamnér and Kirchman, 2015). Se in organic fertilizers is mainly present in organic forms and when organic matter decays, Se is mineralized to selenite and selenate (Borowska and Koper, 2006). The potential amount of Se mineralized from organic amendments can be high enough to influence crop composition (Hamnér and Kirchman, 2015). Positive correlations between organic matter and Se uptake has been shown on mineral soils in Norway (Eich-Greatorex et al., 2007). The study conducted in Poland demonstrated that aboveground winter wheat biomass absorbed and transported selenium more easily from soil treated with farmyard manure at the doses of 20 or 40 Mg/ha, in contrast to the higher ones (Borowska et al., 2012). Binding of iodide to organic material in the soil with pH lower that 6.9 have been reported in several papers and the retention of iodine in soil is often interpreted as binding to these organic components (Johanson, 2000). It was documented that the addition of organic material to the soil reduces the uptake of I by plants. For example, fertilizing oats with peat reduced the uptake of I by 40% or even more, depending on soil type (Moiseyev et al., 1984). However, this binding is reversible so it is possible to get a desorption and plant uptake (Johanson, 2000).

Absorption of trace elements by roots is controlled by the concentration of other elements and their positive or negative interactions, so the uptake of a given element might be improved or depressed by others present in high concentrations in soil (Efremova and Izosimova, 2014). It should be taken into account that at increasing organic wastes application (e.g., sewage sludge), which are often reach in some trace metals, competition or synergy between elements may affect uptake of micronutrients by crops (Hamnér and Kirchman, 2015). Naeem et al. (2012) claimed that the accumulation of Fe, Mn, Cu, and Zn released from organic fertilizer by rice grain was promoted by suitable nitrogen application. The study by Aghili et al. (2014) showed that organic matter amendments to soil can contribute to a better utilization of naturally stocked soil micronutrients, and thereby reduce any need for major external inputs. In the above mentioned experiments, mixing green manure of sunflower to soil mobilized additional Zn of 48 mg/kg soil for transfer to the aboveground wheat biomass, compared to the total Zn of 132 mg/kg soil taken up from plain soil when neither green manure nor $ZnSO_4$ were applied. Green manure amendments to soil also raised the DTPA-extractable Zn in soil.

Few experiments have been performed in order to compare the effects of organic and mineral micronutrient fertilizers on the status of micronutrients in plants. Influence of mineral KI fertilizer and organic seaweed composite on the iodine uptake by Chinese cabbage and lettuce was compared in China (Hong et al., 2008). Available iodine after applying KI fertilizer were apparently faster than those with seaweed composite, but its toxicity in the form of KI was also higher than that in the form of seaweed iodine. Iodine released from seaweed composite maintained relative stability during the whole culture period, demonstrating a long-term efficacy. In addition, the seaweed composite iodine fertilizer is recommended due to its relatively low cost. Research by Aghili et al. (2014) showed that addition of green manure to calcareous soil can raise grain Zn concentration of bread wheat to levels approaching those of only $ZnSO_4$ fertilizer-fed wheat plants. Application of $ZnSO_4$ fertilizer increased grain Zn concentration from 20 to 39 mg/kg and the addition of green manure of sunflower alone to soil raised grain Zn concentration to 31 mg/kg.

In the light of certain studies, combined application of organic and mineral fertilizers seems to be an agronomic practice that will possibly biofortify edible parts of crops with micronutrients. This applies to both the use of organic materials with mineral NPK fertilizers and organic ones with mineral microelement preparations. Substantial increase of micronutrients (Fe, Mn, Zn, Cu) were obtained by integrating farmyard manures with mineral N fertilizers in maize (Ashmaye et al., 2008), spinach (Shaban et al., 2008), and rice (Shaban et al., 2009) production. Barley grain mineral quality could be improved through connected application of organic and mineral NPK fertilizers, especially under water deficit conditions (Farahani et al., 2011). Experiments conducted in Egypt (El-Ghamry et al., 2009) studied the possibility of wheat grain biofortification with micronutrients by farmyard manure and foliar micronutrients application. There was significant effect of the interaction between farmyard manure addition and foliar application of micronutrients and adding farmyard manure with foliar application of the mixed micronutrients (B, Mo, and Zn) was the superior treatment. Another report recommended that the integration of organic (composted rice straw) and inorganic fertilizers (including $ZnSO_4$) management could increase micronutrient (Fe, Mn, and Zn) contents in grain and consequently improve the nutritional quality of rice (Naeem et al., 2012). The study by Aghili et al. (2014) showed that combined addition of green manure and $ZnSO_4$ fertilizer can considerably raise wheat grain Zn concentration in comparison to the separate application of those fertilizers. Adding the two together to soil increased grain Zn concentration even to 54 mg/kg.

Recently, demand for organically grown products has risen steadily because foods produced using natural fertilizers are believed to be more nutritious than conventionally-grown foods, with a better balance of vitamins and minerals. Nevertheless, the scientific community has not conclusively shown that organic products are more nutritious than conventionally grown foods (Winter and Davis, 2006). More concise and precise studies are needed to improve the load of essential microelements in foods by organic fertilizers and also to prevent or avoid the accumulation of toxic or undesirable contaminants.

1.2.3 Chelates

It is well documented that microelements supplemented in the form of chelates result in good bioavailability. The most frequently used carriers of microelements are amino acids whereby nutritive cations are bound with carboxyl groups (Chojnacka et al., 2011). The supply of free metal ions to roots limits their biouptake. Metal complexes in bulk solution and the rhizosphere may play an important role in overcoming the limitations of diffusion and contribute to the biouptake. Metal complexes, if present, will dissociate, resulting in an increased diffusional flux and enhanced metal uptake (Wang et al., 2009). In analyses of metal biouptake from a complexing medium, all the physical (diffusion), chemical (dissociation kinetics of metal complexes), and biological (transport and internalization) processes must be taken into account. Data show that application of a chelating agent such as EDTA in itself affects the mineral uptake of cultivated crops under field conditions. EDTA application changed the mineral composition of plants. Higher phosphorus (P), sulfur (S), iron (Fe) and manganese (Mn) and lower cadmium (Cd) concentrations were determined in the seeds of oilseed rape. No yield effects of residual EDTA were observed for the crop, but the Cd content in seeds was still lower in plots where EDTA had been applied the previous year (Bloem et al., 2017).

It was shown that application of metal-chelate complexes and its dissociation can greatly promote uptake of metal ions into plant roots (Degryse et al., 2006, 2012; Wang et al., 2009). But at the same time, other results proved that the use of chelates could lower metal uptake by plant roots and reduce accumulation of toxic metals in rice (Custos et al., 2014). Application of Fe chelates $EDTANa_2Fe(II)$ increased the Fe content and decreased the Cd content of rice organs. Xylem transport of Cd and redistribution of Cd in leaves by phloem transport can be regulated in rice through the use of Fe chelates that influence Fe availability and Fe-related gene expression. Fe fertilization decreased Cd influx and increased Cd efflux in rice roots (Chen et al., 2017).

In the case of Fe, Zn, which are among the more deficient microelements in human diet, the effectiveness of their complexed/chelated forms is well documented and resulted in higher nutrient density in plants than salts. Fe uptake by the leaves is greater from chelates than from salts. In the soil, the chelates protect the Fe against rapid fixation. Moreover, chelates have a less damaging effect on leaves. For application on Fe-fixing soils, which are generally neutral to alkaline, the stability of the chelate in the soil is important (Roy et al., 2006). A drawback of these preparations is high price. The cost of fertilizer supplementation is 10 times higher as compared with the mineral salts (Chojnacka et al., 2011). Table 1.3 collects chelates of microelements used in the soil fertilizing.

For example the application of Fe-EDDHA affected in the highest Fe content in the fruit body (2799.3 ± 30.7 mg/kg dw) when compared with inorganic form from (Liu et al., 2015). Naik and Das (2008) compared ZnSHH (Zn sulfate heptahydrate) and Zn-EDTA for rice at Pakyong, Sikkim. ZnSHH was applied at 10 and 20 kg/ha as basal or

Table 1.3 Chelated form of nutrients used nowadays by adding to npk fertilizers

No.	Nutrient	Form	Content %
1	Copper	$Na_2CuEDTA$	13
		NaCuHEDTA	9
		Copper polyflavonoids organically bound Cu	5–7
2	Iron	NaFeEDTA	5–11
		NaFeHFDTA	5–9
		NaFeEDDHA	6
		NaFeDTPA	10
		Iron polyflavonoids organically bound Fe	9–10
3	Manganese	Mn-EDTA	5–12
4	Zinc	$Na_2ZnEDTA$	14
		NaZnTA	13
		NaZnHEDTA	9
		Polyflavonoids organically bound Zn	10

Source: Jones, J. B., *Plant Nutrition Manual*, Boca Raton, CRC Press, 1997; Roy, R. N. et al., In: *Sources of Plant Nutrients and Soil Amendments. Ferilizer and Plant Nutrition Biuletin*, Italy, Food and Agriculture Organization of the United Nations, 2006.

in two equal splits (half basal and the rest half at grand tillering stage). Zn-EDTA was applied at 0.5 or 1.0 kg ha-1 in single application as basal; 1 kg/ha was also applied in two equal splits. Zn concentration in rice grain was significantly more (30.3 mg/kg) with 0.5 kg/ha Zn-EDTA than with 10 kg/ha ZuSHH (25.5 mg/kg). Split application was better than a single application in ZuSHH but not in Zn-EDTA. Zn-EDTA was better than Zn-SHH, but more expensive (Prasad et al., 2014). Almendros et al. (2015) compared the influence of different natural and synthetic organic Zn complexes on agronomic biofortification of onion crops grown in two types of soil under greenhouse conditions (Almendros et al., 2015). It was proved that applying Zn organic complexes to an onion crop improved not only productivity, but also Zn concentrations in onions. Applications of Zn-aminolignosulfonate (10 mg Zn/kg) in soil acid and of Zn-DTPA-HEDTA-EDTA at the rate of (10 mg Zn/kg) in Soilcalc produced the highest Zn and soluble Zn concentrations in plants.

Microelements can be supplemented as natural organic complexes or synthetic organic complexes. Utilization of biomass instead of organic molecules as a carrier of micronutrient that is obtained as results of biosorption properties of biomass is becoming a promising alternative for synthetic chelates. Natural biomass possesses many free function groups, mainly carboxyl, and thus can form the same microelements such as in the case of chelates, thus assuring the similar chemism of binding as in the chelates and delivered in the form of nutrients highly available to plants but in more natural and cheaper form (Chojnacka et al., 2011). The advantage of such a solution is lower cost of the biomass compared to organic molecules. High bioavailability of microelements from the biomass preparations was confirmed and maize grains biofortified with micronutrients by enriched biomass of blackcurrant seeds (Samoraj et al., 2015) or biomass of *Spirulina* was obtained (Tuhy et al., 2015).

1.2.4 Biofertilizers

Agronomic biofortification, through the application of fertilizers, has been used to raise nutrients content in plants. However, at high concentrations microelements are toxic and its inorganic form is bound to soil constituents, thus is unavailable to plants, whereas it may be leached under wet fall conditions (Durán et al., 2013). Agronomic strategies to increase the concentrations of mineral elements in edible tissues generally rely not only on the application of mineral fertilizers but also on improvements in the solubilization and mobilization of mineral elements in the soil that can be obtained by application of biofertilizers (Almendros et al., 2015).

Biofertilizers can be descibed as diverse groups of soil-borne microbes, such as root endophytic fungi, mycorrhizal fungi, plant growth-promoting rhizobacteria, and rhizobia that exert positive effects on plant growth and survival through direct and plant-mediated mechanisms. They have been used to stimulate crop production through diverse biofertilization mechanisms, such as biological nitrogen fixation, solubilization of insoluble minerals, production of phytohormones, and biocontrol processes that include phytopathogen antagonism and plant-induced resistance (Olivares et al., 2015). Microorganisms can be used as substitutes for various genetic approaches and chemical fertilizers can improve plant nutrition and health with a decrease in the application of chemical inputs (Shaikh and Saraf, 2017). Usually biofertilizers do not contain a single culture of beneficial microorganisms but a mixture of different beneficial microorganisms.

Beneficial microorganism can be recognized as "effective microorganisms" and "indigenous microorganisms." Both are very much the same in all aspects except origin. The term "indigenous microorganisms" refers to a group of beneficial microbes native to the area; while "effective microorganisms" mean a laboratory-cultured mixture of microorganisms (Kumar and Gopal, 2015). These are used as a microbial mixture that has been developed to improve soil quality and crop yield while simultaneously dramatically reducing organic chemical application (Megali et al., 2014).

The potential of various microbes to enhance plant productivity and yield in cropping systems has been demonstrated in many experiments (Pereg and McMillan, 2015). Another very interesting property is the possibility of increasing the density of nutrients in the edible parts of plants by using our ability to solubilize the insoluble form of micronutrients present in the soil in the retrogradative form. Biofortification of crops through application of PGPRs can be therefore considered a possible supplementary measure that can lead to increased micronutrient concentrations in wheat grains, as well as improving yield. It has been proved that the highest rate of grain nutrient uptake results from the combined use of biofertilization by arbuscular mycorrhizal (AM) fungi (*Glomus mosseae*) and free-living nitrogen-fixing bacteria (*Herbaspirillum seropedicae*) and a moderate level of chemical fertilization. With decreasing the rate of chemical fertilizer use, the efficiency of rice nutrient use increased, which indicates how biofertilizers can be efficient in providing plants with their essential nutrients (Hoseinzade et al., 2016). Zinc solubilization by bacteria has an immense importance in zinc nutrition to plants in calcareous soils of the world. Thus zinc that has been made unavailable can be reverted back to an available form by inoculating soil with a bacterial strain capable of solubilizing the zinc (Bapiri et al., 2012). A number of reviews on Zn (Ramesh et al., 2014) and Fe biofortification are available in the literature, Fe (Ramzani et al., 2016; Bouis and Saltzman, 2017).

AMF showing that a mycorrhiza-friendly approach in agriculture may have great potential in biofertilization of crops and biofortification of foods (Pellegrino and Bedini, 2014). AMF could represent 10% or more of the soil microbial biomass. Mycorrhizal fungi colonize the roots of around 80% of land plant species and agricultural crops, mostly to the mutual benefit of plant host and fungus (Smith and Read, 2008).

Most of field studies testing the effectiveness of inoculation by AMF applied foreign AMF isolates, which are not always optimal for all tested crops since the affinities between host plants and AMF are not always synergistic. The use of an inoculum based on locally sourced AMF would be a suitable choice because of a better adaptation to the prevailing conditions and also because it could avoid the ecological risks of introducing a foreign species. Actually, some studies have shown not only higher plant growth and nutritional performances of locally sourced AMF compared to foreign selected ones but also biofortification of chickpea (*Cicer arietinum* L.) grain in Fe and Zn (Pellegrino and Bedini, 2014). Inoculation by AMF does not always result in biofortification. For example, AMF inoculation may impair the biofortification of lettuce with Se as confirmed by Sanmartín et al. (2014). The reason for that could be the fact that the list of essential minerals for plants is quite similar but not equal to the list for humans. For example, Se, I, Co, and Na are essential for humans but not for most plants. So not all the plants react by increased density of Se even when it is delivered in higher amounts in the soil (Pinto and Ferreira, 2014). What is more, the form of nutrient delivered in the soil solution to the root system strongly affects the level of biofortification. Even when used in the same host plant (e.g., garlic), the addition of AMF to the soil can increase the Se uptake by the roots (Larsen et al., 2006) or have no significant effects (Patharajan and Raaman, 2012). Selenium acquisition by wheat plants through the coinoculation of native selenobacteria strains serves as a selenonanosphere source with arbuscular mycorrhizal fungus (*Glomus claroideum*). When plants were coinoculated with a mixture of selenobacteria strains and *G. claroideum*, selenium content in grain was 23.5% higher (725 mg/kg) than nonmycorrhizal plants (587 mg/kg) (Durán et al., 2013).

1.3 Methods of application

The effectiveness of micronutrient fertilizer application on crop biofortification is influenced not only by the fertilizer type but also by the application method (Mao et al., 2014; Melash et al., 2016; de Valença et al., 2017). In crop plants, micronutrients may be applied to the soil, foliar sprayed, added as seed treatments, or through fertigation (Farooq et al., 2012; Singh and Prasad, 2014; Smoleń et al., 2016).

The decision regarding which method to use ought to depend on the individual nutrient and the fertilizer form (Pankaj et al., 2016). For example, micronutrients that are best foliar applied are Fe and Mn (Narwal et al., 2012) whereas Mo and Ni are not absorbed through the leaves. In turn Zn, B, Cl, and Cu can be applied by both techniques (Dimpka and Bindraban, 2015). Fe, Mn, Zn, Cu, B, Mo can be also supplied through fertigation along with special fertilizers (Pagani et al., 2013). Organic stable fertilizers are spread uniformly in the field and incorporated several days before planting (Piechota et al., 2014). Micronutrient salts used can be applied as a granular material or dissolved in liquid fertilizers (Pagani et al., 2013). Oxides, due to being relatively insoluble, must be finely ground to be effective and more quickly converted to plant-available forms when applied to soil. Chelates generally have higher stability, provide fewer micronutrients, and are also commonly used for foliar application (Pagani et al., 2013). Some micronutrient metals can be complexed with ammonia (Lakshmanan et al., 2005). In addition, because toxicity can occur easily for some micronutrients (such as B), the fertilizer form, placement, and rate should be carefully considered (Pagani et al., 2013).

1.3.1 Fertigation

Fertigation is a method of fertilizer application in which fertilizer is incorporated within the irrigation water by the drip system (Bell and Dell, 2008). In this system fertilizer solution is distributed evenly in irrigation (FERTIGATION = FERTilization + irrIGATION). The availability of nutrients is very high and they are supplied near the active root zone, which results in greater absorption by the crops. It is very important in the case of Fe, when Fe deficiency in calcareous soils is problematic (Kabir et al., 2016) or in case of Cu in nursery mixes high in organic matter content that strongly sorb this element (Hwang et al., 2015). In the fertigation method, liquid fertilizer as well as water soluble fertilizers can be used. By this means, along with using less water and saving fertilizer, time, labor, and energy expenditures are also reduced substantially (Akanda et al., 2012; Bell and Dell, 2008).

The main factors to consider when choosing micronutrient products for a fertigation system are solubility and compatibility (Bell and Dell, 2008). For example, if $Ca(NO_3)_2$ is present in the solution, inorganic sulfates should be avoided. To avoid chemical reaction with some of the macronutrient fertilizers, micronutrients can be applied separately through the irrigation system. Chelated forms of Fe are recommended and FeEDDHA has greater stability than FeEDTA, especially above pH 6.5. Though more expensive than inorganic salts, chelated forms of Cu, Fe, Mn, and Zn are recommended in order to maintain solubility, minimize precipitation, and to achieve more even distribution. Any of the commercial B fertilizers is suitable for fertigation. The use of compound fertilizers containing micronutrients is to be avoided as the quality of the dissolved material varies due to variation in solubility and composition (Bell and Dell, 2008).

The available literature provides many examples of the successful biofortification of edible crop parts through fertigation. In the experiment conducted with wheat in Pakistan (Alam et al., 2000) application of Zn ($ZnSO_4$) together with N (urea) through irrigation increased Zn grain content up to 47,64 mg/kg, that is, by 89% and 45% compared to the control and N treatments respectively. The application of B and Zn (with different levels of NPK) by this method showed a significant effect on the quality of fruits and the yield of tomatos in Bangladesh (Akanda et al., 2012). The study carried out in Poland (Kleibert, 2014) proved that increasing the concentration of manganese used in fertigation significantly influenced the content of Mn in plants of lettuce (*Lactuca sativa* L.). Some authors suggest the use of fertigation as a means of iodine application because their results show that adding iodine to the soil increases its absorption by plants (Ujowundu et al., 2010). Iodination of irrigation water increased the concentration of iodine in spinach in China (Dai et al., 2006), as well as turning out to be an advantageous and cost-effective method of supplying iodine to vegetables (*Telfairia occidentalis, Talinium trangulare, Cucurbita pepo*) commonly consumed in Nigeria (Ujowundu et al., 2010). The application of iodine together with humic substances or organic acids shows further positive effects on I absorption by plants (Smoleń et al., 2016).

A successful example of agronomic biofortification by fertigation was the program realized in the Xinjiang province in China. When potassium iodate (KIO_3) was added to irrigation water (10 kg in a single treatment), the I content of all irrigated crops and foodstuffs substantially increased (Cao et al., 1994; Jiang et al., 1997). Infant mortality in the region declined by 50% and IDD were largely eliminated (Jiang et al., 1997).

The identification of an effective Se method seems to be crucial for better understanding of Se uptake and accumulation, especially in water-stressed crop plants (Nawaz et al., 2014). Selenium transport through xylem and phloem markedly influences the accumulation of ions in plant cells through its interaction with the plasmalemma and metabolic cell processes (Pazurkiewicz-Kocot et al., 2003). A set of experiments with Se (Na_2SeO_4) application by fertigation and other methods was conducted under normal and water-deficit conditions in Pakistan (Nawaz et al., 2014, 2015, 2017). Se fertigation turned out to be a much more viable and effective approach than soil application to increase Se translocation in plants (Nawaz et al., 2014), and as much (Nawaz et al., 2017) or less (Nawaz et al., 2015) profitable method of improving wheat grain than foliar spray. It is worth highlighting that Se fertigation in the same way as foliar spray resulted in the maximum accumulation of Se in wheat shoots and gave the highest net return and cost-benefit ratio under drought stress conditions, as shown in Nawaz et al. (2017) reported.

Higher effectiveness of biofortification achieved by introduction of nutrients through fertigation compared to pre-sowing fertilization was also reported by Smoleń and Sady (2012) and Smoleń et al. (2016). The authors claim that introduction of iodine by fertigation proved to be much more effective for iodine biofortification of spinach than pre-sowing fertilization—by 339% and 498% respectively for KI and KIO_3. Fertilization of this kind could significantly reduce the cost of food fortification by using lower concentrations (for example for I below 0.0004%) for fertigation and might have allowed spinach to be fortified with I on a similar level to that after soil fertilization in a dose of 1 mg I per 1 dm^3 (Smoleń and Sady, 2012). Another very important aspect is that method of application can reduce absorption or synthesis of other undesirable nutrients as well as increasing more valuable ones, as was the case in research by Smoleń et al. (Smoleń and Sady 2012; Smoleń et al., 2016). The application of iodine through fertigation has shown other positive effects, such as increased biomass in leafy vegetables (Dai et al., 2004).

1.3.2 Foliar

Foliar application refers to the spraying of fertilizer solutions containing one or more nutrients on the foliage of growing plants (Mortvedt, 1985). Foliar fertilization with micronutrients often stimulates more nutrient uptake and efficient allocation in the edible plant parts than soil fertilization, especially with cereals and leafy vegetables (Lawson et al., 2015; de Valença et al., 2017). Other advantages of foliar sprays are: application rates are much lower than for soil application, uniform distribution is easily obtained, response to the applied nutrient is almost immediate; therefore, deficiencies can be corrected during the growing season and suspected deficiencies can be more easily diagnosed with spray trials (Mortvedt, 1985). Several downsides concerning this method are also mentioned in the literature: nutrient demand is often high when plants are small and leaf surface is insufficient for foliar absorption, foliar fertilizers can easily be washed off by rain, leaf burn may result if salt concentrations are excessive, it may be too late to correct the deficiency and obtain expected results, there is usually little residual effect from foliar sprays, and extra application costs may be required because more than one spray application may be needed (Mortvedt, 1985).

A number of studies of different fertilizers applied foliarly at various rates did not include measurement of micronutrient concentration in grain (Rengel et al., 1999). Therefore, information available in the literature on the possibilities of increasing micronutrient density in grain via foliar fertilization is limited.

Foliar application has been found to be the most promising fertilization method for increasing zinc content in edible parts of plants (Joy et al., 2015; Yilmaz et al., 1997; de Valença et al., 2017; Zou et al., 2012).

Possibilities of crop enrichment with Zn by foliar spraying seem to be best described in the literature. A large amount of research shows rewarding effects in cereals: wheat (Cakmak, 2008; Mao et al., 2014; Zou et al., 2012), rice (Dhaliwal et al., 2010; Phattarakul et al., 2012; Shivay and Prasad, 2014; Wei et al., 2012), maize (Mao et al., 2014), sorgum (Kumar et al., 2013), and barley (Uddin et al., 2014). For instance, Yilmaz et al. (1997) reported threefold increase of grain Zn concentration (from 9–10 until 30–31 mg/kg d.m.) in some wheat (*Triticum aestivum*) cultivars grains grown on zinc-deficient calcareous soils in Turkey, when 0.4% $ZnSO_4$–$7H_2O$ solution (Zn at 440 g/ha) was sprayed on leaves twice during tillering and stem elongation stages at 15-day intervals. In other research foliar application of $ZnSO_4$ resulted in very significant increases in grain Zn of up to 85% in wheat (Zou et al., 2012) and 25% in rice (Phattarakul et al., 2012), regardless of soil conditions, management practices, and cultivars used. A review of experiments from 10 African countries showed that foliar Zn application increased the Zn concentration in maize, rice, and wheat grains by respectively 30%, 25%, and 63% (Joy et al., 2015).

Cakmak et al. (2010a) also reported that on soils with very low plant-available Zn, foliar application of Zn was also very effective in reducing the phytate (an antinutrient that inhibits zinc bioavailability in humans) concentration in grain.

Among the zinc forms $ZnCl_2$ and $ZnSO_4$, as well as chelated forms of Zn (e.g., Zn-EDTA) are recommended for foliar Zn biofortification (Cakmak, 2008; Wei et al., 2012). $ZnSO_4$ is the most widely applied fertilizer by the farmer due to its high solubility, low cost, and availability on the market (Uddin et al., 2014).

Foliar spray is an effective method of plant biofortification with Se (Nawaz et al., 2017). This method is a popular practical way of producing Se-enriched foods in China (Wu et al., 2015). Chen et al. (2002) reported that the Se concentration in field-grown rice was significantly increased to 0.471 and 0.640 mg/g, respectively, by foliar application of Se-fertilizer at a rate of Se 20g/ha as sodium selenite and sodium selenite. Mao et al. (2014) from China proved that selenium as sodium selenite was effective as a foliar application to winter wheat, increasing it from 25 to 312 μg/kg in wheat grain with Se at 60 g/ha. The results of research by Jiang et al. (2015) showed that foliar spray significantly increased Se uptake in common buckwheat (*Fagopyrum esculentum* M.) grains. Apart from cereals, tea is another popular Se-biofortified product in China. Hu et al. (2003) claimed that, in addition to increased Se concentrations, the number of sprouts, yield, amino-acid content, vitamin content, as well as the sweetness and aroma of tea leaves, were also significantly increased with the Se fertilizer application.

Apart from China, good results in selenium fortification of an Italian rice cultivar via foliar fertilization with sodium selenite were also reported by Giacosa et al. (2014). Nawaz et al. (2017) resulted in the maximum accumulation of Se in shoots of spring wheat through foliar spray (Na_2SeO_4 solution) under drought stress conditions in Pakistan. In addition, this method of Se application gave the highest net return and cost-benefit ratio, as the authors reported. Poggi et al. (2000), who applied selenite and selenate on leaves of potato in Italy, observed greater mobility in the phloem when using selenate, which increased the Se content in this culture. Foliar applications of the different sources of Se resulted in a greater proportion of Se in crops when selenate was applied (Boldrin et al., 2013).

Several research reports referred to Fe foliar application. In experiments conducted in India successful effects in studied cereals were proved. Narwal et al. (2010) observed that foliar application increased wheat grain iron concentration from 1.0 to 2.3 mg/kg. The study by Dhaliwal et al. (2014) indicated that 13.1%–30.3% wheat grain enrichment with Fe is possible through this method. Fang et al. (2008) and Singh et al. (2013) referred to significant increasing of Fe concentration in rice. Kumar et al. (2013) observed an increase of 5%–12% for grain Fe concentration in sorghum on the soils deficient in micronutrients. Data from the study carried out in Australia showed significant increase of Fe in peas grains while treated with different Fe-containing foliar sprays at the time of grain filling in Fe-deficient plants (Kabir et al., 2016). Among foliar-applied Fe fertilizers, $FeSO_4$ and Fe-EDTA seem to be the most useful and efficient in biofortifying Fe in crops (Aciksoz et al., 2010; Kabir et al., 2016; Narwal et al., 2012; Singh et al., 2013; Zhang et al., 2010b).

Some reports from India (Dhaliwal et al., 2014; Narwal et al., 2012) and Pakistan (Ali et al., 2015) revealed that foliar application of Mn in the form of $MnSO_4$ solution increased the grain yield in wheat. In research by Ali et al. (2015) maximum concentration of manganese (105 ppm) was noted while foliar application of manganese at 2% solution were used.

Although foliar application of boron was recommended (Dunn et al., 2005; Hussain et al., 2012), its biofortification potential is poorly desribed (Rehman et al., 2014b). As Rehman et al. (2014b) reported boron foliage application proved an effective way to correct B deficiency in rice. Other reports of Rehman et al. (2014a) documented an increase of B concentrations in rice kernels by even 51.7% through foliar B application. This method was more effective way of biofortication than soil amendment and seed dressing.

The experiments carried out in Poland, Germany, and Italy showed that foliar application of KOI_3 solution might be a useful way to biofortify vegetables with iodine. It was proved in the case of lettuce (Lawson et al., 2015; Smoleń et al., 2011a) and carrot (Smoleń et al., 2011b, Tonacchera et al., 2013), as well as potatoes, carrots, cherry tomatoes, and green salad (Tonacchera et al., 2013). On the other hand, foliar sprays did not lead to a substantial iodine accumulation in the edible parts of kohlrabi (Lawson et al., 2015). Tonacchera et al. (2013) reported that the amount of iodine in plants biofortified through foliar fertilization during the growing season was measured at nearly 50 mg/100 g of vegetable. The cited authors (Tonacchera et al., 2013) concluded that biofortification of vegetables with iodine may contribute to improving the iodine nutritional status of the population without risks of iodine excess. Lawson et al. (2015) claimed that the low iodine doses needed as well as the easy and inexpensive application of foliar sprays may favor its implementation in practice. Therefore, this iodine biofortification approach should be further elaborated, especially for leafy vegetables.

Although a large number of articles have documented successful crop biofortification with micronutrients by foliar spraying, some examples of ineffective application were also noted, as in case of Fe (Aciksoz et al., 2011, Turkey) and Cu (Korzeniowska and Stanisławska-Glubiak, 2011, Poland) in wheat. Poor penetration into leaf tissue of the foliar sprayed Fe along with limited phloem mobility and transport of Fe into grain are said to be the major factors contributing to inefficiency of Fe fertilization in improving seed-Fe concentrations (Welch et al., 2013). The lower Cu content might be explained by the micronutrient dilution effect along with higher yield (Korzeniowska and Stanisławska-Glubiak, 2011; Nawaz et al., 2017). However, foliar applications of Cu fertilizers are occasionally recommended under specific circumstances (Gupta, 1979).

Timing of foliar application of micronutrients seems to be a critical agronomic practice in maximizing grain accumulation of micronutrients. For instance, large cereals grain Zn increases are most likely when foliar Zn fertilizers are applied to plants at a late growth stage (Ozturk et al., 2006; Velu et al., 2014). By optimizing the timing and the solute concentration of foliar Zn application, wheat grain Zn concentration could be further increased, not only in whole grains but also in the endosperm (Cakmak et al., 2010b; Zhang et al., 2010b). Kabir et al. (2016) claimed that flowering was a suitable time for applying foliar sprays to boost Fe in mature peas grains. Studies by Nawaz et al. (2017) reported Se foliar spray at tillering as the most viable and effective method for improving wheat yield in drought-prone areas. Usually the repeated application during vegetation period is needed, as it was noted in case of Fe, which is not readily translocated within plants (Singh et al., 2013).

The foliar application usually brings better results than soil application. In comparison to soil amendment foliar spraying was found to be more effective in increasing Zn in grains of wheat (e.g., Abdoli et al., 2016; Cakmak et al., 2010b; Yilmaz et al., 1997; Zhang et al., 2010b), rice (e.g., Impa and Johnson-Beebout, 2012; Joy et al., 2015; Phattarakul et al., 2012), and maize (Joy et al., 2015), Se in wheat (Nawaz et al., 2017), Fe in wheat (Abdoli et al., 2016; Narwal et al., 2012), as well as Mn in wheat (Abdoli et al., 2016; Ali et al., 2015; Narwal et al., 2012). For instance, it was reported that foliar application of Zn only at 1.2 kg/ha as compared with 5.3 kg/ha in soil application gave a similar grain yield in rice but higher Zn concentration in grain. Zn harvest index for soil and foliar application was similar, but the agronomic efficiency of Zn with foliar application was about four times that for soil application; the rate of Zn application was much lower when applied on foliage (Shivay et al., 2010a,b). Dhaliwal et al. (2010), from India, showed that biofortification recovery (Impa and Johnson-Beebout, 2012) of Zn with foliar application to rice was about eight times that obtained with soil application. At the same time Jiang et al. (2007) claimed that absorption of micronutrients in the case of Zn in rice from the root plays a major role, while mobilization from the leaves plays a minor role.

According to many studies the combination of soil and foliar application is the most effective method for many biofortification pathways (Cakmak et al., 2010a).

The HarvestPlus Zinc Fertilizer Project (called HarvestZinc), explored the potential of various zinc-containing fertilizers for increasing zinc concentration of cereal grains and improving yield in target countries such as India, China, Pakistan, Thailand, Laos, Turkey, Zambia, Mozambique, and Brazil (see www.harvestzinc.org). The results of this project demonstrated that foliar or combined soil+foliar application of zinc fertilizers under field conditions was highly effective in increasing grain, especially in wheat. Zinc-enriched grains were also of great importance for crop productivity resulting in better seedling vigor, denser stands, and higher stress tolerance in potentially zinc-deficient soils (Cakmak, 2012).

It is difficult to disagree with the authors (Cakmak et al., 2010a; Hussain et al., 2012; Ozturk et al., 2006; Yang et al., 2011; Zou et al., 2012), who claim that the most effective method for increasing grain Zn is the soil+foliar application method, while it may even result in about a 3-fold increase in grain Zn concentration. Good results of foliar and soil application interaction in Zn agronomic fortification was also proved in rice (Phattarakul et al., 2012; Wei et al., 2012), barley (Uddin et al., 2014), and maize (Imran and Rehim, 2016). A significant interaction effect of foliar spray Se and soil Se application on Se accumulation in common buckwheat was also indicated (Jiang et al., 2015).

Alternatively, using seeds with high Zn concentrations together with foliar application of Zn is also reported to be an effective way to improve both grain yield and grain Zn concentration (Mohsin et al., 2014; Velu et al., 2014)

A very common farming practice is to combine foliar application of micronutrients with pesticide sprays or with foliar application of primary nutrients (Velu et al., 2014). The inclusion of urea in foliar micronutrient fertilizers often has a positive impact on micronutrient concentration in crops edible parts (Aciksoz et al., 2011). Positive effects of combining application of micronutrients were also noted (Zhang et al., 2010b). However, when two or more materials are combined for foliar application, care must be taken to ensure that the materials are compatible. Many pesticides are incompatible with solutions of micronutrients. Incompatibility means that some chemical or physical change takes place that renders the mixture unusable or harmful. In general, micronutrient solutions should be applied separately unless compatibility is shown (Hlgnett and McClellan, 1985).

Despite the proven effectiveness of foliar fertilization, the technique is often rejected as a sustainable strategy to alleviate micronutrient deficiencies among resource poor populations in Africa because it is costly (Garcia-Banuelos et al., 2014).

1.3.3 Soil application/pre-sowing fertilization

The most common method of crop fertilization with micronutrients is to apply them to the soil either as a broadcast (mixed) treatment prior to tillage or as a band application at planting (Mortvedt,1985). The latter way involves placing fertilizer in bands that may be continuous or discontinuous to the side of the seedling, some distance from it and either on the same level as the seed, above the seed level, or below the seed level (Krishnamurthy et al., 2008). Broadcast applications allow a greater proportion of the soil in the root zone to be affected by the fertilizer. However, this also results in greater reaction of the soil with the applied micronutrient which may reduce its agronomic effectiveness (Mortvedt, 1985). In general, fertilizers applied to soil require the use of higher doses because of relatively low nutrient-use efficiency (Singh, 2007).

Both organic and inorganic fertilizers are used by pre-sowing broadcasting, but the first ones usually require soil cover (Piechota et al., 2014). Inorganic products might be also placed on the soil surface. Surface broadcast applications of inorganic micronutrient sources without subsequent tillage are usually less effective for crops because the metallic micronutrients do not move into the root zone. However, topdressing $ZnSO_4$ after observing Zn-deficiency symptoms in rice was as effective as preplant broadcast $ZnSO_4$ applications in Pakistan (Yoshida et al., 1970). Chelated micronutrients will leach into the root zone after surface application because chelates are not tightly sorbed by soil colloids. Band applications might be more effective than broadcast applications, as in Mn sources (Alley et al., 1978). Care should be taken to place starter fertilizers containing B at the recommended distances away from the seed row because B can be toxic to the seedlings of some crops, even at low rates (Mortvedt, 1985).

Soil based application is considered to increase grain yield rather than its micronutrient content (Narwal et al., 2010). However, the examples of enriching crop with individual micronutrients through this method were noted.

Soil Zn application is, in general, less effective than foliar spraying in the biofortification of cereals grains, as discussed earlier (Section 1.3.2). However, the combination of soil and foliar application often brought better effects than foliar spraying alone (Cakmak et al., 2010a; Phattarakul et al., 2012; Shivay and Prasad, 2014). Application of Zinc alone to soil may improve yield and grain Zn concentration (Abdoli et al., 2016), but this method of enrichment is reported to produce rather small increases in grain Zn concentration (Cakmak et al., 2010b; Yilmaz et al., 1997; Zhang et al., 2010b). Phattarakul et al. (2012) revealed that Zn concentration in brown rice was increased only by 2.4% increase with soil Zn application. In the study by Slaton et al. (2001) soil-applied Zn increased tissue rice Zn concentration by 11.9 mg/kg above that of the control (19.7 mg/kg). A review of experiments from 10 African countries on the impact of Zn-enriched fertilizers showed that soil Zn application increased the Zn concentration in maize, rice, and wheat grains by respectively 23%, 7%, and 19% (Joy et al., 2015). Data from 23 site-year trials in seven countries (China, India, Kazakhstan, Mexico, Pakistan, Turkey, and Zambia) showed that the increase in Zn concentration in wheat grain due to soil application varied from 0.4% to 28.1% (there was negative response at two centers) over no Zn control, Zou et al. (2012) reported. In China, field trials were conducted to investigate the biofortification of micronutrients in the edible parts of winter wheat, maize, soybean, potato, canola, and cabbage (Mao et al., 2014). For Zn, soil-applied zinc sulfate was only found to be effective for increasing the Zn concentration in cabbage leaf and canola seed, with 35 and 61 mg/kg, respectively. As Cakmak et al. (2010a) reported, Zn concentration in grain is, however, not linearly associated with either soil or foliar application of Zn but could also be influenced by initial Zn content of the soil. Soils rich in Zn showed no or little effect on grain yield when Zn was applied (Ram et al., 2015).

Shivay et al. (2013) reported that for soil application, zinc sulfate was better than ZnO. In some soils, the residual effects of a single application of Zn fertilizer can be appreciated over several years (White and Broadly, 2009).

A number of studies showed that soil Se fertilizers have been used successfully to enrich Se contents in a variety of agricultural products in Se-deficient regions (Wu et al., 2015). It has been practiced in Finland (Alfthan et al., 2010), United Kingdom (Lyons, 2010), New Zealand (Curtin et al., 2006), and China (Wu et al., 2015). Many authors agree that the application of soil Se fertilizers increases the total Se and bioavailable Se for plant uptake (Broadley et al., 2010; Hawrylak-Nowak, 2013; Lavu et al., 2012, 2013; Premarathna et al., 2012; Smoleń et al., 2014; Zhao et al., 2005).

Compared with natural biofortification and foliar Se fertilizer application, soil-applied Se fertilizers can be effective under uniform soil conditions (Wu et al., 2015).

One of the most celebrated cases is from Finland (geochemical soil conditions are relatively uniform), where two decades of supplementation of soils nationwide with fertilizers containing inorganic-Se has proven to be a safe and effective way of significantly increasing Se concentrations in most crops grown for human consumption (Alfthan et al., 2010). Thus, Se contents in many indigenous food items have increased over 10-fold (Ekholm et al., 2007; Eurola et al., 1989, 1991, 2004). Similarly, Great Britain has undertaken efforts to develop soil amendment practices with inorganic-Se designed to increase dietary Se intake in the general population via the Se biofortification of food (Adams et al., 2002; Rayman, 2012). In recent years, the Se fertilizer application approach has been commonly used in agricultural production in some regions of China, where crops are generally poor in selenium (Yin and Li, 2011). As some authors reported, the use of soil Se fertilizers can increase the Se concentration in grains, fruits, and vegetables by several 100 times (Jiang et al., 2015; Liu et al., 2011; Mao et al., 2014; Yin and Li, 2011). A study from Malawi also showed the effect of Se fertilization to maize (Chilimba et al., 2012). Yields remained unaffected but grain Se concentrations increased linearly with increased Se application rates.

In the light of some research soil Se application might be more effective than the foliar one. Boldrin et al. (2013) referred that soil application of selenate provided higher Se content in grains, being 450% higher than the foliar application of this Se source. As the authors explained, this result may be related to the longer plant-Se contact time promoted by the soil application. Since foliar application was performed at the flowering stage, possibly the time required for Se transport via phloem from the leaves to the grains was not sufficient to increase the content of this element in the grain.

However, the effect of Se fertilization is not always observed. In the study conducted in Australia by Lyons et al. (2005), Se-enriched fertilizer (soil as well as foliar) did not affect wheat yields or Se concentrations in the grain.

The successful use of inorganic-Se fertilizers is strongly dependent on uniform physical soil conditions with consideration of soil types, soil redox potentials, soil pH (Hartfiel and Bahners, 1988), and the absence of high soil sulfate concentrations and elevated organic matter (Terry et al., 2000).

It is noteworthy that, among the Se sources applied to soil the highest concentrations of this element were provided by selenate. This fact is probably due to the specific adsorption that occurs with selenite on Fe and Al oxide surfaces, which are abundant in tropical soils (Rovira et al., 2008), decreasing Se in the soil solution, and thus its absorption by plants. Furthermore, it is known that selenite in plants is translocated less than selenate (Cartes et al., 2005; Ramos et al., 2010; Rios et al., 2008; Terry et al., 2000).

Although Se-containing fertilizers can be effective for producing Se-enriched crops, excessive bioaccumulation is possible, as Se content in their edible parts has the highest correlation coefficient with soil Se application treatments (Jiang et al., 2015). In addition, downward migration of soluble inorganic Se under variable field conditions can occur, especially in lighter-textured soils (Bañuelos et al., 2016). Hence, Se fertilization strategies must be carefully designed.

Soil Se applications are generally recommended, especially for crops subject to late-season moisture and heat stress (Lyons et al., 2005). One intriguing proposal is to use the Se-rich straw of plants grown on naturally seleniferous soils as a "green manure" in areas with inadequate soil Se concentrations (Terry et al., 2000).

Crops are generally supplied with Cu as a soil application of $CuSO_4$ or as organic fertilizers (Gupta, 1979; Shuman, 1998). The phytoavailability of Cu in many agricultural soils is low, and Cu applied to the soil often becomes rapidly unavailable to plants (Gupta, 1979). Nevertheless, Cu concentrations in the edible parts of cereals, vegetables, and fruits can be increased by soil Cu fertilization (Bunzl et al., 2001; Gupta, 1979; Rengel et al., 1999; Shuman, 1998; Sterrett et al., 1983; Tamoutsidis et al., 2002). Recent pot experiments conducted in Poland (Korzeniowska and Kantek, 2014) have shown the possibility of significantly increasing Cu content in the grain of wheat using soil fertilization with copper. It was also found that a small difference between the deficiency and surplus of Cu in the grain may lead to some excess copper content, especially on the soils with low organic matter content. Results of this and other studies lead to the conclusion that biofortification of crops with copper requires a precise determination of soil fertilization doses under the conditions of field experiments. Cu fertilization must be managed appropriately to ensure that it is adequate but not excessive, as too much Cu can be toxic to both plants and humans (Gupta, 1979; Puig et al., 2007; Shuman, 1998; White and Broadley, 2005).

Application of Fe fertilizers to soil is not an effective strategy for increasing Fe content in edible crop parts. Fe is abundant in mineral soils and the major problem with its acquisition is solubility (Rengel et al., 1999; White and Broadly, 2009). Fe from inorganic fertilizers rapidly becomes unavailable to plant roots through adsorption, precipitation, and oxidation reactions (Rengel et al., 1999). For this reason, Fe-chelates are often used as soil Fe fertilizers to alleviate Fe deficiency in soil (White and Broadly, 2009). According to available literature, both inorganic and chelated Fe fertilizers were found to be ineffective in improving grain-Fe concentrations greatly when applied to soils (Aciksoz et al., 2010, 2011; Rengel et al., 1999).

Soil resources of Mn, natural and added with fertilizers, become unavailable to plants due to oxidation, which is favored by high pH and high oxygen concentration in the soil solution (Norvell, 1988). However, on acid soils, Mn toxicity may occur (Schulte and Kelling, 1999).

Although other application methods (foliar, seed dressing) are reported to be more effective than soil fertilization (Ullah et al., 2016), the possibilities of crop biofortifying with Mn by soil application were recently presented by scientists from Pakistan. Ali et al. (2015) proved that the concentration of manganese was significantly enhanced in wheat plants by the soil application of $MnSO_4$. In the study by Ullah et al. (2016), manganese sulfate application to soil (Mn at 0.5 kg/ha) improved grain yield and grain Mn contents of fine grain aromatic rice by 26%.

Among different practices, soil application is the most prevalent method of B addition, especially in the developed world (Rehman et al., 2014a). However, there is limited research showing influence of soil applied B fertilizers on B concentration in edible crops. Rehman et al. (2014a) reported that soil application of B (B at 1 kg/ha as boric acid) increased B concentrations in rice kernels by 30% on average. Nevertheless, this method was less effective than foliar spraying and seed treatment.

Crops absorption and accumulation of iodine might be increased by applying iodine-containing salts or iodine-rich organic materials (e.g., seaweed) to soils, however, this method is reported to be less effective than foliar application and fertigation (Lawson et al., 2015; Smoleń et al., 2016). The pot experiments (under controlled conditions) for iodine soil fertilization showed characteristic response patterns depending on the oxidation state of the element (I^-/IO_3^-) as well as the applied iodine dose and the plant species examined (Dai et al., 2004; Hong et al., 2008; Muramatsu et al., 1989). Applicable I concentrations in the range of 5–25 mg/kg soil without yield impairment have been reported (Dai et al., 2004; Hong et al., 2008). In the field trial conducted in China (Mao et al., 2014) soil applied potassium iodate (at 590 g/ha) was only effective in increasing I concentration in cabbage leaf (by 98%), and biofortification of the other crops (winter wheat, maize, soybean, potato, canola) was not possible. Iodine being nonmobile is not concentrated in the seed (Johnson, 2003; Zia et al., 2015), therefore, seed crops such as rice (and wheat) cannot be considered a good source of dietary iodine (Fordyce et al., 2000; Tsukada et al., 2008). Iodine (I) biofortification of butterhead lettuce and kohlrabi by means of soil application was investigated in field experiments on a sandy loam soil in Germany (Lawson et al., 2015). The study showed that the supply of iodine to the soil in trial plots fertilized with potassium iodide (KI) and potassium iodate (KIO_3) directly before planting increased the iodine concentration in the edible plant parts. The desired iodine content (50–100 μg/100 g fresh mass) was obtained or exceeded at a fertilizer rate of I-IO_3^- at 7.5 kg/ha without a significant yield reduction or impairment of the marketable quality. In contrast, supplying KI at the same rate resulted in a much lower iodine enrichment and clearly visible growth impairment. In the experiment, soil-applied iodine was phytoavailable only for a short period of time. This result leads to the conclusion that long-term effects of a one-time iodine soil fertilization could not be observed (Lawson et al., 2015). It has been suggested that, because human dietary I requirements are quite low, I fertilizers might be added to large areas of agricultural production from airplanes (Graham et al., 2007).

Application of micronutrients to soil together with macronutrients fertilizers may increase their biofortification efficiency (Aciksoz et al., 2010, 2011; Lakshmanan et al., 2005; Shi et al., 2010). The combined application of organic inputs and mineral micronutrient fertilizers has the potential to alleviate overall micronutrient shortage (de Valença et al., 2017).

1.3.4 *Seed treatment*

Crops may be fertilized with micronutrients through seed treatments, which refer to the application of one or more elements to seeds. Amounts which may be applied as a seed treatment are very limited (Mortvedt, 1985).

Seeds may be treated with micronutrients either by soaking in nutrient solution of a specific concentration for a specific duration (seed priming) or by coating with micronutrients and invigoration is a relatively new term and has been interchangeably used for both methods of seed treatment (Farooq et al., 2012).

In seed priming, seeds are partially hydrated to allow metabolic events to occur without actual germination, and then re-dried (near to their original weight) to permit routine handling (Bradford, 1986). Such seeds germinate faster than non-primed seeds (Farooq et al., 2009). In micronutrient seed priming (nutripriming), micronutrients are used as osmotica (Imran et al., 2004; Singh, 2007). Primed seeds usually have better and more synchronized germination (Farooq et al., 2009), owing simply to less imbibition time (Brocklehurst and Dearman, 2008; McDonald, 2000; Taylor et al., 1998) and build-up of germination-enhancing metabolites (Basra et al., 2005).

Seed coating generally refers to the application of finely-ground solids or liquids containing dissolved or suspended solids to form a more or less continuous layer covering the natural seed coat; it includes pelleting and many other seed treatments (Scott, 1989). Strictly speaking, seed pelleting involves the addition of inert materials to modify seed shape and size for precision planting, while in seed coating, useful materials such as microorganisms, plant growth regulators, nutrients and other chemicals are adhered around the seed with the help of some sticky material. However, both of these terms are used interchangeably.

The success and effectiveness of seed coating with micronutrients depends on the nutrient used, coating material, soil type, moisture and fertility status, and the nutrient:seed ratio (Halmer, 2008).

Seed priming and seed coating with fertilizers is a strategy to apply micronutrients in precise amounts and locations (Duffner et al., 2014). Several reports indicated the potential of seed treatments in improving crop growth and yields (Marcar and Graham, 1986;, Sherrell, 1984; Wilhelm et al., 1988). Less research is concerned with the possibility of increasing the content of micronutrients in the edible parts of plants; increased nutritional values of them are rarely found (Duffner et al., 2014).

In the study by Harris et al. (2007) seed priming in 1% $ZnSO_4$ solution (for 16 h) substantially improved crop growth, grain yield, and grain Zn content in maize. The same team of scientists in other experiments (Harris et al., 2008) proved that in addition to increased yield, seed priming with Zn increased grain zinc content by 12% in wheat (mean of three trials) and by 29% in chickpea (one trial). Ajouri et al. (2004) reported 708% increase of Zn content in barley grains due to seed priming in zinc sulfate (10 mg/kg). In a trial by Johnson et al. (2005) on chickpea, lentil, rice, and wheat, seed priming with Zn increased grain Zn contents in all tested crops by 1066, 1160, 580, and 900% over untreated control, respectively, having no effect on grain yields. Shivay et al. (2008) showed increased Zn concentrations in rice grain due to application of ZnO-coated urea by 4.38–48.15% over untreated control depending on application rate (0.5–2.0% w/w).

Johnson et al. (2005) also reported that priming seeds in B (boric acid) solution increased grain B content in chickpea, lentil, rice, and wheat grains by 900, 1566, 700, and 2122% respectively. However in pigeonpea, B application through seed treatment (4 g/kg seed) was more effective and economical in increasing seed yield by 10.53% compared with the control; soil application (10 kg/ha) increased yield by 5.26% (Malla et al., 2007). Although seed priming with B is the most convenient and cost-effective method of B application, solution concentration is of vital significance and must be tested and optimized before field application, as Farooq et al. (2012) suggested.

Priming wheat seeds in $MnSO_4$ solutions significantly improved growth, grain yield and grain Mn contents in the study by Khalid and Malik (1982). Grain yield and grain Mn contents increased linearly with increasing priming solution concentration up to a maximum of 0.2% $MnSO_4$ solution for 12 h. Increased grain yield and grain Mn content in wheat from priming with $MnSO_4$ has also been observed in other studies by Marcar and Graham (1986).

MacLeod and Gupta (1995) proved that concentrations of Se in harvested soybean seed increased with increasing rates of Se applied to seed (soaking with sodium selenite at 83–830 mg/kg). Seed treatment with the higher rate of Se produced soybean Se concentrations greater than 10 mg/kg. Accumulation of selenium in seeds of haricot bean through pre-sowing seed-treatment confirmed Rodionova (2001). Nawaz et al. (2017) reported the great increase of Se in wheat shoot due to Se seed priming (75 µM Se solution of Na_2SeO_4, soaking for 24 h at 25°C).

Micronutrient application through seed treatment as a biofortification method performed better or similar to soil application (Slaton et al., 2001), but rather worse than foliar spraying (Johnson et al., 2005; MacLeod and Gupta, 1995; Nawaz et al., 2017). Combined application of micronutrients as seed priming and foliage spray may produce additional increase in their content in target crop organs, as noted in Zn in maize grains (Mohsin et al., 2014; Pankaj et al., 2016).

Despite the beneficial effects of seed treatments, some studies have indicated that this method may not be effective in fulfilling micronutrient requirements of different crops, especially in case of severe soil deficiency. For example, in kidney beans seed priming with Zn alone did not fulfill crop Zn requirements (Rasmussen and Boawn, 1969). Furthermore, seed damage and germination inhibition by seed dressing at higher nutrient concentrations may occur (Roberts, 1948).

Studies to date indicate that seed treatment with micronutrients has the potential not only to meet crop micronutrient requirements, and thus, to improve seedling emergence, stand establishment, and yield, but also to enrich the edible parts of crops with micronutrients. Seed priming or seed coating seems to be a pragmatic, inexpensive, and easy method of micronutrient delivery, especially by small landholders in developing countries (Farooq et al., 2012; Johnson et al., 2005). Several suggestions and recommendations for further work are given by Farooq et al. (2012). These concern developing techniques using a range of micronutrient sources at varying concentrations and durations, optimizing the temperature range, oxygenation requirements, and water potential, using commercially-available fertilizers for seed coating and priming osmoticum appraising large-scale field trials using nutriprimed seeds, integrating inoculation and micronutrient seed invigoration, and storage potential of nutriprimed seeds.

1.4 Other agricultural practices affecting micronutrient concentrations in crops

A fertilizer strategy represents a rapid and effective way for biofortification of food crops (Cakmak, 2010). However, other agricultural practices, such as application of macronutrients, crop rotation, intercropping, tillage, and water management, may also influence micronutrient content in crops. Unfortunately, there are relatively few studies of those treatments that consider micronutrients.

1.4.1 Macronutrients application

Application of macronutrient fertilizers is an agricultural practice that can have significant positive or negative effects on the accumulation of micronutrients in plants.

A positive N-Zn interaction in cereals was reported by a number of researchers (Lakshmanan et al., 2005). This is due to improvement in root uptake and translocation of Zn due to nitrogen (Kutman et al., 2010). Xu et al. (2012) reported that grain Zn concentration in winter wheat increased with an increase in N application rate; Zn concentration (mg/kg) was 21.5, 25.1, 30.9, and 37.0 with N at 0, 99, 198, and 297 kg/ha. Kutman et al. (2011) also reported that Zn concentration in wheat grain increased with high rates of N application. Nitrogen fertilization represents an important agronomic practice in increasing grain Fe (Aciksoz et al., 2010, 2011). Aciksoz et al. (2011) reported that when the plant N status improved by soil N application, grain concentration of Fe increased by up to 47%, whereas the application of Fe fertilizers either in inorganic ($FeSO_4$) or chelated form (e.g., Fe-EDTA, Fe-EDDHA or Fe-citrate) had only a small positive impact. In the study by Shi et al. (2010) N fertilization increased iron (Fe), zinc (Zn), and copper (Cu) density in wheat grain compared to the control. Increase of N application rate from 130 to 300 kg N/ha, however, did not further increase the three micronutrient densities in grain. The authors (Shi et al., 2010) also proved that micronutrient concentrations were usually highest in the bran and lowest in the flour. High N application increased Zn and Cu densities in all milling fractions and increased Fe concentration in shorts and bran but not in flour. N application did not affect the manganese (Mn) concentration in grain.

It is well recognized that Zn interact inversely with P fertilization (Subba Rao and Rupa, 2003). Zhang et al. (2012) reported that as the P application rate increased from 0 to 400 kg ha^{-1}, the Zn concentration in wheat grain decreased from 29.5 to 13.0 mg/kg. Reduced Zn concentration in wheat grain due to P application has been reported by a number of workers (Goh et al., 1997; Grant et al., 2002; Ryan et al., 2008). Possible reasons for reduced uptake of Zn due to application of large amounts of P were reported. These include: decreased concentration of Zn in soil solution (Norvell et al., 1987), enhanced shoot growth resulting in dilution of Zn concentration (Loneragan and Webb, 1993), and reduced mycorrhizal (VAM) infection resulting in reduced Zn uptake (Loneragan and Webb, 1993). Huang et al. (2000) pointed out that in Zn-deficient plants, expression of genes decoding a high affinity P transport protein breaks down leading to P accumulation in plants.

Liming of acid soils is a common practice in agriculture (Tyler and Olsson, 2001). Liming significantly increases grain yields of crops (Fageria, 2002), however, decreases uptake of all micronutrients except Mo (Fageria et al., 1997). Most important in the context of liming would be changes in the solubility, or soil solution concentrations, of elements (Tyler and Olsson, 2001). Not only pH itself, but also the increased HCO^{-}_{3} or Ca^{2+} concentration of the soil solution may interact with solubility and uptake of elements.

Proper management of macronutrient fertilization has the potential to enhance the nutritional quality of crop food, including micronutrient accumulation.

1.4.2 *Crop rotation*

Crop rotation or the practice of growing different types of crops sequentially in a recurrent sequence has long been known to have a number of benefits for crop yield, nutrition, and other agronomic parameters (Bullock, 1992; Stockdale and Watson, 2011). Crop residues and the use of cover crops and green manures are often considered a means of increasing available N to a following crop although they are also likely to have effects on micronutrient availability (Watson et al., 2012). The inclusion of crops such as legumes, which affect soil pH, are likely to affect micronutrient availability. For example, long-term cultivation of legumes can lead to increased plant-available Mn through lowering the pH in the soil (Williams and David, 1976). The micronutrient concentration of crops has been shown to be influenced by perennial legume crops such as alfalfa in the rotation (Turmel et al., 2009) and whether the preceding crop forms mycorrhizal associations (Grant et al., 2010). The study conducted in Poland by Fordoński et al. (2015) revealed a tendency toward an increased accumulation of nitrogen, phosphorus, calcium, copper, iron, and zinc in winter oilseed rape seeds grown after bean, while seeds of winter oilseed rape grown after spring wheat were characterized by the lowest content of macronutrients and micronutrients. The positive effect of pea and soybean as preceding crops on the content of some micronutrients in spring wheat grain was verified by Woźniak and Makarski (2012).

1.4.3 *Intercropping*

Intercropping, or the growing of two or more species together at one time, is widespread (Watson et al., 2012). It relies on the two crops having complementary rather than competing traits and thus the ability to use resources more efficiently than a single species can (Willey, 1979). While the benefits of intercropping are widely accepted in terms of yield and resource use efficiency there has been relatively little consideration of their potential benefits for managing micronutrients (Zuo and Zhang F., 2009). Legume/cereal intercrops, such as chickpeas intercropped with wheat or barley, can facilitate uptake of Fe, Zn, and Mn compared to sole crops (Gunes et al., 2007; Zhang et al., 2010a). Mechanisms by which dicots and gramineous species grown together can facilitate increased Fe and Zn uptake and possible management options to optimize micronutrient uptake in intercropping have been reviewed by Zhang et al. (2010a). In Europe, species mixtures are much more common in grassland than in many other cropping systems. Høgh Jensen and Søegaard (2012) illustrate the ability of grass- legume mixtures to buffer micronutrient supply under different N regimes compared with monocultures by showing that micronutrient contents of legumes remained relatively constant between single stand and mixtures but grass micronutrient contents were more subject to change. The experiments conducted by Głowacka (2013) indicated that strip cropping can be an effective agricultural practice for plant biofortification. Strip cropping reduced Mn content in maize, did not significantly affect Zn content, and increased accumulation of Cu and Fe. The content and uptake of the elements by maize depended on the position of the row in the strip and on the adjacent plant species. Placement next to beans resulted in higher Fe and Zn content, while placement next to barley increased Cu content.

The studies presented suggest that a rational intercropping system of nutrient-efficient species may be one of a number of approaches to produce more biofortified crops.

1.4.4 Tillage

The tillage system may have an indirect effect on micronutrient content in crops. Reduced tillage is known to increase soil compaction (Larney and Kladivko, 1989; Prasad and Power, 1991), which can create serious problems for root proliferation (Busscher and Sojka, 1987). An increased soil bulk density with no tillage as compared to conventional tillage was proved (Hill and Curse, 1985). A large number of researchers in the United States reported accumulation of P in surface soil in no-tillage plots (Follet and Peterson, 1988; Weil et al., 1988). This can lead to reduced Zn uptake (Lavedo et al., 2001). Stipesevic et al. (2009) reported that in winter wheat Zn concentration in the plant tissue at the beginning of heading did not differ due to tillage treatments in the first 2 years, but in the third year it was 11.7 mg/kg in the conventional tillage plots and only 6.4 mg/kg in the zero till plots.

1.4.5 Water management

Water management seems to be crucial factor for crop biofortification as low soil moisture condition may reduce micronutrient uptake by plants

(Halvorson, 2006). If soil water becomes limiting, as it frequently does under dryland or rainfed conditions, nutrient availability to plants can be affected (Taylor et al., 1983). Gunes et al. (2007) reported that drought stress applied under greenhouse conditions reduced the accumulation of micronutrients, including Zn, in shoots of wheat and chickpea, but enhanced Zn accumulation by lentil. Unfortunately, no data on seed Zn concentrations were given by the authors for this drought experiment. Khan et al. (2003) compared the effects of imposed drought conditions on growth and Zn uptake of two drought-tolerant chickpea cultivars with different Zn-efficiencies grown under conditions of severe to marginal Zn deficiency. Water stress reduced seed Zn only in the Zn-efficient cultivar under marginal Zn deficiency, whereas the stress slightly increased Zn density in the seeds of the other cultivar under severe Zn-deficiency conditions. In all other treatment combinations, there was no significant effect on seed Zn concentration.

Water regime is of particular concern in rice cultivation, as it determines the aerobic/anaerobic conditions (Schulin et al., 2009). Kirk and Bajita (1995) observed that submerged conditions as obtained in the conventional lowland rice cultivation result in increased H^+ extrusion by rice roots, which increases Zn availability. Under prolonged submergence, Fe could get precipitated as plaques of ferric hydroxide (Zhou et al., 2007), which are primarily lepidocrocite or goethite and have a high capacity to bind metal ions, such as Zn^{2+} and Cu^{2+}, resulting in their reduced uptake by rice roots (Chen et al., 1980). Fe deficiency is observed in rice nurseries and in rice grown under upland conditions, when rains fail and irrigation is delayed (Pal et al., 2008; Reddy and Siva Prasad, 1986). Zn deficiency could be a hidden hunger in cereals such as pearl millet and sorghum, which are mostly grown under dryland agriculture conditions (Prasad et al., 2014).

Micronutrient fertilizers might be applied through irrigation systems, as discussed in Section 1.3.1.

1.5 Obstacles and disadvantages

Concentration of micronutrients in food products can be understood as a density that expresses the amount of nutrient per unit of grain dry weight and is a more important measure of micronutrient supply in grain destined for human food than micronutrient content (the total amount of nutrient per seed or plant) (Rengel et al., 1999). Unfortunately, the density cannot be understood as the total amount of nutrient that will be efficiently undertaken and used, since the total amount of nutrients are not delivered in available form. Bioavailability is defined as the amount of a nutrient that is potentially available for absorption from a meal and once absorbed, utilizable for metabolic processes in the body. Plant foods contain substances such as antinutrients (phytic acid or phytin, fiber [e.g., cellulose, hemicellulose, lignin, cutin, suberin, etc.], certain tannins and other polyphenolics, oxalic acid, hemagglutinins [e.g., lectins], goitrogens, and heavy metals [e.g., Cd, Hg, Pb, etc.]) that influence the bioavailability of these nutrients to humans, so it is necessary to demonstrate the efficacy of micronutrient enrichment of plant foods toward improving the nutritional health of targeted populations (Welch, 2002; Welch and Graham, 2005).

It is difficult to program the places/tissues where the microelements will be accumulated in plants by agronomic fortification. It has often happened that some parts of plants are removed during the food processing, which results in significant nutrient loss. For example milling caused a 27% loss of Se due to the removal of Se located in bran and germ of durum wheat, the pasta-making process and the cooking process resulted in a loss of Se, mainly as selenite, which was about 7% (Poblaciones et al., 2014). At the same time food processing often reduces the amount of antinutrients and thus effects an increase in the bioavailability of micronutrients. For example, soaking cereals in water can reduce the presence of phytate, which enhances the bioavailability of Fe, Zn, and Ca (Hotz and Gibson, 2007). Cooking may improve nutritional value by decreasing concentration of antinutrients, such as phytate or tannins, and increasing concentration of other components such as protein and starch. At the same time it was reported that freezing and cooking caused a decrease of about 30% in grain Zn concentration and a 17%-increase in phytate:Zn ratios (ratios greater than 15 were associated with Zn deficiency) (Poblaciones and Rengel, 2016). At the same time some nutrients such as Se, Fe, Mn, and Cu are resistant and hardly lost during the wheat grain milling and bread production—making wheat more suitable for agronomic biofortification (Lyons et al., 2005). In addition to tailored food-processing techniques, the main technique to ensure that targeted micronutrients end up in the food being consumed is breeding for crop varieties that allocate micronutrients in the edible part of the crop (genetic biofortification) (de Valença et al., 2017).

A major drawback of the fertilization strategy for plant biofortification is the frequent need for regular applications, which makes this approach costly, difficult in logistic terms (heavy and bulky products), and potentially negative for the environment. Taking into account all the these limitations inherent to the agronomic biofortification through fertilizer application, it is important to explore more cost-effective and long-term strategies to improve micronutrient density in edible plant portions. Nonetheless, it has been advocated that this strategy should be combined with other biofortification approaches, particularly when the phytoavailability of minerals can restrict their concentration in the edible plant portions (Carvalho and Vasconcelos, 2013).

1.6 Prospects and challenges

It was reported by IFA that one-third of world's population is deficient in zinc. It has been recognized that the concentration of a nutrient in a food is not necessarily a reliable indicator of the value of that food as a source of the nutrient. It is even possible to improve the nutritional quality of plant foods and their products, for example, through agronomic practices described in this chapter, alhough the soil-to-plant and plant-to-human transfer of mineral nutrients is a very complex process. That is why the development of biofortified plant foods must rely on a holistic approach focusing on the following three concepts:

1. nutrient phytoavailability
2. nutrient accumulation in edible tissues
3. nutrient bioavailability (Pinto and Ferreira, 2015)

Proper balanced and designed fertilizing of soils can improve human health. It is important to modify agronomic practices, mainly through plant fertilization, that may influence nutrients content in the crops in order to maintain if not increase the concentration of micronutrients in plants (Bilski et al., 2012). Several issues should be taken into account when choosing fertilizing strategy, such as

- right source—to match fertilizer type to crop needs
- right rate—to match amount of fertilizer to crop needs
- right time—to make nutrients available when crops need them
- right place—to keep nutrients where crops can use them

One new strategy is to use the delivered nutrients in a way that minimizes the loss of macro- and micronutrients in the soil. The use of novel products, such as "designer fertilizers" dedicated to specific kinds of plants, with composition adapted to soil, are possible ways to mitigate nutrient depletion in food products. The new idea is to deliver all nutrients necessary for proper growth in one spherical granule, designed so as to release nutrients, in order, adapted to the requirements of specific plants, since the nutritional needs of plants are different in specific phases. Coating (for example by natural polymers) improves the controlled release of nutrients into the soil. As the coating dissolves, nutrients gradually permeate through tiny pores. The thickness of the coating governs the rate of nutrient release. This kind of attitude would limit the loss of nutrients in soil, because most of the released nutrients from such fertilizer formulations would be taken by plant root system (Saeid and Chojnacka, 2017).

Another significant issue in successful fortification is the availability to humans of nutrients in biofortified foods. As has been proved in many scientific papers, fortification as an increase of the density of nutrients in the edible parts of plants is possible with very good results. At the same time, little is still known about the relative merits of biofortification in terms of nutrient bioaccessibility and bioavailability, and much depends on the biochemical nature of the nutrient, which can promote or delay uptake and determine how efficiently different nutrients are transported through the blood, stored, and utilized. Many more experiments should be done that includes all stages of nutrients starting from the fertilizers and ending in the human body. Probably material flow analysis would be suitable to investigate the fate of nutrients delivered to the plant or seeds in the form of fertilizers (Díaz-Gómez et al., 2017).

1.7 Conclusions

Agronomic approaches such as application of micronutrients to plant growth media, through micronutrient fertilizer application to the soil and/or foliar application directly to the leaves of the crop seems to be a very cost-effective, fast, and practical approach to improve micronutrient concentration in cereal crops. Such approaches to the malnutrition problem become an alternative in reference to salt supplementation. Presented in this chapter solutions of utilization of different kind of biomass that can serve as a carrier of micronutrients seems to be an answer, particularly for developing countries, through the application of some cheap materials that would serve as micronutrient fertilizers, in forms available to plants, and would be considered as non-toxic from an environmental health point of view. What is more, application of biofertilizers could reduce the need for application of NPK fertilizers. Different methods of application (fertigation, foliar, soil application/pre-sowing fertilization, seed treatment) and other agricultural practices, such as macronutrient application, crop rotation, intercropping, tillage, and water management can also affect micronutrient concentration.

Acknowledgments

This project is financed in the framework of grant PBS 2/A1/11/2013 titled: "Phosphorus renewable raw materials—a resource base for new generation of fertilizers," attributed by the National Center for Research and Development.

This project is financed in the framework of grant entitled: "Cultivated plants and natural products as a source of biologically active substances assign to the production of cosmetic and pharmaceutical products as well as diet supplements," (no BIOSTRATEG2/298205/9/NCBR/2016) attributed by the National Center for Research and Development.

References

Abdoli, M., Esfandiari, E., Sadeghzadeh, B., and Mousavi S. B. 2016. Zinc application methods affect agronomy traits and grain micronutrients in bread and durum wheat under zinc-deficient calcareous soil. *Yyü Tar Bil Derg Yuzuncu Yil University Journal of Agricultural Sciences* 26(2):202–214.

Aciksoz, S. B., Yazici A., and Cakmak, I. 2010. Effect of nitrogen and iron fertilizers on grain concentration of iron in wheat. *19th World Congress of Soil Science, Soil Solutions for a Changing World,* August 1–6, Brisbane, Australia, pp. 7–8.

Aciksoz, S. B., Yazici, A., Ozturk, L., and Cakmak, I. 2011. Biofortification of wheat with iron through soil and foliar application of nitrogen and iron fertilizers. *Plant and Soil* 349:215–225.

Adams, C. L., Hambidge, M., Raboy, V. et al. 2002. Zinc absorption from a low-phytic acid maize. *American Journal of Clinical Nutrition* 76:556–559.

Adegoke, A. A., Awolusi, O. O., and Stenström, T. A. 2016. Organic fertilizers: Public health intricacies. In: Larramendy, M. (Ed.). Organic Fertilizers—From Basic Concepts to Applied Outcomes, Rijeka, Croatia: InTech. https://www.intechopen.com/books/organic-fertilizers-from-basic-concepts-to-applied-outcomes/organic-fertilizers-public-health-intricacies.

Aghili, F., Gamper, H. A., Eikenberg, J. et al. 2014. Green manure addition to soil increases grain zinc concentration in bread wheat. *PLOS ONE* 9(7):e101487.

Ajouri, A., Asgedom, H., and Becker, M. 2004. Seed priming enhances germination and seedling growth of barley under conditions of P and Zn deficiency. *Journal of Plant Nutrition and Soil Science* 167:630–636.

Akanda, M. A. R, Ahamad, M. S., Rahman, M. S., Halim, G. M. A. and Hasan, M. M. 2012. Performance evaluation of fertigation and micronutrients on fruit yield and quality of summer tomato (Lycopersicon esculentum L.). *Bangladesh Journal of Agricultural Research* 37(3):449–456.

Alam, S. M., Iqbal, Z. and Latif, A. 2000. Effect of P and Zn application by fertigation on P use efficiency and yield of wheat. *Tropical Agricultural Research and Extension* 3(2):115–119.

Alfthan, G., Aspila, P., Ekholm, P. et al. 2010. Nationwide supplementation of sodium selenite to commercial fertilizers: History and 25-year results from the Finnish selenium monitoring programme. In: Thompson, B. and Amoroso, L. (Eds.). *Combating Micronutrient Deficiencies: Food-Based Approaches*, Italy: FAO, pp. 312–337.

Ali, A. U., Sarwar, G., Tahir, M. A., and Noorka, I. R. 2015. Improvement of human health through biofortification of manganese in wheat (Triticum aestivum L.) crops. *International Journal of Medicine & Applied Health* 3(1):1–6.

Alley, M. M., Rich, C. I., Hawkins, G. W., and Martens, D. C. 1978. Correction of Mn deficiency in soybeans. *Agronomy Journal* 70:35–38.

Almendros, P., Obrador, A., Gonzalez, D., Alvarez, J. M. 2015. Biofortification of zinc in onions (Allium cepa L.) and soil Zn status by the application of different organic Zn complexes. *Scientia Horticulturae* 186:254–265.

Arsic, B., Dimitrijevic, D., Kostic, D. 2016. 1-Mineral and vitamin fortification. *Nutraceuticals* 4:1–40.

Ashmaye, S. H., Shaban, Kh. A., and Abd El-Hader, M. G. 2008. Effects of mineral nitrogen, sulphur, organic and bio-fertilizer on maize productivity in saline soil of Sahl El-Tina. *Minufiya Journal of Agricultural Research* 33(1):195–209.

Bañuelos, G. S., Arroyo, I. S., Dangi, S. R., and Zambrano, M. C. 2016. Continued selenium biofortification of carrots and broccoli grown in soils once amended with Se-enriched S. pinnata. *Frontiers in Plant Science* 7:1251.

Bapiri, A., Asgharzadeh, A., Mujallali, H., Khavazi, K., Pazira, E. 2012. Evaluation of Zinc solubilization potential by different strains of Fluorescent Pseudomonads. *Journal of Applied Sciences and Environmental Management* 16(3):295–298.

Barrameda-Medina, Y., Blasco, B., Lentini, M. et al. 2017. Zinc biofortification improves phytochemicals and amino-acidic profile in Brassica oleracea cv. Bronco. *Plant Science* 258:45–51.

Basra, S. M. A., Farooq, M., Tabassum, R., and Ahmad, N. 2005. Physiological and biochemical aspects of seed vigor enhancement treatments in fine rice (Oryza sativa L.). *Seed Science and Technology* 33:623–628.

Bell, R. W. and Dell, B. 2008. *Micronutrients for Sustainable Food, Feed, Fibre and Bioenergy Production*. Paris, France: International Fertilizer Industry Association.

Bilski, J., Jacob, D., Soumaila, F., Kraft, C., and Farnsworth, A. 2012. Agronomic biofortification of cereal crop plants with Fe, Zn, and Se, by the utilization of coal fly ash as plant growth media. *Advances in Bioresearch* 3:130–136.

Bloem, E., Haneklaus, S., Haensch, R., Schnug, E. 2017. EDTA application on agricultural soils affects microelement uptake of plants. *Science of The Total Environment* 577:166–173.

Bogaard, A., Fraser, F., Heaton, T. H. E. et al. 2013. Crop manuring and intensive land management by Europe's first farmers. *Proceedings of the National Academy of Sciences of the United States of America* 110(31):12589–12594.

Boldrin, P. F., Faquin, V., Ramos, S. J., Boldrin, K. V. F., Avila, F. W., and Guilherme L. R. G. 2013. Soil and foliar application of selenium in rice biofortification. *Journal of Food Composition and Analysis* 31:238–244.

Borowska, K. and Koper, J. 2006. The effect of manure on the selenium content in soil and potato tubers. *Polish Journal of Environmental Studies* 15(2):17–19.

Borowska, K., Koper, J., and Kozik, K. 2012. Dynamics of changes in selenium content in soil and winter wheat affected by long-term organic fertilization. *Society of Ecological Chemistry and Engineering Serie A* 19(11):1341–1348.

Bouis, H. E., Hotz, C., McClafferty, B., Meenakshi, J. V., and Pfeiffer, W. H. 2011. Biofortification: A new tool to reduce micronutrient malnutrition. *Food and Nutrition Bulletin* 32:S31–S40.

Bouis, H. E. and Saltzman A. 2017. Improving nutrition through biofortification: A review of evidence from HarvestPlus, 2003 through 2016. *Global Food Security* 12:49–58.

Bradford, K. J. 1986. Manipulation of seed water relations via osmotic priming to improve germination under stress conditions. *HortScience* 21:1105–1112.

Brigide, P., Canniatti-Brazaca, S. G., Silva, M. O. 2014. Nutritional characteristics of biofortified common beans. *Food Science and Technology* 34(3):493–500.

Broadley, M. R., Alcock, J., Alford, J. et al. 2010. Selenium biofortification of high-yielding winter wheat (*Triticum aestivum L.*) by liquid or granular Se fertilisation. *Plant and Soil* 332:5–18.

Brocklehurst, P. A. and Dearman, J. 2008. Interaction between seed priming treatments and nine seed lots of carrot, celery and onion. II. Seedling emergence and plant growth. *Annals of Applied Biology* 102:583–593.

Bullock, D. G. 1992. Crop rotation. *Critical Reviews in Plant Science* 11:309–326.

Bunzl, K., Trautmannscheimer, M., Schramel, P., and Reifenhäuser, W. 2001. Availability of arsenic, copper, lead, thallium, and zinc to various vegetables grown in slag-contaminated soils. *Journal of Environmental Quality* 30:934–939.

Businelli, D., D'Amato, R., Onofri, A., Tedeschini, E., and Tei, F. 2015. Se-enrichment of cucumber (*Cucumis sativus L.*), lettuce (*Lactuca sativa L.*) and tomato (*Solanum lycopersicum* L. Karst) through fortification in pre-transplanting. *Scientia Horticulturae* 197:697–704.

Busscher, W. J. and Sojka, R. E. 1987. Enhancement of sub-soiling effect on soil strength by conservation tillage. *Transactions of the American Society of Agricultural Engineers* 30(4):0888–0892.

Cakmak, I. 2008. Enrichment of cereal grains with zinc: Agronomic or genetic biofortification. *Plant and Soil* 302:1–17.

Cakmak, I. 2010. Biofortification of cereals with zinc and iron through fertilization strategy. *19th World Congress of Soil Science, Soil Solutions for a Changing World,* August 1–6, *Brisbane,* Australia, pp. 4–6.

Cakmak, I. 2012. HarvestPlus zinc fertilizer project: HarvestZinc. *Better Crops* 96(2):17–19.

Cakmak, I., Kalayci, M., Kaya, Y. et al. 2010b. Biofortification and localization of zinc in wheat grain. *Journal of Agricultural and Food Chemistry* 58:9092–9102.

Cakmak, I., Pfeiffer, W. H. and McClafferty, B. 2010a. Biofortification of durum wheat with zinc and iron. *Cereal Chemistry* 87(1):10–20.

Cao, X.-Y., Jiang, X.-M., Dou, Z.-H. et al. 1994. Iodination of irrigation water as a method of supplying iodine to a severely iodine-deficient population in XinJiang, China. *Lancet* 344:107–110.

Cartes, P., Gianfreda, L., and Mora, M. L., 2005. Uptake of selenium and its antioxidant activity in ryegrass when applied as selenate and selenite forms. *Plant and Soil* 276:359–367.

Carvalho, S. M. P. and Vasconcelos, M. W. 2013. Producing more with less: Strategies and novel technologies for plant-based food biofortification. *Food Research International* 54:961–971.

Chen, C. C., Dixon, J. B., and Turner, F. T. 1980. Iron coatings on rice roots: Mineralogy and quantity influencing factors. *Soil Science Society of America Journal* 44:635–639.

Chen, L., Yang, F., Xu, J. et al. 2002. Determination of selenium concentration of rice in China and effect of fertilization of selenite and selenate on selenium content of rice. *Journal of Agricultural and Food Chemistry* 50:5128–5130.

Chen, Z., Tang, Y.-T., Zhou, C. et al. 2017. Mechanisms of Fe biofortification and mitigation of Cd accumulation in rice (Oryza sativa L.) grown hydroponically with Fe chelate fertilization. *Chemosphere* 175:275–285.

Chilimba, A. D. C., Young, S. D., Black, C. R., Meacham, M. C., Lammel, J., and Broadley, M. R. 2012. Agronomic biofortification of maize with selenium (Se) in Malawi. *Field Crops Research* 125:118–128.

Chojnacka, K., Mikulewicz, M., Cieplik, J., 2011. Biofortification of food with microelements. *American Journal of Agricultural and Biological Sciences* 6 (4):544–548.

Coyne, M. S. and Mikkelsen, R. 2015. Soil microorganisms contribute to plant nutrition and root health. *Better Crops* 99(1):18–20.

Curtin, D., Hanson, R., Lindley, T. N., and Butler, R. C. 2006. Selenium concentration in wheat (*Triticum aestivum*) grain as influenced by method, rate, and timing of sodium selenite application. *New Zealand Journal of Crop and Horticultural Science* 34:329–339.

Custos, J. M., Moyne, C., Treillon, T., and Sterckeman, T., 2014. Contribution of Cd-EDTA complexes to cadmium uptake by maize: A modeling approach. *Plant Soil* 374:497–512.

Da Silva, P. H. M., Poggiani, P., and Laclau, J. P. 2011. Applying sewage sludge to Eucalyptus grandis plantations: Effects on biomass production and nutrient cycling through litterfall. *Applied and Environmental Soil Science* 2011:11.

Dai, J.-L., Zhu, Y.-G., Zhang, M., and Huang, Y.-Z. 2004. Selecting iodine-enriched vegetables and the residual effect of iodate application to soil. *Biological Trace Element Research* 3:265–276.

Dai, J. L., Zhang, M., Hu, Q. H., Huang, Y. Z., Wang, R. Q., and Zhu, Y. G., 2009. Adsorption and desorption of iodine by various Chineses oils : II. Iodide and iodate. *Geoderma* 153:130–135.

Dai, J. L., Zhu, Y. G, Huang, Y. Z., Zhang, M., and Song, J. L. 2006. Availability of iodide and iodate to Spinach in relation to total iodine in soil solution. *Plant and Soil* 289:301–308.

Das, S. K. 2014. Role of micronutrient in rice cultivation and management strategy in organic agriculture—a reappraisal. *Agricultural Sciences* 5:765–769.

de Valença, A. W., Bake, A., Brouwer, I. D., and Giller, K. E. 2017. Agronomic biofortification of crops to fight hidden hunger in sub-Saharan Africa. *Global Food Security* 12:8–14.

Degryse, F., Shahbazi, A., Verheyen, L., and Smolder, E., 2012. Diffusion limitations in root uptake of cadmium and zinc, but not nickel, and resulting bias in the Michaelis constant. *Plant Physiology* 160:1097–1109.

Degryse, F., Smolders, E., and Merckx, R., 2006. Labile Cd complexes increase Cd availability to plants. *Environmental Science & Technology* 40:830–836.

Dhaliwal, S. S., Sadana, U. S., Khurana, M. P. S., Dhadli, H. S., and Manchanda, J. S. 2010. Enrichment of rice grains through ferti-fortification. *Indian Journal of Fertilisers* 6(7):28–35.

Dhaliwal, S. S., Shukla, A. K., Manchanda, J. S., and Kumar, D. 2014. Screening of wheat cultivars and fertifortification with zinc, manganese and iron in low fertility soils of Punjab. *Vegetos* 27:139–145.

Díaz-Gómez, J., Twyman, R. M., Zhu, C. et al. 2017. Biofortification of crops with nutrients: Factors affecting utilization and storage. *Current Opinion in Biotechnology* 44:115–123.

Dimpka, C. O. and Bindraban, P. 2015. Fortification on micronutrients for efficient agronomic production. *Agronomy for Sustainable Development* 36:1–26.

Duffner, A., Hoffland, E., Stomph, T. J., Melse-Boonstra, A., and Bindraban, P. S. 2014. Eliminating zinc deficiency in rice-based systems. *VFRC Report 2014/2*. Virtual Fertilizer Research Center, Washington, DC.

Dunn, D., Stevens, G., and Kending, A. 2005. Boron fertilization of rice with soil and foliar application. *Crop Management* 4:1–7.

Durán, P., Acuña, J. J., Jorquera, M. A. et al. 2013. Enhanced selenium content in wheat grain by co-inoculation of selenobacteria and arbuscular mycorrhizal fungi: A preliminary study as a potential Se biofortification strategy. *Journal of Cereal Science* 57:275–280.

Efremova, M. and Izosimova, A. 2014. Contamination of agricultural soils with heavy metals. In: Jakobsson C. (Ed.). *Sustainable Agriculture*. Uppsala: Baltic University Press, pp. 250–252.

Eghball, B., Wienhold, B. J., Gilley, J. E., and Eigenberg, R. A. 2002. Mineralization of manure nutrients. *Journal of Soil and Water Conservation* 57:470–473.
Eich-Greatorex, S., Sogn, T. A., Øgaard, A. F., and Aasen, I. 2007. Plant availability of inorganic and organic selenium fertiliser as influ-enced by soil organic matter content and pH. *Nutrient Cycling in Agroecosystems* 79:221–231.
Ekholm, P., Reinivuo, H., Mattila, P. et al. 2007. Changes in the mineral and trace element contents of cereals, fruits and vegetables in Finland. *Journal of Food Composition and Analysis* 20:487–495.
El Sayed Hameda, E. A., Amen, El-Sh. A., EI-Morsy, A. H., and Tolba M.H. 2012. Effects of foliar spraying with microelements and different fertilizer sources on quality and yield of Pisum sativum L. plant. *International Research Journal of Agricultural Science and Soil Science* 2(1):17–24.
El-Ghamry, A. M., Abd El-Hamid, A. M., and Mosa, A. A. 2009. Effect of farmyard manure and foliar application of micronutrients on yield characteristics of wheat grown on salt affected soil. *American-Eurasian Journal of Agricultural and Environmental Sciences* 5(4):460–465.
Eurola, M., Ekholm, P., Ylinen, M., Koivistoinen, P., and Varo, P. 1989. Effects of selenium fertilization on the selenium content of selected Finnish fruits and vegetables. *Acta Agriculturae Scandinavica* 39:345–350.
Eurola, M. H, Ekholm, P. I, Ylinen, M. E., Koivistoinen, P. E., and Varo, P. T. 1991. Selenium in Finnish foods after beginning the use of selenite supplemented fertilisers. *Journal of the Science of Food and Agriculture* 56:57–70.
Eurola, M., Hietaniemi, V., Kontturi, M. et al. 2004. Selenium content of Finnish oats in 1997–1999: Effect of cultivars and cultivation techniques. *Agricultural and Food Science* 13:46–53.
Fageria, N. K. 2002. Influence of micronutrients on dry matter yield and interaction with other nutrients in annual crops. *Pesquisa Agropecuária Brasileira* 37(12):1765–1772.
Fageria, N. K., Baligar, V. C., and Jones, C. A. 1997. *Growth and Mineral Nutrition of Field Crops*, 2nd ed. New York, NY: M. Dekker.
Fang, Y., Wang, L., Xin, Z., Zhao, L., An, X., and Hu, Q. 2008. Effect of foliar application of zinc, selenium, and iron fertilizers on nutrients concentration and yield of rice grain in China. *Journal of Agricultural and Food Chemistry* 56:2079–2084.
Farahani, S. M., Chaichi, M. R., Mazaheri, D., Afshari, R. T., and Savaghebi, Gh. 2011. Barley grain mineral analysis as affected by different fertilizing systems and by drought stress. *Journal of Agricultural Science and Technology* 13: 315–326.
Farooq, M., Basra, S. M. A., Wahid, A., Khaliq, A., and Kobayashi, N. 2009. Rice seed invigoration. In: Lichtfouse, E. (Ed.). *Sustainable Agriculture Reviews*. Netherlands, Springer: pp. 137–175.
Farooq, M., Wahid, A., and Siddique, K. H. M. 2012. Micronutrient application through seed treatments–A review. *Journal of Soil Science and Plant Nutrition* 12(1):125–142.
Follet, R. F. and Peterson, G. A. 1988. Surface soil nutrient distribution as affected by wheat fallow tillage system. *Soil Science Society of America Journal* 52:141–147.
Fordoński, G., Pszczółkowska, A., Krzebietke, S., Olszewski, J., and Okorski, A. 2015. Yield and mineral composition of seeds of leguminous plants and grain of spring wheat as well as their residual effect on the yield and chemical composition of winter oilseed rape seeds. *Journal of Elementology* 20(4):827–838.

Fordyce, F. M., Johnson, C. C., Navaratna, U. R., Appleton, J. D., and Dissanayake, C. B. 2000. Selenium and iodine in soil, rice and drinking water in relation to endemic goitre in Sri Lanka. *Science of the Total Environment* 263:127–141.

Garcia-Banuelos, M. L., Sida-Arreola, J. P., and Sanches, E. 2014. Biofortification–Promising approach to increasing the content of iron and zinc in staple food crops. *Journal of Elementology* 19(3):865–888.

Giacosa, A., Faliva, M. A., Perna, S., Minoia, C., Ronchi, A., and Rondanelli, M. 2014. Selenium fortification of an Italian rice cultivar via foliar fertilization with sodium selenate and its effects on human serum selenium levels and on erythrocyte glutathione peroxidase activity. *Nutrients* 6:1251–1261.

Głowacka, A. 2013. Uptake of Cu, Zn, Fe and Mn by maize in the strip cropping system. *Plant Soil and Environment* 59(7):322–328.

Goh, T. B., Banerjee, M. R., Tu, S., and Burton, D. L. 1997. Vesicular arbuscular mycorrhizae-mediated uptake and translocation of P and Zn by wheat on a calcareous soil. *Canadian Journal of Plant Science* 77:339–346.

Gondek, K., Kopeć, M., and Głąb, T. 2013. Sewage sludge as a source of microelements regarding fodder value of spring wheat grain. *Ecological Chemistry and Engineering Serie A* 20(9):975–985.

Gonzali, S., Kiferle, C., and Perata, P. 2017. Iodine biofortification of crops: Agronomic biofortification, metabolic engineering and iodine bioavailability. *Current Opinion in Biotechnology* 44:16–26.

Graham, R. D., Welch, R. M., Saunders, D. A. et al. 2007. Nutritious subsistence food systems. *Advances in Agronomy* 92:1–74.

Grant, C. A., Bailey, L. D., Harapiak, J. T., and Flore, N. A. 2002. Effect of phosphate source, rate, and cadmium content and use of *Penicillium bilaii* on phosphorus, zinc and cadmium concentrations in durum wheat grain. *Journal of the Science of Food and Agriculture* 82:301–308.

Grant, C. A., Monreal, M. A., Irvine, R. B., Mohr, R. M., McLaren, D. L., and Khakbazan, M. 2010. Preceding crop and phosphorus fertilization affect cadmium and zinc concentration of flaxseed under conventional and reduced tillage. *Plant and Soil* 333:337–350.

Gunes, A., Inal, A., Adak, M. S. et al. 2007. Mineral nutrition of wheat, chickpea and lentil as affected by mixed cropping and soil moisture. *Nutrient Cycling in Agroecosystems* 78(1):83–96.

Gupta, U. C. 1979. Copper in agricultural crops. In: Nriagu, J. O. (Ed.). *Copper in the Environment*. New York, NY: John Wiley, pp. 255–287.

Gupta, U. C. and Lipsett, J. 1981. Molybdenum in soils, plants and animals. *Advances in Agronomy* 34:73–115.

Halmer, P. 2008. Seed technology and seed enhancement. *Acta Horticulturae* 771:17–26.

Halvorson, A. D. 2006. Nutrient-water interaction. In: Lal, R. (Ed.). *Encyclopedia of Soil Science*, vol. 2, 2nd ed. pp. 1161–1163.

Hamnér, K. and Kirchmann, H. 2015. Trace element concentrations in cereal grain of long-term field trials with organic fertilizer in Sweden. *Nutrient Cycling in Agroecosystems* 103:347–358.

Harris, D., Rashid, A., Miraj, G., Arif, M., and Shah, H. 2007. On-farm seed priming with zinc sulphate solution–a cost-effective way to increase the maize yields of resource-poor farmers. *Field Crops Research* 10:119–127.

Harris, D., Rashid, A., Miraj, G., Arif, M., and Yunas, M. 2008. 'On-farm' seed priming with zinc in chickpea and wheat in Pakistan. *Plant and Soil* 306:3–10.

Hartfiel, W. and Bahners, N. 1988. Selenium deficiency in the Federal Republic of Germany. *Biological Trace Element Research* 15:1–12.

Hawrylak-Nowak, B. 2013. Comparative effects of selenite and selenate on growth and selenium accumulation in lettuce plants under hydroponic conditions. *Plant Growth Regulation* 70:149–157.

Hazra, G. 2016. Different types of eco-friendly fertilizers: An overview. *Sustainability in Environment* 1(1):54–70.

Hill, R. M. and Curse, R. M. 1985. Tillage effects on bulk density and soil strength of two mollisols. *Soil Science Society of America Journal* 49:1270–1273.

Hlgnett, T. P. and Mcclellan, G. H. 1985. Sources and production of micronutrient fertilizers. In: Vlek, P. L. G. (Ed.). *Micronutrients in Tropical Foods*. Netherlands: Springer, pp. 237–259.

Høgh Jensen, H. and Søegaard, K. 2012. Robustness in the mineral supply from temporary grasslands. *Acta Agriculturae Scandinavica, Section B. Soil and Plant Science* 62:79–90.

Hong, C.-L., Weng, H.-X., Qin, Y.-C., Yan, A.-L., and Xie, L.-L. 2008. Transfer of iodine from soil to vegetables by applying exogenous iodine. *Agronomy for Sustainable Development* 28:575–583.

Hoseinzade, H., Ardakani, M. R., Shahdi, A, Rahmani, H. A., Noormohammadi G., and Miransari, M. 2016. Rice (Oryza sativa L.) nutrient management using mycorrhizal fungi and endophytic Herbaspirillum seropedicae. *Journal of Integrative Agriculture* 15:1385–1394.

Hotz, C. and Gibson, R. S. 2007. Traditional food-processing and preparation practices to enhance the bioavailability of micronutrients in plant-based diets. *Journal of Nutrition* 136:1079–1100.

Hu, Q., Xu J., and Pang, G. J. 2003. Effect of Se on increasing the antioxidant activity of tea leaves harvested during the early spring tea producing season. *Journal of Agricultural and Food Chemistry* 51:3379–3381.

Huang, C., Barker, S. J., Langridge, P., Smith, F. W., and Graham, R. D. 2000. Zinc deficiency up-regulation expression of high-affinity phosphate transporter genes in both P deficient and sufficient barley. *Plant Physiology* 124:415–422.

Hussain, M., Khan, M. A., Khan, M. A., Farooq, M., and Farooq, S. 2012. Boron application improves growth, yield and net economic return of rice. *Rice Science* 19:259–262.

Hwang, B.-R., Kim, E.-J., Yang, J.-S., and Baek, K. 2015. Extractive and oxidative removal of copper bound to humic acid in soil. *Environmental Science and Pollution Research* 22:6077–6085.

Impa, S. M. and Johnson-Beebout, S. E. 2012. Mitigating zinc deficiency and achieving high grain Zn in rice through integration of soil chemistry and plant physiology research. *Plant and Soil* 361:3–41.

Imran, M., Neumann, G., and Römheld, V. 2004. *Nutrient Seed Priming Improves Germination Rate and Seedling Growth Under Submergence Stress at Low Temperature.* International Research on Food Security, Natural Resource Management and Rural Development, Cuvillier Verlag Göttingen.

Imran, M. and Rehim, A. 2016. Zinc fertilization approaches for agronomic biofortification and estimated human bioavailability of zinc in maize grain. *Archives of Agronomy and Soil Science* 63(1):106–116.

Jayalath, N., Fitzpatrick, R. W., Mosley, L., and Marschner, P. 2016. Type of organic carbon amendment influences pH changes in acid sulfate soils in flooded and dry conditions. *Journal of Soils and Sediments* 16:518–526.

Jiang, W., Strik, P. C., Lingna, J., van Keulen, H., Ming, Z., and Stomph, T. J. 2007. Uptake and distribution of root-applied or foliar applied 65 Zn after flowering in aerobic rice. *Annals of Applied Biology* 150:383–391.

Jiang, X. M., Cao, X. Y., Jiang, J. Y. et al. 1997. Dynamics of environmental supplementation of iodine: Four years' experience of iodination of irrigation water in Hotien, Xinjiang, China. *Archives of Environmental Health* 52(6):399–408.

Jiang, Y., Zeng, Z. H., Bu, Y. et al. 2015. Effects of selenium fertilizer on grain yield, Se uptake and distribution in common buckwheat (Fagopyrum esculentum Moench). *Plant, Soil and Environment* 61(8):371–377.

Johanson, K. J. 2000. Iodine in soil. *Technical Report TR-00-21*. Svensk Arnbranslehantering AB Swedish Nuclear Fuel and Waste Management, Stockholm, Sweden.

Johnson, C. C. 2003. The geochemistry of iodine and its application to environmental strategies for reducing risks from iodine deficiency disorders. *British Geological Survey Commissioned Report, CR/03/057N*, http://nora.nerc.ac.uk/10724/1/CR03057N.pdf (accessed 10 July 2014).

Johnson, S. E., Lauren, J. G., Welch, R. M., and Duxbury, J. M. 2005. A comparison of the effects of micronutrient seed priming and soil fertilization on the mineral nutrition of chickpea (*Cicer arietinum*), lentil (*Lens culinaris*), rice (*Oryza sativa*) and wheat (*Triticum aestivum*) in Nepal. *Experimental Agriculture* 41:427–448.

Jones, C. and Jacobsen, J. 2009. Micronutrients: Cycling, testing and fertilizer recommendations. *Nutrient Management Module* 7:1–16.

Jones, J. B.,Jr. 1997. *Plant Nutrition Manual*. Boca Raton, FL: CRC Press.

Joy, E. J. M., Stein, A. J., Young, S. D., Ander, E. L., Watts, M. J., and Broadley, M. R. 2015. Zinc-enriched fertilisers as a potential public health intervention in Africa. *Plant and Soil* 389:1–24.

Kabata-Pendias, A. 2010. *Trace Elements in Soils and Plants*, 4th ed. Boca Raton, FL: CRC Press.

Kabir, A., Paltridge, N., and Stangoulis, J. 2016. Chlorosis correction and agronomic biofortification in field peas through foliar application of iron fertilizers under Fe deficiency. *Journal of Plant Interactions* 11(1):1–4.

Khalid, B. Y. and Malik, N. S. A. 1982. Presowing soaking of wheat seeds in copper and manganese solutions. *Communications in Soil Science and Plant Analysis* 13:981–986.

Khan, H. R., McDonald, G. K., and Rengel, Z. 2003. Zinc fertilization improves water use efficiency, grain yield and seed Zn content in chickpea. *Plant and Soil* 249(2):389–400.

Kirk, G. J. D. and Bajita, J. B. 1995. Root induced iron oxidation, pH changes and zinc solubilisation in the rhizosphere of lowland rice. *New Phytologist* 131:129–137.

Kizos, T. 2014. Effect of manganese nutrition on content of nutrient and yield of lettuce (*Lactuca sativa* L.) in hydroponic. *Ecological Chemistry and Engineering Serie S* 21(3):529–537.

Kizos, T., Veikontis, G., and Marín-Guirao, J. I. 2010. Comparison of organic and integrated farming systems: The case of Sultana table grapes in Korinthos, Greece. *Journal of Sustainable Agriculture* 35(1):7–47.

Korzeniowska, J. and Kantek, K. 2014. Biofortification of wheat grain with copper through soil fertilization. *Environmental Protection and Natural Resources* 4(62):23–27.

Korzeniowska, J. and Stanisławska-Glubiak, E. 2011. The effect of foliar application of copper on content of this element in winter wheat grain. *Polish Journal of Agronomy* 4:3–6.

Krishnamurthy, V. N., Gowariker, S., Paranjape, K., and Dhanorkar, M. 2008. *The Fertilizer Encyclopedia*. Hoboken, NJ: John Willey and Sons, pp. 83–84.

Kumar, A. A., Anuradha, K., and Ramaiah, B. 2013. Increasing grain Fe and Zn concentration in sorghum: Progress and way forward. *Journal of Semi-Arid Tropical Agricultural Research* 11:1–5.

Kumar, B. L. and Gopal, D. V. R. S. 2015. Effective role of indigenous microorganisms for sustainable environment. *3 Biotech* 5(6):867–876.

Kutman, U. B., Yildiz, B., and Cakmak, I. 2011. Improved nitrogen status enhances zinc and iron concentrations both in the whole grain and the endosperm fraction of wheat. *Journal of Cereal Science* 53:118–125.

Kutman, U. B., Yildiz, B., Oztruk, L., and Cakmak, I. 2010. Biofortification of dutrum wheat with zinc through soil and foliar application of nitrogen. *Cereal Chemistry* 87:1–9.

Lakshmanan, R., Prasad, R., and Jain, M. C. 2005. Yield and uptake of micronutrients by rice as influenced by duration of variety and nitrogen utilization. *Archives of Agronomy and Soil Science* 51:1–14.

Larney, F. J. and Kladivko, E. J. 1989. Soil strength properties under four tillage systems at three long term study sites in Indiana. *Soil Science Society of America Journal* 53:1539–545.

Lavedo, R. S., Porcelli, C. A., and Alvarez, R. 2001. Nutrient and heavy metal concentration distribution in corn, soybean and wheat as affected by tillage systems in the Argentine Pampas. *Soil and Tillage Research* 62:55–60.

Lavu, R. V. S., De Schepper, V., Steppe, K., Majeti, P. N. V., Tack F., and Du Laing, G. 2013. Use of selenium fertilizers for production of Se-enriched kenaf (Hibiscus cannabinus): Effect on Se concentration and plant productivity. *Journal of Plant Nutrition and Soil Science* 176:634–639.

Lavu, R. V. S., Du Laing, G., Van de Wiele, T. et al. 2012. Fertilizing soil with selenium fertilizers: Impact on concentration, speciation, and bioaccessibility of selenium in leek (*Allium ampeloprasum*). *Journal of Agricultural and Food Chemistry* 60:10930–10935.

Lawson, P. G., Daum D., Czauderna, R., Meuser, H., and Härtling, J. W. 2015. Soil versus foliar iodine fertilization as a biofortification strategy for field-grown vegetables. *Frontiers in Plant Science* 6:450.

Li, B., Wei, M., Shen, A., Xu, J., Zhang, H., and Hao, F. 2009. Changes of yields, soil properties and micronutrients as affected by 17-yr fertilization treatments. *Journal of Food, Agriculture and Environment* 7(3–4):408–413.

Liu, H., Xu, J., Li, X. et al. 2015. Effects of microelemental fertilizers on yields, mineral element levels and nutritional compositions of the artificially cultivated Morchella conica. *Scientia Horticulturae* 189:86–93.

Liu, X., Yang, Y., Deng, X., Li, M., Zhang, W., and Zhao, Z. 2017. Effects of sulfur and sulfate on selenium uptake and quality of seeds in rapeseed (Brassica napus L.) treated with selenite and selenate. *Environmental and Experimental Botany* 135:13–20.

Liu, Y., Li, F., Yin, X. B., and Lin, Z. Q. 2011. *Plant-based biofortification: From phytoremediation to Se-enriched agriculture products*. In: Sharma, S. K. and Mudhoo, A. (Eds.). Green Chemistry for Environmental Sustainability, Boca Raton, FL: CRC Press, pp. 341–356.

Loneragan, J. F. and Webb, M. J. 1993. Interaction between Zn and other nutrients affecting the growth of plants. In: Robson, A. D. (Ed.). *Zn in Soils and Plants.* Dordrecht, Netherlands: Kluwer Academic.

Lyons, G. 2010. Selenium in cereals: Improving the efficiency of agronomic biofortification in the UK. *Plant and Soil* 332:1–4.

Lyons, G. H., Genc, Y., Stangoulis, J. C., Palmer, L. T., and Graham, R. D. 2005. Selenium distribution in wheat grain, and the effect of postharvest processing on wheat selenium content. *Biological Trace Element Research* 103:155–168.

MacLeod, J. A. and Gupta, U. C. 1995. Effect of selenium seed treatment on selenium concentrations in soybeans. *Canadian Journal of Soil Science* 75:287–291.

Malla, R. M., Padmaja, B., Malathi, S., and Jalapathi, R. L. 2007. Effects of micronutrients on growth and yield of pigeonpea. *Journal of Semi-Arid Tropical Agricultural Research* 5:1–3.

Mao, H., Wang, J., Wang, Z., Zan, Y., Lyons, G., and Zou, C. 2014. Using agronomic biofortification to boost zinc, selenium, and iodine concentrations of food crops grown on the loess plateau in China. *Journal of Soil Science and Plant Nutrition* 14(2):459–470.

Marcar, N. E. and Graham, R. D. 1986. Effect of seed manganese content on the growth of wheat (Triticum aestivum) under manganese deficiency. *Plant and Soil* 96:165–173.

McCauley, A., Jones, C., and Jacobsen, J. 2009. Soil pH and organic matter. *Nutrient Management Module* 8:1–12.

McDonald, M. B. 2000. *Seed priming.* In: Black, M. and Bewley, J. D. (Eds.). *Seed Technology and Its Biological Basis*, Sheffield, England: Sheffield Academic Press, pp. 287–325.

Megali, L., Glauser, G., and Rasmann, S. 2014. Fertilization with beneficial microorganisms decreases tomato defenses against insect pests. *Agronomy for Sustainable Development* 34(3):649–656.

Melash, A. A., Mengistu, D. K., and Aberra, D. A. 2016. Linking agriculture with health through genetic and agronomic biofortification. *Agricultural Sciences* 7:295–307.

Mofunanya, A. A. J., Ebigwai, J. K., Bello, O. S., and Egbe, A. O. 2015. *Comparative study of the effects of organic and inorganic fertilizer on nutritional composition of Amaranthus spinosus L. Asian Journal of Plant Sciences* 14(1):34–39.

Mohsin, A. U., Ahmad, A. U. H., Farooq, M., and Ullah, S. 2014. Influence of zinc application through seed treatment and foliar Spray on growth, productivity and grain quality of hybrid maize. *Journal of Animal and Plant Sciences* 24:1494–1503.

Moiseyev, I. T., Tikhomirov, F. A., Perevezentsev, V. M., and Rerikh, L. A. 1984. Role of soil properties, interspecific plant differences, and other factors affecting the accumulation of radioactive iodine in crops. *Soviet Soil Science* 16:60–66.

Mortvedt, J. J. 1985. Micronutrient fertilizers and fertilization practices. In: Vlek, P. L. G. (Ed.). *Micronutrients in Tropical Foods.* Netherlands: Springer, pp. 221–235.

Mouritsen, O. G. 2013. *Seaweeds, Edible, Available and Sustainable.* Chicago, IL: University of Chicago Press.

Muramatsu, Y., Uchida, S., Sumiya, M., Ohmomo, Y., and Obata, H. 1989. Tracer experiments on transfer of radioiodine in the soil-rice plant system. *Water, Air, and Soil Pollution* 45:157–171.

Naeem, S. S., El-habet, H. B. I., El- Namaky, R. A., and El-Salamouni, M. H. 2012. Effect of organic, inorganic fertilizers and storage periods on grain yield and nutritional value of two Egyptian rice cultivars. *Journal of Agricultural Science, Mansoura University* 3(12):1153–1168.

Naik, S. K. and Das, D. K. 2008. Relative performance of chelated Zn and zinc sulphate for low-land rice (Oryza sativa L). *Nutrient Cycling in Agroecosystems* 81:219–227.

Narwal, R., Dahiya, R., Malik, R., and Kala, R. 2012. Influence of genetic variability on zinc, iron and manganese responses in wheat. *Journal of Geochemical Exploration* 121:45–48.

Narwal, R., Malik, R., and Dahiya, R. 2010. Addressing variations in status of a few nutritionally important micronutrients in wheat crop. *19th World Congress of Soil Science, Soil Solutions for a Changing World, August 1–6, Brisbane*, pp. 1–3.

Nawaz, F., Ahmad, R., Ashraf, M. Y., Waraich, E. A., and Khan, S. Z. 2015. Effect of selenium foliar spray on physiological and biochemical processes and chemical constituents of wheat under drought stress. *Ecotoxicology and Environmental Safety* 113:191–200.

Nawaz, F., Ashraf, M. Y., Ahmad, R., Waraich, E. A., and Shabbir, R. N. 2014. Selenium (Se) regulates seedling growth in wheat under drought stress. *Advances in Chemistry* 2014:7.

Nawaz, F., Ashraf, M. Y., Ahmad, R., Waraich, E. A., Shabbir, R. N., and Hussain, R. A. 2016. Selenium supply methods and time of application influence spring wheat (*Triticum aestivum* L.) yield under water deficit conditions. *Journal of Agricultural Science* 155:1–14.

Norvell, W. 1988. Inorganic reactions of manganese in soils. In: Graham, R., Hannan, R. and Uren, N. (Eds.). *Manganese in Soils and Plants*. Dordrecht: Kluwer Academic Publishers, pp. 155–173.

Norvell, W. A., Dabkowska, N., and Cary, E. 1987. Effect of phosphorus and zinc fertilization on the solubility of Zn^{2+} in two alkaline soils. *Soil Science Society of America Journal* 51:584–588.

Olivares, F. L., Aguiar, N. O., Rosa, R. C. C., and Canellas, L. P. 2015. Substrate biofortification in combination with foliar sprays of plant growth promoting bacteria and humic substances boosts production of organic tomatoes. *Scientia Horticulturae* 183:100–108.

Ozturk, L., Yazici, M. A., Yucel, C. et al. 2006. Concentration and localization of zinc during seed development and germination in wheat. *Physiologia Plantarum* 128:144–152.

Pagani, A., Sawyer, J. E., and Mallarino, A. 2013. Site-specific nutrient management-for nutrient management planning to improve crop production, environmental quality, and economic return. Micronutrient Management, Chap. 7. *NRCS, Iowa State University*.

Pal, S., Datta, S. P., Rattan, R. K., and Singh, A. K. 2008. Diagnosis and amelioration of iron deficiency under aerobic rice. *Journal Journal of Plant Nutrition* 31:919–940.

Pandey, V. J., Dev, S. M., and Jayachandran U. 2016. Impact of agricultural interventions on the nutritional status in South Asia: A review. *Food Policy* 62:28–40.

Pankaj, S. C. and Dewangan, P. K. 2016. Biofortification: An alternative for zinc and iron deficiency in cereals—A review. *International Journal of Advanced Research* 4(5):618–631.

Patharajan, S. and Raaman, N. 2012. Influence of arbuscular mycorrhizal fungi on growth and selenium uptake by garlic plants. *Archieves of Phytopathology and Plant Protection* 45:138–151.

Pazurkiewicz-Kocot, K., Galas, W., and Kita, A. 2003. The effect of selenium on the accumulation of some metals in Zea mays L. plants treated with indole-3-acetic acid. *Cellular and Molecular Biology Letters* 8:97–103.

Pellegrino, E. and Bedini, S. 2014. Enhancing ecosystem services in sustainable agriculture: Biofertilization and biofortification of chickpea (Cicer arietinum L.) by arbuscular mycorrhizal fungi. *Soil Biology and Biochemistry* 68:429–439.

Pereg, L. and McMillan, M. 2015. Scoping the potential uses of beneficial microorganisms for increasing productivity in cotton cropping systems. *Soil Biology and Biochemistry* 80:349–358.

Phattarakul, N., Rerkasem, B., Li, L. J. et al. 2012. Biofortification of rice grain with zinc through zinc fertilization in different countries. *Plant and Soil* 361:131–141.

Piechota, T., Kowalski, M., Sawinska, Z., and Majchrzak, L. 2014. Assessment of one operation strip tillage and in row liquid organic manure injection in maize. *Fragmenta Agronomica* 31(1):74–82.

Pinto, E. and Ferreira, I. M. P. L. V. O. 2015. Cation transporters/channels in plants: Tools for nutrient biofortification. *Journal of Plant Physiology* 179:64–82.

Poblaciones, M. J. and Rengel, Z. 2016. Soil and foliar zinc biofortification in field pea (Pisum sativum L.): Grain accumulation and bioavailability in raw and cooked grains. *Food Chemistry* 212:427–433.

Poblaciones, M. J., Rodrigo, S., Santamaría, O., Chen, Y., and McGrath, S. P. 2014. Agronomic selenium biofortification in Triticum durum under Mediterranean conditions: From grain to cooked pasta. *Food Chemistry* 146:378–384.

Poggi, V., Arcioni, A., Filippini, P., and Pifferi, P. G. 2000. Foliar application of selenite and selenate to potato (Solanum tuberosum): Effect of a ligand agent on selenium content of tubers. *Journal of Agricultural and Food Chemistry* 48:4749–4751.

Prasad, R. and Power, J. F. 1991. Crop residue management. *Advances in Soil Science* 5:205–251.

Prasad, R, Shivay, Y. S., and Kumar, D. 2014. Agronomic biofortification of cereal grains with iron and zinc. In: Sparks, D. L. (Ed.). *Advances in Agronomy*, vol. 125. Burlington: Academic Press, pp. 55–91.

Premarathna, L., McLaughlin, M. J., Kirby, J. K., Hettiarachchi, G. M., Stacey, S., and Chittleborough, D. J. 2012. Selenate-enriched urea granules are a highly effective fertilizer for selenium biofortification of paddy rice grain. *Journal of Agricultural and Food Chemistry* 60:6037–6044.

Puig, S., Andrés-Colás, N., García-Molina, A., and Peñarrubia, L. 2007. Copper and iron homeostasis in Arabidopsis: Responses to metal deficiencies, interactions and biotechnological applications. *Plant, Cell and Environment* 30:271–290.

Ram, H., Sohu, V. S., Cakmak, I. et al. 2015. Agronomic fortification of rice and wheat grains with zinc for nutritional security. *Current Science* 109:1–6.

Ramesh, A., Sharma, S. K., Sharma, M. P., Yadav, N., and Joshi, O. P. 2014. Inoculation of zinc solubilizing Bacillus aryabhattai strains for improved growth, mobilization and biofortification of zinc in soybean and wheat cultivated in Vertisols of central India. *Applied Soil Ecology* 73:87–96.

Ramos, S. J., Faquin, V., Guilherme, L. R. G., et al. 2010. Selenium biofortification and antioxidant activity in lettuce plants fed with selenate and selenite. *Plant, Soil and Environment* 56:584–588.

Ramzani, P. M. A., Khalid, M., Naveed, M., Ahmad, R., and Shahid, M. 2016. Iron biofortification of wheat grains through integrated use of organic and chemical fertilizers in pH affected calcareous soil. *Plant Physiology and Biochemistry* 104:284–293.

Rasmussen, P. E. and Boawn, L. C. 1969. Zinc seed treatment as a source of zinc for beans. *Agronomy Journal* 61:674–676.

Rayman, M. P. 2012. Selenium and human health. *Lancet* 379:1256–1268.

Reddy, C. K. and Siva Prasad, G. V. S. 1986. Varietal response to iron chlorosis in upland rice. *Plant and Soil* 94:285–292.

Rehman, A., Farooq, M., Ata Cheema, Z., Nawaz, A., and Wahid, A. 2014b. Foliage applied boron improves the panicle fertility, yield and biofortification of fine grain aromatic rice. *Journal of Soil Science and Plant Nutrition* 14(3):723–733.

Rehman, A., Farooq, M., Nawaz, A., and Ahmad, R. 2014a. Influence of boron nutrition on the rice productivity, kernel quality and biofortification in different production systems. *Field Crops Research* 169:123–131.

Rengel, Z., Batten, G. D., and Crowley, D. E. 1999. Agronomic approaches for improving the micronutrient density in edible portions of field crops. *Field Crops Research* 60:27–40.

Ribeiro, A. R., Gonçalves, A., Bandarra, N. et al. 2016. Natural fortification of trout with dietary macroalgae and selenised-yeast increases the nutritional contribution in iodine and selenium. *Food Research International* in Press.

Rietra, R. P. J. J., Heinen, M., Dimpka, C., and Bindraban, P. S. 2015. Effects of nutrient antagonism and synergism on fertilizer use efficiency. *VFRC Report 2015/5*. Virtual Fertilizer Research Centre, Washington, DC.

Rios, J. J., Rosales, M. A., Blasco, B., Cervilla, L. M., Romero, L., and Ruiz, J. M. 2008. Biofortification of Se and induction of the antioxidant capacity in lettuce plants. *Scientia Horticulturae* 116:248–255.

Roberts, W. O. 1948. Prevention of mineral deficiency by soaking seed in nutrient solution. *Journal of Agricultural Science* 38:458–468.

Rodionova, V. N. 2001. *Accumulation of selenium and chromium in seeds of haricot bean.* In: Horst, W. J. et al. (Eds.). *Plant Nutrition—Food Security and Sustainability of Agro-Ecosystems*, Netherlands: Kluwer Academic Publishers, pp. 474–475.

Roe, E. 1998. Compost utilization for vegetable and fruit crops. *Hortscience* 33:934–937.

Rosado, J. L., Hambidge, K. M., Miller, L. V., Garcia, O. P., and Westcott, J. 2009. The quantity of zinc absorbed from wheat in adult women is enhanced by biofortification. *Journal of Nutrition* 139:1920–1925.

Rovira, M., Gimenez, J., Martinez, M. et al. 2008. Sorption of selenium (IV) and selenium (VI) onto natural iron oxides: Goethite and hematite. *Journal of Hazardous Materials* 150:279–284.

Roy, R. N., Finck, A., Blair, G. J., and Tandon, H. L. S. 2006. Plant nutrition for food security. A guide for integrated nutrient management. In: *Sources of Plant Nutrients and Soil Amendments. Ferilizer and Plant Nutrition Biuletin*, Chap. 5. Italy: Food and Agriculture Organization of the United Nations.

Ruel, M. T., Alderman H., and The Maternal and Child Nutrition Study Group. 2013. Nutrition-sensitive interventions and programmes: How can they help to accelerate progress in improving maternal and child nutrition? *Lancet* 382:536–551.

Rutkowska, B., Szulc, W., Sosulski, T., and Stępień, W. 2014. Soil micronutrient availability to crops affected by long-term inorganic and organic fertilizer applications. *Plant, Soil and Environment* 60(5):198–203.

Ryan, M. H., McInerney, J. K., Record, I. R., and Angus, J. F. 2008. Zinc bioavailability in wheat grain in relation to phosphorus fertilizer, crop sequence and mycorrhizal fungi. *Journal of the Science of Food and Agriculture* 88:1208–1216.

Saeid, A. and Chojnacka, K. 2017. *Fertlizers: Need for new strategies* In: Unni, M. R. and Sarathchandran, C. (Eds.). *Organic Farming: New Methods, Advancements and Future*, Elsevier.

Saha, S., Mandal, B., Hazra, G. C., et al. 2015. Can agronomic biofortification of zinc be benign for iron in cereals? *Journal of Cereal Science* 65:186–191.

Saltzman, A., Birol, E., Bouis, H. E., et al. 2013. Biofortification: Progress toward a more nourishing future. *Global Food Security* 2:9–17.

Samoraj, M., Tuhy, Ł., Baśladyńska, S., and Chojnacka, K. 2015. Biofortification of maize grains with micronutrients by enriched biomass of blackcurrant seeds. *Open Chemistry* 13:1236–1244.

Sanmartín, C., Garmendia, I., Romano, B., Díaz, M., Palop, J. A., and Goicoechea, N. 2014, Mycorrhizal inoculation affected growth, mineral composition, proteins and sugars in lettuces biofortified with organic or inorganic selenocompounds. *Scientia Horticulturae* 180:40–51.

Schulin, R., Khoshgoftarmanesh, A., Afyuni, A., Nowack, B., and Frossard, E. 2009. Effects of soil management on zinc uptake and its bioavailability in plants. In: Banuelos, G. S. and Lin, Z.-Q. (Eds.). *Development and uses of Biofortified Agricultural Products*. CRC Press, Taylor and Francis Group, pp. 95–114.

Schulte, E. E. and Kelling, K. A. 1999. Soil and applied manganese. In: Understanding Plant Nutrients. *Cooperative Extension Publications, University of Wisconsin-Extension*, pp. 1–4.

Schulz, R. and Rornheld, V. 1997. Recycling of municipal and industrial organic wastes in agriculture: Benefits, limitations, and means of improvement. In: Ando, T. et al. (Eds.). *Plant Nutrition—For Sustainable Food Production and Environment*. Berlin: Kluwer Academic Publishers, pp. 581–586.

Scott, J. M. 1989. Seed coatings and treatments and their effects on plant establishment. *Advances in Agronomy* 42:43–83.

Shaban, K. A., Khafaga, E. E., and Hoda, S. S. 2008. Effect of organic manure and mineral N on some soil properties and spinach productivity under saline soil conditions. *Journal of Agricultural Science, Mansoura University* 33(5):3865–3879.

Shaban, K. A., Mahmoud, A. A., Mansour, A., and Abd El-Kader, M. G. 2009. Biofertilizer and organic manure affects rice productivity in newly reclaimed saline soil. *Dynamic Soil, Dynamic Plant* 3(1):55–60.

Shaikh, S. and Saraf, M. 2017. Biofortification of Triticum aestivum through the inoculation of zinc solubilizing plant growth promoting rhizobacteria in field experiment. *Biocatalysis and Agricultural Biotechnology* 9:120–126.

Shen, H., Starr, J., Han, J. et al. 2016. The bioaccessibility of polychlorinated biphenyls (PCBs) and polychlorinated dibenzo-p-dioxins/furans (PCDD/Fs) in cooked plant and animal origin foods. *Environment International* 94:33–42.

Sherrell, C. G. 1984. Effect of molybdenum concentration in the seed on the response of pasture legumes to molybdenum. *New Zealand Journal of Agricultural Research* 27:417–423.

Shi, R., Zhang, Y., Chen, X. et al. 2010. Influence of long-term nitrogen fertilization on micronutrient density in grain of winter wheat (Triticum aestivum L.). *Journal of Cereal Science* 51:165–170.

Shivay, Y. S., Kumar, D., Prasad, R., and Ahlawat, L. P. S. 2008. Relative yield and zinc uptake by rice from zinc sulphate and zinc oxide coatings onto urea. *Nutrient Cycling in Agroecosystems* 80:181–188.

Shivay, Y. S. and Prasad, R. 2014. Zinc deficiency in humans and its amelioration. *Indian Journal of Community Health* 26(Supplement S2).

Shivay, Y. S., Prasad, R., and Pal, M. 2013. Zinc fortification of oats grain and straw through zinc fertilization. Agricultural Research 2:375–381.

Shivay, Y. S., Prasad, R., and Rahal, A. 2010a. Genotypic variation for productivity zinc utilization efficiencies, and kernel quality in aromatic rices under low available zinc conditions. *Journal of Plant Nutrition* 33:1835–1848.

Shivay, Y. S., Prasad, R., and Rahal, A. 2010b. Studies on some nutritional quality parameters of organically or conventionally grown wheat. *Cereal Research Communications* 38:342–352.

Shuman, L. M. 1998. Micronutrient fertilizers. *Journal of Crop Production* 1:165–195.

Silva, G. T. A., Matos, L. V., de Oliveira Nóbrega, P., Campello. E. F. C., and Silva de Resende, A. 2008. Chemical composition and decomposition rate of plants used as green manure. *Scientia Agricola (Piracicaba, Brazil)* 65(3):298–305.

Singh, M. K. and Prasad, S. K. 2014. Agronomic aspects of zinc biofortification in rice (*Oryza sativa* L). *Proceedings of the National Academy of Sciences, India Section B: Biological Sciences* 84(3):613–623.

Singh, M. V. 2007. *Efficiency of seed treatment for ameliorating zinc deficiency in crops. Proceedings of Zinc Crops Conference,* May 24 -26, Istanbul, Turkey.

Singh, P., Dhaliwal, S. S., and Sadana, U. S. 2013. Iron enrichment of paddy grains through ferti-fortification. *Journal of Research Punjab Agricultural University* 50:32–38.

Slaton, N. A., Wilson-Jr, C. E., Ntamatungiro, S., Norman, R. J., and Boothe, D. L. 2001. Evaluation of zinc seed treatments for rice. *Agronomy Journal* 93:152–157.

Smith, S. E. and Read, D. J. 2008. *Mycorrhizal Symbiosis,* 3rd ed. London: Academic Press.

Sterrett, S. B., Reynolds, C. W., Schales, F. D., Chaney, R. L., and Douglass, L. W. 1983. Transplant quality, yield, and heavy-metal accumulation of tomato, muskmelon, and cabbage grown in media containing sewage sludge compost. *Journal of the American Society for Horticultural Science* 108:36–41.

Smoleń, S., Kowalska, I., and Sady, W. 2014. Assessment of biofortification with iodine and selenium of lettuce cultivated in the NFT hydroponic system. *Scientia Horticulturae* 166:9–16.

Smoleń, S., Ledwożyw-Smoleń, I., and Sady, W. 2016. The role of exogenous humic and fulvic acids in iodine biofortification in spinach (*Spinacia oleracea* L.). *Plant and Soil* 402:129–143.

Smoleń, S., Rożek, S., Ledwożyw-Smoleń, I., and Strzetelski. P. 2011a. Preliminary evaluation of the influence of soil fertilization and foliar nutrition with iodine on the efficiency of iodine biofortification and chemical composition of lettuce. *Journal of Elementology* 16:613–622.

Smoleń, S., Rożek, S., Strzetelski, P., and Ledwożyw-Smoleń, I. 2011b. Preliminary evaluation of the influence of soil fertilization and foliar nutrition with iodine on the effectiveness of iodine biofortification and mineral composition of carrot. *Journal of Elementology* 16:103–114.

Smoleń, S. and Sady, W. 2012. Influence of iodine form and application method on the effectiveness of iodine biofortification, nitrogen metabolism as well as the content of mineral nutrients and heavy metals in spinach plants (Spinacia oleracea L.). *Scientia Horticulturae* 143:176–183.

Stipesevic, B., Jug, D., Jug, I., Tolimir, M., and Cvijovic, M. 2009. Winter wheat and soybean zinc uptake in different soil tillage systems. *Cereal Research Communications* 37:305–310.

Stockdale, E. and Watson, C. 2011. Can we make crop rotations fit for a multi-functional future? Aspects of *Applied Biology* 113:119–126.

Subba Rao, A. and Rupa, T. R. 2003. Importance of Zn x P interaction in crop production. *Fertility News* 48(4):69–82.

Tamoutsidis, E., Papadopoulos, I., Tokatlidis, L., Zotis, S., and Mavropoulos, T. 2002. Wet sewage sludge application effect on soil properties and element content of leaf and root vegetables. *Journal of Plant Nutrition* 25:1941–1955.

Taylor, A. G., Allen, P. S., Bennett, M. A., Bradford, J. K., Burris, J. S., and Misra, M. K. 1998. Seed enhancements. *Seed Science Research* 8:245–256.

Taylor, H. M., Jordan, W. R., and Sinclair, T. T. 1983. Limitation to Efficient Water use in Crop Production American Society of Agronomy. Madison WI: Crop Society of America, and Soil Science Society of America.

Teas, J., Pino, S., Critchley, A., and Braverman, L. E. 2004. Variability of iodine content in common commercially available edible seaweeds. *Thyroid* 14(10):836–841.

Tennakoon, N. A. and Bandara, S. D. S. 2003. Nutrient content of some locally available organic materials and their potential as alternative sources of nutrients for coconut. *Cocos* 15:23–30.

Terry, N., Zayed, A. M., de Souza, M. P., and Tarun, A. S. 2000. Selenium in higher plants. *Annual Review of Plant Physiology and Plant Molecular Biology* 51:401–432.

Tonacchera, M., Dimida, A., De Servi, M. et al. 2013. Iodine fortification of vegetables improves human iodine nutrition. *Journal of Clinical Endocrinology and Metabolism* 98(4):E694–E697.

Tontisirin, K., Nantel, G., Bhattacharjee, L. 2002. Food-based strategies to meet the challenges of micronutrient malnutrition in the developing world. Proceedings of the Nutrition Society 61(2):243–250.

Tsukada, H., Takeda, A., Tagami, K., and Uchida, S. 2008. Uptake and distribution of iodine in rice plants. *Journal of Environmental Quality* 37:2243–2247.

Tuhy, L., Samoraj, M., Witkowska, Z., and Chojnacka, K. 2015. Biofortification of maize with micronutrients by Spirulina. *Open Chemistry* 13:1119–1126.

Turmel, M.-S., Entz, M. H., Bamford, K. C., and Thiessen Martens, J. R. 2009. The influence of crop rotation on the mineral nutrient content of organic vs. conventionally produced wheat grain: Preliminary results from a long-term field study. *Canadian Journal of Plant Science* 89:915–919.

Tyler, G. and Olsson, T. 2001. Plant uptake of major and minor mineral elements as influenced by soil acidity and liming. *Plant and Soil* 230:307–321.

Uddin, M. N., Kaczmarczyk, A., and Vincze, E. 2014. Effects of Zn fertilization on hordein transcripts at early developmental stage of barley grain and correlation with increased Zn concentration in the mature grain. *PLOS ONE* 9(9):e108546.

Ujowundu, C. O., Ukoha, A. I., Agha, C. N., Nwachukwu, N., Igwe, K. O. and Kalu, F. N. 2010. Effects of potassium iodate application on the biomass and iodine concentration of selected indigenous Nigerian vegetables. *African Journal of Biotechnology* 9(42):7141–7147.

Ullah, A., Farooq, M., Nadeem, A., Rehman, A., Asad, S. A., and Nawaz, A. 2016. Manganese nutrition improves the productivity and grain biofortification of fine grain aromatic rice in conventional and conservation production systems. *Paddy and Water Environment* 15:1–10.

Uyanöz, R. 2007. The effects of different bio-organic, chemical fertilizers and their combination on yield, macro and micro nutrition content of dry bean (Phaseolus vulgaris L.). *International Journal of Agricultural Research* 2(2):115–125.

Velu, G., Ortiz-Monasterio, I., Cakmakb, I., Hao, Y., and Singh, R. P. 2014. Biofortification strategies to increase grain zinc and iron concentrations in wheat. *Journal of Cereal Science* 59:365–372.

Wang, F., Wang, Z., Kou, C., Ma, Z., and Zhao, D. 2016. Responses of wheat yield, macro- and micro- nutrients, and heavy metals in soil and wheat following the application of manure compost on the North China Plain. *PLOS ONE* 11(1):e0146453.

Wang, P., Zhou, D. M., Luo, X. S., Li, L. Z. 2009. Effects of Zn-complexes on zinc uptake by wheat (Triticum aestivum) roots: A comprehensive condsideration of physical, chemical and biological processes on biouptake. *Plant Soil* 316:177–192.

Warman, P. R. 2005. Soil fertility, yield an nutrient contents of vegetable crops after 12 years of compost or fertilizer amendments. *Biological Agriculture and Horticulture* 23:85–96.

Watson, C. A., Öborn, I., Edwards, A. C. et al. 2012. Using soil and plant properties and farm management practices to improve the micronutrient composition of food and feed. *Journal of Geochemical Exploration* 121:15–24.

Wei, Y., Shohag, M. J. I., and Yang, X. 2012. Biofortification and bioavailability of rice grain zinc as affected by different forms of foliar zinc fertilization. *PLOS ONE* 7(9):e45428.

Weil, R. R., Bendetto, P. W., Sikora, L. J., and Bandel, V. A. 1988. Influence of tillage practices on phosphorus distribution and forms in three ultisols. *Agronomy Journal* 80:503–509.

Welch, R. M. 2002. Breeding strategies for biofortified staple plant foods to reduce micronutrient malnutrition globally. *Journal of Nutrition* 132(3):495S–499S.

Welch, R. M. and Graham, R. D. 2005. Agriculture: The real nexus for enhancing bioavailable micronutrients in food crops. *Journal of Trace Elements in Medicine and Biology* 18:299–307.

Welch, R. M., Graham, R. D., and Cakmak, I. 2013. Linking agricultural production practices to improving human nutrition and health. *Second International Conference on Nutrition, FAO and WHO*, pp. 1–39.

White, P. J. and Broadley, M. R. 2005. Biofortifying crops with essential mineral elements. *Trends in Plant Science* 10:586–593.

White, P. J. and Broadley, M. R. 2009. Biofortification of crops with seven mineral elements often lacking in human diets -iron, zinc, copper, calcium, magnesium, selenium and iodine. *New Phytologist* 182:49–84.

Wilhelm, N. S., Graham, R. D., and Rovira, A. D. 1988. Application of different sources of manganese sulphate decreases take-all (Gaeumannomyces graminis var. tritici) of wheat grown in a manganese deficient soil. *Australian Journal of Agricultural Research* 39:1–10.

Willey, R. W. 1979. Intercropping: Its importance and research needs. Competition and yield advantages. Part 1. *Field Crop Abstracts* 1–10.

Williams, C. H. and David, D. J. 1976. Effects of pasture improvement with subterranean clover and superphosphate on the availability of trace metals to plants. *Australian Journal of Soil Research* 14:85–93.

Winter, C. K. and Davis, S. F. 2006. Organic food. *Journal of Food Science* 71:117–124.

Woźniak, A. and Makarski, B. 2013. Content of minerals, total protein and wet gluten in grain of spring wheat depending on cropping systems. *Journal of Elementology* 18(2):297–305.

Wu, Z., Bañuelos, G. S., Lin, Z. et al. 2015. Biofortification and phytoremediation of selenium in China. *Frontiers in Plant Science* 6:136.

Xu, Y.-F., Yue, S.-C., Zhang, Y.-Q. et al. 2012. Grain and shoot Zn accumulation in winter wheat affected by nitrogen management. *Plant and Soil* 361:153–163.

Yang, X. E., Chen, W. R., and Feng, Y. 2007. Improving human micronutrient nutrition through biofortification in the soil-plant system: China as a case study. *Environ Geochem Health* 29(5):413–428.

Yang, X. W., Tian, X. H., Gale, W. J., Cao, Y. X., Lu, X. C., and Zhao, A. Q. 2011. Effect of soil and foliar zinc application on zinc concentration and bioavailability in wheat grain grown on potentially zinc deficient soils. *Cereal Research Communications* 39:535–543.

Yilmaz, A., Ekiz, H., Torun, B. et al. 1997. Effect of different zinc application methods on grain yield and zinc concentration in wheat cultivars grown on zinc- deficient calcareous soils. *Journal of Plant Nutrition* 20(4–5):461–471.

Yin, X. B. and Li, F. 2011. The standardization in Se biofortification. In: Bañuelos, G. S., Lin, Z. Q., Yin, X. B., and Duan, N. (Eds.). Se Global Perspectives of Ion Human, Animals and the Environment. *Hefei: University of Science and Technology of China Press*, pp. 113–114.

Yoldas, F., Ceylan, S., Mordogan, N., and Esetlili, B. C. 2011. Effect of organic and inorganic fertilizers on yield and mineral content of onion (Allium cepa L.). *African Journal of Biotechnology* 10:11488–11492.

Yoshida, S., McLean, G. W., Shafi, M., and Mueller, K. E. 1970. Effects of different methods of zinc applications on growth and yields of rice in a calcareous soil, West Pakistan. *Soil Science and Plant Nutrition* 16:147–149.

Zhang, F., Shen, J., Zhang, J., Zuo, Y., Li, L., and Chen, X. 2010a. Rhizosphere processes and management for improving nutrient use efficiency and crop productivity: Implications for China. *Advances in Agronomy* 107:1–32.

Zhang, Y., Shi, R., Rezaul, K. M., Zhang, F., and Zou, C. 2010b. Iron and zinc concentrations in grain and flour of winter wheat as affected by foliar application. *Journal of Agricultural and Food Chemistry* 58:12268–12274.

Zhang, Y. Q., Deng, Y., Chen, R. Y. et al. 2012. The reduction in zinc concentration of wheat grain upon increased phosphorus-fertilization and its mitigation by foliar Zn application. *Plant and Soil* 361:143–152.

Zhao, C. Y., Ren, J. H., Xue, C. Z., and Lin, E. 2005. Study on the relationship between soil Se and plant Se uptake. *Plant and Soil* 277:197–206.

Zhao, F. J. and McGrath, S. P. 2009. Biofortification and phytoremediation. *Current Opinion in Plant Biology* 12:373–380.

Zhou, X. B., Shi, W. M., and Zang, L. H. 2007. Iron plaque outside roots affects selenite uptake by rice (Oryza sativa L.) grown in solution culture. *Plant and Soil* 290:17–28.

Zia, M. H., Watts, M. J., Gardner, A., and Chenery, S. R. 2015. Iodine status of soils, grain crops, and irrigation waters in Pakistan. *Environmental Earth Sciences* 73:7995–8008.

Zou, C. Q., Zhang, Y. Q., Rashid, A. et al. 2012. Biofortification of wheat with zinc through zinc fertilization in seven countries. *Plant and Soil* 361:119–130.

Żuk-Gołaszewska, K., Żeranńska, A., Krukowska, A., and Bojarczuk, J. 2016. Biofortification of the nutritional value of foods from the grain of *Triticum durum* desf. by an agrotechnical method: A scientific review. *Journal of Elementology* 21(3): 963–975.

Zuo, Y. and Zhang, F. 2009. Iron and zinc biofortification strategies in dicot plants by intercropping with gramineous species. A review. *Agronomy for Sustainable Development* 29:63–71.

chapter two

Advances in food fortification with vitamins and co-vitamins

Malgorzata Korzeniowska, Aneta Wojdylo, and Angel Antonio Carbonell Barrachina

Contents

Fortification or enrichment is, generally, the practice of deliberately increasing the content of an essential micronutrient, that is, vitamins and minerals, in a food, to improve the nutritional quality of the food supply, and provide a public health benefit with minimal risk (Allen et al., 2006). The World Health Organization (WHO) underlines also that food fortification is the process of the micronutrient addition to foods *"but in relatively small quantities"* to maintain or improve the quality of the diet of a specific group, a community, or a population. First, examples of the procedures of food fortification with vitamins were noted in the United States and Switzerland at the beginning of the twentieth century, and then spread throughout the world after World War II. Vitamin and co-vitamin fortification was introduced to the specific group of food products following incidences of the recognized micronutrient deficiencies, leading to malnutrition and significant impact on local communities' health status. Vitamin deficiencies, due to insufficient intake or poor absorption, frequently induce diseases with characteristic symptoms. Of the lipid-soluble vitamins, deficiencies in vitamins A, D, and K cause xerophthalmia, rickets in children, and hemorrhagic diarrhea, respectively, with the first being more common, especially in developing countries. Of the water-soluble vitamins, deficiencies in vitamins B1, B2, B6, B12, niacin, folate, pantothenic acid, and biotin cause beriberi, angular stomatitis, neuritis, megaloblastic anemia, pellagra, defects in the formation of the neural tube, feet burning syndrome, and hair loss, respectively (Schellack et al., 2015). Over the last decades, fortification of foods has become a public health measure for preventing deficiencies of vitamins dissolved in lipids, such as A, D, or those well dissolved in water, especially B12, thiamin, and folic acid.

Food can be fortified with vitamins in several ways:

1. *Mass fortification*, by fortifying foods that are widely consumed by the general population
2. *Targeted fortification*, by fortifying foods designed for specific population subgroups, such as complementary foods for young children or rations for displaced populations
3. *Market-driven fortification*, to allow food manufacturers to voluntarily fortify foods available in the market

Mass fortification is nearly always mandatory, while targeted fortification can be either mandatory or voluntary depending on the public health significance of the problem, and finally market-driven fortification is always voluntary but governed by regulatory limits. The choice between mandatory or voluntary food fortification depends on national circumstances. For example, in Australia and New Zealand vitamins can only be added to food with the permission of the Food Standards Code agreed on by The Ministerial Forum on Food Regulation. Food manufacturers can add vitamins to food in response to an actual or potential population health need, outlined in the Fortification of Food with Vitamins and Minerals Policy Guidelines.

Within the European Union all issues connected with food fortification are stated in the EU Parliament Regulation (EC) No 1925/2006 from 20 December 2006 on the addition of vitamins and minerals and of certain other substances to foods. European regulations are based on and supported by European Food Standard Authority EFSA documents (EFSA, 2006). However, selected countries introduced and led complex fortification programmes to prevent their population from malnutrition and minimize the incidence of serious health and development problems. Besides, there is no one general, clear guideline on nutrients that can be fortified or that are permissible under law throughout the world.

Anyway, fortification procedures cover a higher number of food products and also a wider selection of vitamins. Prior to the implementation of any substance to the fortification program, all its physical, chemical, and safety characteristics should be examined and accepted by the respective agency. The fortificant must be stable and safe, sufficiently well absorbed from the food vehicle, and able to improve the micronutrient status of the target population. The level of consumption required in order for fortification to be effective must be compatible with a healthy diet.

The most frequently consumed fortified foods in Europe are beverages, carbonated and cordial beverages, beverage powders (including instant teas, instant powders, or chocolate powders), soft drinks (including fruit juices and fruit juice drinks, squashes, and sports drinks), energy drinks and isotonic sports drinks, children's foods, breakfast cereals and ready-to-eat breakfast cereals, cereal bars, fats/oils, margarines, fat spreads, butter, sweet foods (including biscuits, chocolates, and marmalade), breads and buns, and milks and dairy products (Hennessy et al., 2013).

As fortification is optional for industries, they use labels to attract consumer attention and use fortification as a marketing tool. Consumers can be led to choose products based on their contents of added nutrients rather than on their overall nutritional quality. Vitamins are added to foods by manufacturers for a number of purposes, including to restore them when content has been reduced during manufacturing, storage, or handling procedures or to provide a similar nutritional value to foods for which they are intended as alternatives. Only vitamins normally found in and consumed as part of the diet and considered essential nutrients should be allowed to be added to foods, although this does not mean that their addition is necessary. Vitamins may not be added to unprocessed foodstuffs, including, but not limited to, fruit, vegetables, meat, poultry and fish, as well as to beverages containing more than 1.2% volume alcohol with some exceptions (Regulation (EC) No 1925/2006).

General criteria for fortification are as follows:

- Nutrient deficiency should be widespread.
- The vehicle food must be consumed by the target group.
- High consumption of fortified food will not lead to toxicity.
- Addition of micronutrient should not change the taste, color, flavor, texture, and shelf-life of the food.
- The nutrient in the food being fortified has to be stable.
- Combinations of certain nutrients, such as vitamins and minerals, present simultaneously in the same food can improve their utilization, e.g. vitamin C and iron.

- The food product should be regularly and centrally controlled and monitored.
- The cost of fortification should be affordable for the population.

According to the FAO report for the year 2015, there are still about 795 million undernourished people in the world (FAO et al., 2015). Thus, it is very important to continue intensive work to overcome all challenges in food fortification, which include: creation of better community awareness about benefits of food fortification; encouraging private sector, governments, and international agencies to cooperate and make commitments for investing in food fortification; increase the availability of fortified foods to vulnerable populations; develop uniform law and regulatory aspects; and also develop technologies that will produce food in the future.

2.1 Vitamin A

Carotenoids are naturally occurring polyenes synthesized in plants and certain microorganisms and are pigments used by plants and animals in numerous physiological processes. They are organic pigments found in the chloroplasts of plants responsible for red, orange, and yellow fruit and vegetable colors. Carotenoids can be divided into two major subgroups based on their molecular configuration. One group is the *carotenes* and the other group is the *xanthophylls*, which are very similar in chemical structure except that the xanthophylls have oxygen atoms. Only few of the over 600 known carotenoids are capable of metabolic conversion to the essential nutrient vitamin A (retinol) in vertebrates. The most well-known and important precursor of vitamin A in the human diet is β-carotene, a naturally occurring pigment with a red to orange hue in fruit and vegetables. Carotene (1 molecule) is converted into vitamin A (2 molecules) in the liver. It also has antioxidant properties and may help in preventing cancer and other diseases. Vitamin A also gives rise to a number of other metabolites which, along with their analogs, are known as retinoids.

Vitamin A is an essential lipid-soluble nutrient that is required in small amounts by humans for the normal functioning of the visual system, the maintenance of cell function for growth, epithelial cellular integrity and repair, production of myelin (nerve coating) and other membranes, immune system function enhancement and reproduction especially for embryonic development. Recommended daily intakes of vitamin A for adult men and women are 1,000 and 800 μg, respectively, with an extra allowance for pregnant or lactating women. It is assumed that every 6 μg of β-carotene has the activity of 1 μg of retinol (vitamin A). Dietary requirements for vitamin A are normally provided as a mixture of preformed retinol, which is present in animal source foods, and provitamin A carotenoids, which are supplied by foods of plant origin, and which have to be converted into retinol by tissues such as the intestinal mucosa and the liver to be utilized by cells. Deficiency of vitamin A led to night blindness and xerophthalmia, growth retardation, dry skin, diarrhea, and vulnerability to infection. Nevertheless, clinical data suggest that lack of vitamin A is an important determinant of child survival and safe motherhood.

The best sources of vitamin A are animal raw materials, in particular, liver, eggs and dairy products, which contain vitamin A in the form of retinol, that can be easily used by the body. It is not surprising then that the risk of vitamin A deficiency is strongly inversely related to intakes of vitamin A from animal foods. In fact, it is difficult for children and people on specific diets (limited diets, vegetarians, vegans, etc.) to meet their requirements for vitamin A. In a mixed diet, the conversion rate of β-carotene to retinol is approximately 12:1, while the conversion of the other provitamin-A carotenoids to retinol is less efficient (24:1).

Vitamin A is readily destroyed upon exposure to heat, light, or air. Thus, cooking and processing of some carotenoid-rich foods can cause nutrients to be leached. However, various food preparation techniques, such as cooking, grinding, and the addition of oil, can improve the absorption of food carotenoids. The most stunning example is lycopene, which can be obtained more easily from canned and cooked tomatoes than from fresh ones. Synthetic β-carotene in oil, which is widely used in vitamin A supplements, has a conversion rate to retinol of 2:1, and the synthetic forms of β-carotene commonly used to fortify foods a conversion rate of 6:1.

The choice of a vitamin A fortificant is largely governed by the characteristics of the food vehicle, as well as various technological, regulatory and religious considerations. As preformed vitamin A (retinol) is an unstable compound, in commercial preparations it is esterified, usually with palmitic or acetic acid, to the more stable corresponding esters. Retinyl acetate and retinyl palmitates, along with provitamin A (β-carotene), are thus the main commercial forms of vitamin A that are available and permitted by the fegulations for use as food fortificants. The intense orange color of β-carotene makes it unsuitable for use as a fortificant in many foods, but it is widely used to give an orange-yellow color to margarines and beverages. Since vitamin A is fat-soluble, it is easily added to fat-based or oily foods. When the food vehicle is either dry or a water-based liquid, an encapsulated form of the vitamin is needed. Based on this distinction, vitamin A fortificants can be divided into two categories:

1. Oily forms that can be incorporated directly into fat-based foods or emulsified into water-based ones (e.g., milk)

2. Dry forms that can be dry-mixed into foods or dispersed in water, depending on whether they are cold-water dispersible or non-cold water dispersible

Pure vitamin A and β-carotene in solution are unstable when exposed to ultraviolet light, oxygen, or air. Thus all forms of vitamin A, oily or dried, are protected by antioxidants to prolong their shelf-life. Further protection can be provided by the use of airtight packaging. For example, the loss of vitamin A in sealed cans of oil is minimal, but losses from fortified cereals, fortified sugar, or oil can be as high as 40%, depending on ambient conditions and storage times. Opaque packaging is indispensable for maintaining stability in vitamin A-fortified oil. The fat-soluble forms of retinol are about one half to one third as expensive as the dry forms.

An important issue related to food fortification is that some nutrients added simultaneously to food vehicle can adversely interact with each other. Therefore, for vitamin A fortification strategy it is *important to avoid iron addition* or to use protective technologies, such as microencapsulation of nutrients with protective coatings.

Data collected on Philippine children showed that vitamin A fortification of margarine had positive effects on child mortality. Wheat flour fortified with vitamin A and fed as buns for 30 weeks reduced the number of children with low liver stores of the vitamin by 50% (Solon et al., 2000). Promising data on increasing vitamin A levels in daily diet were obtained in Central America by implementation of national programs of sugar fortification with vitamin A (Arroyave et al., 1981).

Wheat and maize flour fortification is a preventive food-based approach to improving the micronutrient status of populations over time that can be integrated with other interventions in efforts to reduce vitamin and mineral deficiencies identified as public health problems (WHO et al., 2009). While fortification of flour with vitamin A has been initiated in a few countries, questions remain about the cost of adding vitamin A to flour, as well as the stability of vitamin A in flour and flour products.

The study by Uchendu et al. (2012) of the stability of vitamin A in selected bread made from commercial fortified wheat flavor indicates that mean stability is better in bread than in flour. This might be due to the additional vitamin A contents of butter/margarine and sugar used in baking the bread. On the other hand, the stability losses in cookies have been estimated at 30–50%. which is within the normal range of stability of vitamin A in dry fortified products (Mahmood et al., 2008). Regarding the stability of vitamin A in baked products such as bread, biscuits, and cake baked under moderate conditions, Butt et al. (2007) revealed that 80% to 100% of the vitamin A survives the baking process. Storage of cookies at ambient temperature significantly reduced vitamin A contents. Additionally, sensory evaluation of fortified cookies was carried out. Vitamin A showed no effect on color and flavor of analyzed cookies. Significant variations in color and flavor of cookies were observed only with respect to storage intervals. Color and flavor are significantly affected due to the Maillard reaction (Bender, 1996). The color changes during storage might be due to acceleration of the Maillard reaction. Absorption of moisture contents during storage stimulates the Maillard reaction in cookies. High amounts of fat in cookies increases vitamin A absorption in the human body, as vitamin A absorption is in direct proportion to fat content. Cookies are also comparatively cheap and liked by all age groups and classes of society; cookies, therefore, are considered the best product for the fortification purpose with vitamin A as retinyl acetate or retinyl palmitate form.

Gomes Ribeiro et al. (2015) fortified different pumpkin purees with pro-vitamin A and investigated the effects of several styles of home cooking on the retention and bioaccessibility of pro-vitamin A during in-vitro digestion. Retention of pro-vitamin A carotenoids after boiling and steaming was relatively high (>78%), although the impact of cooking style varied among the genotypes. Although transfer of the pro-vitamin A carotenoids from cooked pulp to mixed micelles during simulated digestion was relatively inefficient, total β-carotene equivalents in the bioaccessible fraction of digested pulp from one genotype appeared to have the potential to provide children 4–8 years of age consuming 100 ×g cooked pumpkin with more than 40% of the daily EAR of vitamin A. Future research with this pro-vitamin A rich food should focus on methods to increase release of pro-vitamin A from pulp.

Vitamin A is not naturally present in plant materials, which is why oils, especially refined oils, should be fortified with retinal palmitate or acetate at a level of at least 60 IU/g. The methods of fortifying vegetable oils are well established, fairly simple, and easy to implement at low cost. In Brazil, vitamin A added to oil was well absorbed when provided with a rice-based diet, and it significantly increased plasma retinol and liver stores (Dutra de Oliveira et al., 1994). Margarine and other hydrogenated oil products were among the first fortified food ever. Vitamin A fortification of margarine (from 1 to 15 mg/kg) is either a mandatory or a voluntary practice in many countries (Johnson, 1998). In the Philippines, product of a blend of coconut oil and hardened palm oil is fortified with 25 mg/kg vitamin A plus 3.5 mg/kg of β-carotene (Solon et al., 1996).

Milk is considered to be a good source of vitamin A. However, during processing, especially fat content standardization and thermal treatment, a significant amount of vitamin A is lost. Therefore, vitamin A should be added to milk and dairy products from which fat has been removed. In USA and Canada, vitamin A fortification is mandatory, according to the regulations, for liquid low and skim milk with the amount not less than 2000 IU (Murphy and Newcomer, 2001), but voluntary for whole fat milk. Petrogianni et al. (2014) proved that extra fortification of phytosterol-enriched milk with vitamin A is effective enough to reduce serum total cholesterol, low density lipoproteins, and apolipoprotein-B levels, as well as to maintain plasma β-carotene level. Dried milk and flavored milk powders are often fortified with vitamin A. In order to protect vitamin A against oxidation and isomerization, the addition of antioxidants should be carried out in nonfat dry milk (Kurzer, 2013). Thus, combined fortification with vitamin A and D, along with vitamin C (ascorbic acid) and E (α-tocopherol) seems to be the most appropriate method of milk and dairy product fortification.

Ilic and Ashoor (1988) showed that yogurt fortified with 10,000 IU of vitamin A provided at least 100% of the US RDI, without any deteriorative effects of this fortification on physicochemical and sensory characteristics of yogurt. Yeh (2017) proved that skim milk fortification with high level of vitamin A (3000–6000 IU) could have a negative effect on flavor, especially due to developing faint carrot flavor in oil-soluble fortified skim milks. Morover, high dosage of vitamin A results in potential toxic action, thus it is recommended to use β-carotene to fortify dairy products (Gahruie et al., 2015). β-carotene is used also as a color-enhancing agent to some milk products, such as butter, as well as plant butters and spreads.

Microencapsulation of vitamin A palmitate is another way to preserve the active substance from losses during processing and storage (Goncalves et al., 2016), and this technique can be successfully applied to powdered milk (Kurzer, 2013), yogurt and pudding (Donhowe et al., 2014), peanut butter and spread (Galvez et al., 2006), and almond butter (Roman et al., 2012).

Meat and meat products are not considered to be a good source of β-carotene; however, its concentration can be increased by dietary supplementation (Bou et al., 2009), especially in poultry meat. Application of β-carotene to processed meat can be often difficult because of its chemical instability and possible effects on the color of the muscle and final product (Decker and Park, 2010).

Vitamin A, as a lipid-soluble compound, is not eliminated from the body by the urinary system but is rather stored in the liver, where it may eventually reach toxic levels. According to the Good Manufacture Practice, a concentration of vitamin A higher than 6,000 IU is considered harmful. Adverse physiological effects have been associated with both acute hypervitaminosis A and chronic high intake. The routine consumption of a large amount (app. 150,000 μg daily) of vitamin A for at least several months can result in a various toxic symptoms including liver damage, bone abnormalities and joint pain, headaches, vomiting, and skin desquamation. β-Carotene and other provitamin A carotenoids are of less concern in terms of potential toxicity (they are not toxic *per se*), not being active forms of the vitamin and because at high doses they are absorbed less efficiently, but the blood plasma may contain a high enough concentration of the pigment to impart a yellowish color to the skin, known as carotenemia. Furthermore, the synthesis of vitamin A from β-carotene and other provitamin A carotenoids is strictly regulated in the body. Hypervitaminosis A has never been reported as a result of provitamin A supplementation.

2.2 *Vitamin D*

Vitamin D (calciferol), as a derivative of sterols, is a lipid soluble compound found in two forms: naturally formed vitamin D3 (cholecalciferol), and its synthetic analogue vitamin D2 (ergocalciferol), which differs only by the side chain to the sterol skeleton (Holick, 1999). Vitamin D3 is synthesized in the human skin from its precursor, 7-dehydrocholesterol, initiated by the ultraviolet radiation from sunlight. Vitamin D, despite the form, can also be supplied to the body via diet. Calciferol is an essential factor for the regulation of minerals metabolism, especially Ca and P. It also plays many roles in cell differentiation and in the secretion and metabolism of hormones, including parathyroid hormone and insulin. Vitamin D deficiency is spotted mostly in populations from regions with lower sun exposure, infants and young children and the elderly. Recently, due to the drastic change of life style, far fewer outdoor activities combined with hours spent with electronic devices and under stress, calciferol deficiency occurs also in the highly developed countries. Severe vitamin D deficiency leads to muscular weakness and bone pain, disorders, deformities and diseases (calcification of the bone matrix), such as rickets in infants and children, and osteomalacia in adults and elderly (Thacher and Clarke, 2011), which in fact contributes to osteoporosis (brittle and porous bone due to the loss of bone tissue) (Spiro and Buttriss, 2014). Low vitamin D level in the body is also associated with poor Ca intakes. Dietary supplementation of vitamin D has to be correlated with higher fat consumption, otherwise deficiency of calciferol may occur due to poor absorption of vitamin D. Moreover, some experiments showed that vitamin A might antagonise the actions of vitamin D at the molecular level (Rohde et al., 1999). Recommended daily intake for cholecalciferol is established on 15 μg for adults, 20 μg for people older than 70 and 10 μg for children, especially in case of inadequate sunlight exposure. However, the EU Regulation no 1169/2011/EC (2014) set up the daily reference intake of calciferol at 5 μg/day. Vitamin D is naturally present in relatively few types of foods, such as salt-water fish (salmon, sardines), fish liver oil, eggs, and mushrooms. Vitamin D is quite stable in food rich in lipids and fat solutions; however, it is very sensitive to oxygen and moisture. Most of the low-heat cooking techniques as well as short pasteurization or sterilization will not reduce the level of calciferol immensely, but all processing required contact with air and minerals will degrade significant amount of vitamin D.

Food fortification with vitamin D was one of the first in history and it is still ongoing in many countries. Both forms of vitamin D, either D2 or D3, are approved in food fortification. The two forms are characterized by similar biological activity in the human body. Generally, vitamin D is added to food as a dried antioxidatively stabilized form, which protects its activity even in the presence of minerals. Tocopherol is among the most widely used antioxidants in the commercial preparations. Because children are the most susceptible population group to vitamin D deficiency, fortification procedure is mainly carried out for milk and other dairy products, including dried milk powder and evaporated milk. It is often fortified with vitamins A and D together, mostly for bone health, because Ca promotes bone strength and vitamin D helps the body absorb Ca. In some countries fortification is mandatory, for example in both the United States and Canada the infant formula must be fortified with vitamin D reaching 40–100 IU/100 kcal in the United States and 40–80 IU/100 kcal in Canada (U.S. NA et al., 2010). Moreover, in Canada milk is also fortified by law with 35–40 IU/100 mL, the same as margarine at ≥530 IU/100 g. Almost all of the U.S. milk supply is voluntarily fortified with 100 IU/cup (U.S. NA et al., 2010). In Europe all issues connected with vitamin fortification are regulated by regulation no 1925/2006/EC. Generally, food fortification is voluntary across the European union. However, some countries, such as Finland, introduced in 2003 mandatory addition of vitamin D to fluid milk products (0.5 μg/100 mL) and margarines and butter (10 μg/100 g), France got an authorization to fortify vegetable oils (10 μg/100 g), milk and dairy products (1 and 1.25 μg/100 g), and the Netherlands fortified fat spreads (3 IU/g) (Dhaussy, 2014; Hennessy et al., 2013).

Ready-to-eat breakfast cereals often contain added vitamin D, as do some brands of orange juice, yogurt, margarine, and other food products.

However, eggs are one of the best sources of calciferol, many successful studies have been done on dietary fortification of chicken egg yolk with both vitamin D3 (D3) and 25-hydroxyvitamin D3 (25(OH)D3) (Browning and Cowieson, 2014). Biofortification was also claimed as an effective way to increase D3 and 25(OH)D3 concentration in pork (Cashman et al., 2015).

Dairy foods such as cheese and ice cream, are generally not fortified; however, recently some works on the increase of the retention of vitamin D3 in cheddar cheese were carried out (Tippetts et al., 2012), as well as on the stability of vitamin D encapsulated during cheese ripening (Banville et al., 2000). Kazmi et al. (2007) proved that cheddar type cheese, ice cream, and yogurt can be used as viable vehicles of vitamin D3.

Hypovitaminosis D is one of the most important public health concerns occurring in all racial, gender, and age subpopulations with almost no geographical boundaries. Naturally, the vitamin D supply depends mostly on cutaneous synthesis upon exposure to solar UV beam, at wavelengths of 290–315 nm. However, environmental, cultural, and social as well as individual factors can all influence the amount of UV beam reaching the skin and hence the amount of calciferol synthesis. Many countries have established a mandatory fortification program for several staple food items, whereas in some countries, fortification with vitamin D is voluntary.

Jakobsen and Knuthsen (2013) investigated the retention of vitamin D3 and D2 in bread. For bread baked,as recommended in the recipe, the retention of vitamin D3 in rye bread at 69% was lower than in wheat bread at 85%. A similar observation was made for vitamin D2, although the retention was slightly higher, 73% and 89%. Rye bread has a lower pH than wheat bread, which might be part of the explanation for the lower retention due to the known acidic isomerisation of vitamin D to isotachysterol.

Being a lipid-soluble vitamin, calciferol is not simply utilized and removed from the body by urination. Therefore, excess levels of vitamin D results in toxic effects with nonspecific symptoms, such as anorexia, weight loss, polyuria, and heart arrhythmias. Extende vitamin D deficiency, which is primarily related to the role of free 1,25-dihydroxycholecalciferol in the regulation of plasma Ca (Reichel et al., 1989), leads to vascular and tissue calcification, with the heart, blood vessels, and kidneys subsequent damage (hypercalcaemia) (Norman, 1996). Moreover, some data showed evidence of a negative impact of high concentrations of vitamin D on kidney, bone, the central nervous system and the cardiovascular system (Holmes and Kummerow, 1983). For vitamin D the tolerable upper intake level was set by EFSA in 2012 at 100 µg/day for adults including pregnant and lactating women, and adolescents for ages 11–17 years, at 50 µg/day for children aged 1–10 years, and at 25 µg/day for infants.

2.3 Vitamin E

Vitamin E in foods derives from two classes of compounds, tocopherols and tocotrienols, consisting of a hydroquinone nucleus and an isoprenoid side chain. Tocopherols have a saturated side chain, whereas the tocotrienols have an unsaturated side chain containing three double bonds. Vitamin E activity is found in four main forms of tocopherol: α, β, γ, and δ. Among them α -tocopherol expresses the highest biological activity and, thus, it is the predominant vitamin E active compound used in feedstuffs (Freiser and Jiang, 2009). Vitamin E is essential for growth, immune function enhancement, red-blood cell production, tissue integrity, reproduction, disease prevention (including coronary heart diseases and cancers), and antioxidant function in biological systems. Moreover, tocopherol improves absorption and metabolism of vitamin K by the body. Low fat diets or poor retention of vitamin E may lead to deficiency syndromes, such as muscle weakness and atrophy, vision problems, and unsteady walking. Long-term deficiency may also cause liver and kidney problems. Recommended daily intake of vitamin E is set on 15 mg α-tocopherol equivalents. Muscle foods, including fatty fishes, shrimp, red and white meat, are the most important sources of vitamin E. Tocopherols are also found in green leafy vegetables, oils, nuts, and eggs.

Supplementation of animal diets, mostly with α-tocopheryl acetate, can make muscle foods even better sources of vitamin E. European regulation permits vitamin E fortification with D-α-tocopherol, DL-α-tocopherol, D-α-tocopheryl acetate, DL-α-tocopheryl acetate, and D-α-tocopheryl acid succinate. However, meat and meat products are mostly fortified with α-tocopheryl acetate, primarily due to its high antioxidant activity, which effects the protection of feedstuffs as well as reduced lipid and protein oxidation in cell membranes (Delles et al., 2014). As a result of such supplementation, higher concentration of α-tocopherol was found in mitochondria and microsomes of porcine, poultry, and cattle muscles. The increase can be obtained both by using long-term lower dietary doses and by short-term supplementation with high levels of the vitamin in the diet (Wen et al., 1997). Vitamin E supplementations increase tocopherol concentration in animal products, including eggs, milk, and meat, and prolong their shelf life. Moreover, vitamin E fortification improves quality of meat including color, flavor, texture, increased water holding capacity, and reduced incidence of PSE (pale, soft, and exudative meat) development in poultry and pigs (Zhang et al., 2012). Vitamin E fortification through dietary supplementation of α-tocopheryl acetate is a common practice used for poultry (chickens, rabbits), pigs, ruminants (cows, goats), fish, and sea creatures. Numerous studies show that the addition of 200 mg α-tocopheryl acetate per kilogram of animal feed can double the amount of tocopherol in rabbit meat (Tres et al., 2010; Zhang et al., 2012), while dietary fortification with 250 mg α-tocopheryl acetate/kg resulted in higher than threefold elevation of tocopherol concentration in meat (Ebeid et al., 2013). Higher concentration of vitamin E in meat was also found in turkey (Mercier et al., 1998). Sloan (2000) reported that specially designed feeding strategies have been successfully used to produce eggs, beef, and chicken with up to seven times the normal level of vitamin E.

Fortification of animal diet with vitamin E significantly delayed lipid oxidation in meat, organs and fat, despite the type of dietary fat, as well as strongly reducing off-flavor and N-nitrosamine formation in final products. Dietary α-tocopheryl acetate improves the oxidative stability of raw (Lo Fiego et al., 2004), cooked (Dal Bosco et al., 2001), and stored meat (Castellini et al., 1999).

The addition of vitamin E to fat-rich diets of cows prevented the drop in milk fat yield, and improved resistance to oxidation (Bell et al., 2006). Supplementation with Se and vitamin E alleviated milk fat depression and improved antioxidant status in blood of cows. Moreover, Se combined with vitamin E improved the nutritional quality of milk fat by better balance between fatty acids (Zhao et al., 2008).

Zsédely et al. (2008) found the natural form of vitamin E (D-α-tocopheryl), an oil industry by-product, to be more efficient in improving the oxidative stability of rabbit meat than its synthetic form (DL-α-tocopheryl acetate). Tres et al. (2008) found that cooking reduced α-tocopheryl by 9% in rabbit meat. As concerns meat physicochemical characteristics, studies have reported increased water holding capacity (Dal Bosco and Castellini, 1998) or reduced shear value (Castellini et al., 1998) in meats from animals fed a 200 mg α-tocopheryl acetate/kg supplement. WHC, L*a*b* color, and oxidative stability were all preserved better during 30-day frozen storage with the same supplementation dose (Dal Bosco and Castellini, 1998). As reported in pigs (Monahan et al., 1994), dietary α-tocopheryl acetate has been found to stabilize the surface color of both raw (α-tocopheryl acetate in drinking water [Corino et al., 1999]) and cooked rabbit meat (Castellini et al., 1998) and also raw hamburger, while also improving oxidative stability, appearance, and texture, both on 1 and 7 days storage at + 4 °C (Dalle Zotte et al., 2000).

The synergistic effects of simultaneous dietary supplementation with vitamins E and C was found to increase content of both vitamins and to decrease lipid oxidation (Selim et al., 2008), but only when high dose of vitamin C (500 mg/kg) together with low dose of vitamin E (40 mg/kg) was added to the diet (Lo Fiego et al., 2004).

Vitamin E can also be applied directly into processed meat, with highly positive effects on slowing down lipid oxidation and preventing the formation of warmed-over-flavor during thermal processing and storage (Kim and Choi, 2012). α-tocopherol was proven to be stable during processing. Bolger et al. (2016) stated no effects of frying and grilling on vitamin E level in breakfast style poultry sausages. Contradictory data exist on the effect of storage on α-tocopherol level in meat products. Gerling and Ternes (2014) stated that storage of salami-type sausages did not change vitamin E level; however, it was proved that long-term frozen storage had a deteriorative impact on vitamin E in beef burgers, chicken frankfurters (Rosli et al., 2006), and beef frankfurters (Rosli et al., 2010). Bolger et al. (2017) pointed out that vitamin E fortification of comminuted meat products can be used as an innovative method for nutritious food development. Nevertheless, Meineri et al. (2013) claimed that dietary supplementation of pigs with vitamin E is more effective in reducing the production of carcinogenic substances, that is, N-nitrosamine, than addition during processing.

2.4 Vitamin K

The compounds expressing vitamin K activity generally contain a 2-methyl-1,4-naphthoquinone nucleus with a lipophilic side chain at position 3. Until now, more than 100 substances with vitamin K activity have been discovered but only three of them play physiological role. Vitamin K1 (α-phylloquinone) found in green plants, vitamin K2 (menaquinones) synthesized by bacteria, and menadione, a synthetic compound (which cannot be applied to food products). Vitamin K can be produced by gut bacteria from supplied food but in insufficient amounts (approximately half of required vitamin K). The physiological role of vitamin K is the formation of vitamin K-dependent coagulation proteins synthesized in the liver, which impact blood circulation and reduce the risk of haemorrhage or bleeding. Vitamin K is also essential for the synthesis of a number of proteins produced in extra-hepatic tissues and is one of the nutrients that promote bone synthesis. New-born babies can sometimes suffer vitamin K deficiency, as can people who do not absorb fat, because vitamin K is fat soluble. Those with liver disease may require more vitamin K. Fresh green vegetables, as well as green spices such as parsley, basil, cilantro, sage, and oregano are the most excellent sources for vitamin K.

However, it is allowed to fortify food with phylloquinone (phytomenadione), although the practice is still not very common. Generally, dairy products are considered to be a good delivery system for vitamin K because of the strong links between the natural levels of Ca and vitamin D, which can act synergistically with vitamin K. One example of vitamin K fortification is provided by Knapen et al. (2015) for a menaquinone-fortified yogurt drink (28 µg vitamin K *per* yogurt drink). The study showed that consumption of vitamin K fortified dairy product (along with the addition of n-3 PUFA, vitamin D and C, Ca and Mg) improves status and markers of vascular health, as well as significantly increased vitamin K level from 0.28 to 1.94 ng/mL.

Vitamin K is a fairly stable nutrient in most types of processing. Vitamin K in oils, but probably not in vegetables, is reduced by exposure to light. The hydrogenation process used to stabilize and solidify liquid fats damages a significant amount of vitamin K.

2.5 Vitamin B1

Vitamin B1 (thiamin), a water-soluble chemical compound, 3-[(4-amino-2-methyl-5-pyrimidinyl)methyl]-5-(2-hydroxyethyl)-4-methylthiazolium, present in plants in free form, while in animal-based foods is present in the biologically active phosphorylated forms of thiamin mono-, di-, and triphosphate (Combs, 2012). Vitamin B1 is a cofactor for several key enzymes responsible for carbohydrate metabolism (enables carbohydrate to be used as an energy source), defence mechanisms (Martin et al., 2003), and is also directly involved in neural function. Thiamin deficiency leads to disorders in brain function (Wernicke-Korsakoffs psychosis), diarrhea, muscle atrophy, as well as occurrence dry and wet beriberi disease connected with impairment of nerve system and heart functions. Vitamin B1 deficiency occurs in many regions, especially among populations with a high carbohydrate intake (white rice). Moreover, the presence of thiamin antagonists in food, especially thiaminase, occurring in raw fish can break down vitamin B1 level in the body and cause beriberi in some people. Thiamin is generally supplied by the consumption of legumes and vegetables, as well as nuts and seeds. Unfortunately, a high percentage of thiamin is lost during raw materials processing, such as milling of cereals, baking, cooking in water, and operating in alkaline solutions, storing especially under exposure on high temperature, light and air, or oxygen (Martinez-Villaluenga et al.; 2009, Mihhalevski et al., 2013). Additionally, alcohol can reduce the availability of thiamin to the body. Therefore, thiamin deficiency can be a problem in both developing and developed countries. Thus, the fortification of white rice and white wheat flour with thiamin is popular or even mandatory in many regions. For example, the Australian fortification program mandates the addition of minimum 0.64 mg thiamin hydrochloride per 100 g bread-making flour (Tiong et al., 2015). The European Union Regulation approved the fortification of food with thiamin hydrochloride and thiamin mononitrate. Recommended daily intake of vitamin B1 highly depends on carbohydrate consumption, but generally for children balanced on 0.5-1.2 mg, for men it varies between 0.9 mg and 1.1 mg, while for women from 0.7 mg to 0.8 mg.

Whole grain cereals are typically rich in thiamin. However, the scutellum and germ are removed during milling, which results in the production of grains and flour with lower thiamin content. Thiamin found in food is sensitive to pH and high temperatures but is stable between pH 2.0 and 4.0, though unstable in alkaline solutions. Other studies (Tiong et al., 2015) reported that heat during baking causes loss of endogenous thiamin that ranges from 20% to 56%. Bread samples (white and whole meal) showed significantly lower thiamin content than their respective proofed dough samples, because the heat during baking elicited thermal degradation of thiamin. White bread had 18% lower thiamin than its proofed dough and whole meal bread 15%. Even though baking caused thiamin loss, the results suggested that endogenous thiamin in yeast contributed to higher thiamin level in bread than its corresponding flour.

Among foods of animal origin, thiamin-fortified fish sauce has been already approved in southeast Asia as a good source of vitamin B1 (Whitfield et al., 2017). Due to the susceptibility of thiamin to heat treatment Riccio et al. (2006) recommended fortification of meat products, such as burgers and ham, with 25 μg/g of vitamin B1 to assure a designed concentration to the desired substance.

Vitamin B1 is a good example of complex interaction, particularly absorption of thiamin with presence of folic acid and vitamin B12. None of the toxicity evidence is known in relations to dietary intake of vitamin B1.

2.6 *Vitamin B2*

Vitamin B2 [riboflavin, 7,8-dimethyl-10-(1′-D-ribityl)isoalloxazine] is a water-soluble compound normally isolated or synthesized as a yellowish-orange amorphous solid. It is a precursor of nucleotides such as flavin mononucleotide and flavin adenine dinucleotide, which act as coenzymes in various metabolic pathways and in energy production. Riboflavin deficiency occurs rarely in isolation, and is associated with lack of one or more of the other B-group vitamins. Symptoms of riboflavin deficiency are non-specific and may include weakness, fatigue, mouth pain, burning eyes and itching, and inflammation of the tongue and lips. More advanced deficiency is characterized by dermatitis, cracking and dryness of the lips and corner of the mouth (cheilosis), and angular stomatitis, brain dysfunction and microcytic anemia. Riboflavin deficiency also reduces the absorption and utilization of Fe for haemoglobin synthesis leading to the incidence of anemia. However, riboflavin is widely distributed in food of plant and animal origin, the only sources that contain more than 2 mg/100 g are yeast and liver. Vitamin B2 is also present in milk, egg white, fish roe, and leafy vegetables. Recommended daily intake of riboflavin varies between 1.3–1.7 mg for men and 1.0–1.2 mg for women.

Riboflavin, like other water-soluble vitamins, can be lost in processing, especially during cooking in water. It is susceptible to ultraviolet radiation (sunlight), thus a particularly important loss of this vitamin can occur in milk packed in transparent containers exposed to sunlight during or after delivery. The formation of riboflavin derivatives increases the loss of vitamin C in food. Moreover, riboflavin derived flavo-coenzymes are involved in the biosynthesis of niacin-containing coenzymes from tryptophan, conversion of the 5′-phosphates of vitamin B6 to pyridoxal 5′-phosphate and dehydrogenation of 5,10-methylene-tetrahydrofolate to the 5′-methyl product, with the vitamin B12-dependent formation of methionine and sulfur amino metabolism. Thus, the presence of riboflavin, within the vitamin B complex, is an essential condition of normal regulation and function of the organism.

The forms allowed for food fortification are riboflavin and riboflavin sodium 5'-phosphate. One of the challenges of food fortification with vitamin B2 is achieving a designed level of fortification without changing the sensory properties off the food item. Sensory characteristics play an important role in determining the amount of micronutrient added to food, the amount of riboflavin added to corn flour can be limited by the extent of acceptable to consumers color changes. This problem seems to be smaller when fortifying grains, flakes, and cereal-based products, to which riboflavin is routinely added during processing. Fortification of food with riboflavin is common in Australia and New Zealand, especially for hot and cold beverages containing grains and nuts (ANZ Food Standards, 2009). Multiple-micronutrient fortification, including vitamin B2, of nondairy-based beverages is mostly performed in many countries dealing with malnutrition (Aaron et al., 2015). However, a wide selection of carbonated beverages fortified with vitamin complex is typically offered on the market in highly developed regions (Mehansho et al., 1989).

An increased concentration of vitamin B2 in fermented dairy products can be achieved by biofortification with the specific strains of lactic acid bacteria (*Propionibacterium freudenreichii*) able to produce significant amount of riboflavin (LeBlanc et al., 2006).

Toxicity is not a problem for riboflavin, thus upper intake limits (UL) have not been defined.

2.7 Vitamin B3

Vitamin B3 (niacin or nicotinic acid), as a functional group of the coenzymes, nicotinamide adenine dinucleotide and its phosphate, is essential for oxidative processes. Deficiency results in pellagra (occurrence of symmetrically pigmented rash on skin exposed to sunlight) and is associated with a heavily cereal-based diet that is low in bioavailable niacin, tryptophan, and other micronutrients needed for the synthesis of niacin and tryptophan. Niacin is unique among vitamins due to the possible body synthesis of vitamin B3 from supplied tryptophan with the conversion ratio of 60 mg tryptophan to 1 mg of niacin. Niacin is widely distributed in plant and animal foods. The main sources are baker's yeast, animal and dairy products, cereals, legumes. and leafy green vegetables. However, not all niacin in food may be equally available to the body, because some is rather tightly bound to other food constituents and not easily released. Recommended daily intake of niacin varies between 14–20 mg niacin equivalents for men and 10–14 mg niacin equivalents for women.

Niacin depletion is a risk where diets rely heavily on refined grains or grain products and have little variety. Severe deficiency, pellagra, is mostly found in people who consume diets that are deficient in bioavailable niacin and low in tryptophan, such as corn- or sorghum-based diets and alcohol abusers. Vitamin B3 deficiency can also be spotted by changes in the mucosa of the digestive tract, leading to oral lesions, vomiting and diarrhea, and neurological symptoms such as depression, fatigue, loss of memory, and dementia. Fortification with nicotinic acid nicotinamide is allowed in the EU for such products as biscuits, breakfast cereals, bread, pasta, and hot and soft drinks. The latests are mostly fortified with niacin along with other vitamins.

Because niacin is water soluble, losses can occur by discarding water containing the dissolved vitamin.

High doses of nicotinic acid used in the hyperlipidaemia treatment caused a burning or itching sensation in the face, arms, and chest. The Scientific Committee for Food in the European Union has proposed a UL for nicotinic acid of 10 mg/day (UL in the US 35 mg/day) and a separate, much higher, UL for niacinamide of 900 mg/day. The latter thus poses no safety limitations in common food fortification practice.

2.8 Vitamin B5

Vitamin B5 is also known as D-pantothenic acid. This vitamin plays a crucial role in the breakdown of fats and carbohydrates, as well as protein metabolism, by constituting two important enzymes, coenzyme A and acyl carrier protein. Pantothenic acid is also critical to the production of red blood cells and cholesterol, as well as sex and stress-related hormones. Moreover, it helps to absorb other vitamins, particularly B2 and therefore maintain the digestive tract in good condition. Pantothenic acid is widely distributed in nature and is present in a wide variety of foods including meat, vegetables, cereal grains, legumes, eggs, and milk. Deficiency is, therefore, rare, but may include symptoms such as fatigue, insomnia, depression, irritability, vomiting, stomach pains, burning feet, and upper respiratory infections. It is water soluble, heat sensitive, and can be degraded in both acid and alkaline conditions. Recommended daily intake varied between 4 mg and 7 mg. According to the European legislation following forms of the chemical can be incorporated in food vehicles: calcium D-pantothenate, sodium D-pantothenate, and dexpanthenol. Foods that are routinely fortified with vitamin B5 includes breakfast cereals, pasta, and hot and soft drinks. In Canada fortification with pantothenic acid is mandatory for simulated meat products, simulated poultry meat products, meat product extenders, and poultry product extenders (D.03.002, FDR, 2017). Promising results for panthotenic acid fortification by dietary modification has been claimed for eggs by Leeson and Caston (2003), who found doubled amounts of active vitamin B5, as well as by Zang et al. (2011).

2.9 Vitamin B6

Vitamin B6 is a mixture of three related forms, pyridoxine (or pyridoxol), pyridoxal, pyridoxamine, and three phosphorylated and then oxidized forms of 5′-phosphates; interconversion is possible among all forms (Bender, 1989). Vitamin B6 plays an essential role as a carbonyl-reactive coenzyme to various enzymes involved in the metabolism of many amino acids. It is also involved in the formation of chemicals responsible for transmission of impulses in brain and nerves, and in red blood cell formation. Recommended daily intake of vitamin B6 for men varies between 1.0 and 1.9 mg, for women 0.8–1.4 mg, while for children reaches 2.2 mg. Vitamin B6 deficiency alone is relatively rare, but occurs most often in association with deficiencies of the other B group vitamins. The most typical symptoms of vitamin B6 deficiency are sleeplessness, irritability, and weakness. However, deeper lack of pyridoxine-related compounds in diet can lead to retarded growth, dermatitis, skeletal changes, and anemia, while changes in neurotransmitters, such as dopamine, serotonin, noradrenaline, tryptamine, tyramine, histamine, GABA and taurine, affect brain and nerve system functions and can lead to depression and convulsions.

The forms of vitamin B6 found in food are pyridoxine, mainly in vegetables, and pyridoxal and pyridoxamine, mainly in foods from animal sources. Vitamin B6 is water soluble and can be lost by discarding water while cooking. It is also sensitive to light, air, or oxygen, and to alkaline conditions. Food can be fortified with pyridoxine hydrochloride, pyridoxine 5'-phosphate, and pyridoxine dipalmitate. Berendsen et al. (2016) claimed that only 11% of the total vitamin B6 intake in the Netherlands came from fortified foods. An example of a good source of vitamin B6 and B12 is a group of the fortified soy-based meat substitutes (Tucker et al., 2010). According to Riccio et al. (2006), thermally processed meat products should be fortified with vitamin B6 in order to be used as a valuable source of pyridoxine.

No adverse effects associated with vitamin B6 consumption from food have been reported; however, this does not mean that there are no potential negative effects resulting from high intakes. Thus, maximum level has been set for vitamin B6 intake of 100 mg for adults and 30–40 mg for children.

2.10 Vitamin B9

Vitamin B9 (folate, folacin, or folic acid) is present in food in many forms of pteroylglutamic acid. It plays a crucial role in the synthesis and methylation of nucleotides that intervene in cell multiplication and tissue growth. Folacin, like vitamin B12, is involved in the formation of the genetic material of newly forming cells and in protein formation. The combination of severe folate deficiency and vitamin B12 deficiency can result in megaloblastic anemia. A relatively high intake of refined cereals, genetic disorders of folic acid metabolism, infection with *Giardia lamblia*, bacterial overgrowth, usage of certain medications, and overconsumption of alcohol lead to folate deficiency. Low intakes of folate can cause serious birth defects, such as neural tube defects in newborn infants, and also lead to defective lining of the gut, adversely affecting absorption of many nutrients, to prolonged bleeding and increased risk of cardiovascular diseases, cancer, and impaired cognitive function in adults. Recommended daily intake of vitamin B9 is set on 200 µg for both men and women, with double the amount for pregnant women.

The main sources of dietary folate are leafy green vegetables, fruits, yeast, and liver; however, the availability of folacin in food depends on the chemical form, but also on product acidity, the amount of dietary fiber and the amount of carbohydrate.

Folate can be introduced to food via a fortification procedure in form of pteroylmonoglutamic acid. Folacin is water soluble and easily lost in discarded cooking water. It is also sensitive to heat, air and oxygen, and to alkaline conditions. No adverse health effects were discovered in relation to the consumption of folic acid. However, there has been some concern that high folic acid intake could mask or exacerbate neurological problems, such as pernicious anemia, in people with low intakes of vitamin B12 (Johnson, 2007), and also raised the prostate cancer risk, especially while consuming food fortified with synthetic folic acid (Wien et al., 2012). This has led to a reluctance to fortify with folic acid in some countries. This concern is particularly pertinent to those individuals who derive folic acid from both supplements and a range of fortified foods, as it is the case in many industrialized countries.

Hoffpauer and Bonnette (1998) discussed manufacturing concerns with respect to folic acid fortification. In considering riboflavin and folic acid, the authors noted that the stability of these two vitamins continues to be a problem in an environment unprotected from heat and light. However, there is a large body of evidence regarding the stability of folic acid added to cereal-grain products. Numerous reports have described the stability of folic acid in fortified breads, vitamin-minerals premixes, fortified flour, and grains and during baking applications (Gregory, 1989). Based on the WHO recommendation, between 1.5 and 2.2 µg/100 g of folic acid is routinely added to wheat flour in many regions, including North and Latin America, as well as Arabic countries (Allen et al., 2006). Moreover, in the United States, fortification of breads, cereals, flours, cornmeals, pastas, rice, and other grain products, with folic acid is required by law (US FDA, 1996). The high degree of stability of folic acid in foods of high moisture content has also been demonstrated (Day and Gregory, 1983). Thus, to date, there appear to be no data supporting the concept that overages are needed because folic acid is unstable when added to cereal-grain products.

Dairy and meat products are generally not good sources of foliates. Thus, fortification with folic acid can be beneficial for plain and fruit-flavored yogurt. Boeneke and Aryana (2008) proved that the addition of up to 400 µg of folic acid had no impact on the physicochemical and sensory attributes of strawberry-flavored-yogurt; however, post-pasteurization fortification of lemon-flavored-yogurt resulted in lower sensory scores and higher syneresis values (Boeneke and Aryana, 2008).

Folate fortification can be successfully carried out on processed meat products, such as cooked sausage (Caceres et al., 2008) and hamburgers (Galan et al., 2010), to ensure coverage of 100% of the RDA (2.4 mg folic acid/100 g of ready to eat product).

2.11 Vitamin B12

Vitamin B12 (cobalamin) is a cofactor in the synthesis of an essential amino acid, methionine. Its metabolic role is closely linked to that of folate because they share an enzyme, methionine synthase, which is necessary for cell metabolism and survival. Deficiency of this vitamin can, thus, impair the use of folate and causes neurological deterioration, megaloblastic anemia, elevated plasma homocysteine, and possibly impaired immune function. In infants and young children, it can also cause severe developmental delays.

Vitamin B12 is synthesized by microorganisms in the gut of animals and is subsequently absorbed and incorporated into animal tissues. Products from herbivorous animals (i.e., meat, eggs, milk) are thus the only source of the vitamin for humans. Consequently, intakes are very low or close to zero in many economically disadvantaged population groups, or among those who avoid animal products for religious or other reasons. There is high risk of deficiency in strict vegetarians and even lacto-ovo vegetarians, who may have lower plasma concentrations of the vitamin compared with meat consumers. The recommended daily intake is 2 μg for both men and women.

The fortification procedure covers the addition of cyanocobalamin or hydroxocobalamin. Among plant-based foods, bread would be a good product for fortification with natural [hydroxocobalamin (OHCbl, natural form), synthetic (cyanocobalamin (CNCbl, chemically modified form)], or *in situ*-produced vitamin B12. Knowledge of the stability of added vitamin B12 in bread is limited and the retention of *in situ*-produced vitamin B12 in bread making has not been studied. Added CNCbl was stable, whereas 20%–30% of added OHCbl was lost during the baking steps in straight- and sponge-dough processes. Malt medium containing active vitamin B12 produced in situ by *Propionibacterium freudenreichii* was successfully used in the straight- and sour-dough processes (Edelmann et al., 2016).

Eggs can also be fortified with vitamin B12, mostly by the dietary modification of hens fodder. Leeson and Caston (2003) succeded in increasing cyanocobalamin level in eggs by almost four times, whereas Zang et al. (2011) found it increased by ten times; however, in both cases, a high amount of the vitamin in premix was required. Red meat is the major dietary source of vitamin B12, providing over two thirds of the daily requirement in one 100 g serving (Cosgrove et al., 2005). Thus fortification of meat products with cyanocobalamin is not necessary.

As vitamin B12 is typically found in animal products, vegetarians and vegans usually suffer from this micronutrient deficiency. Thus, food designed for those groups of consumers, such as meat analogs substitutes, and alternatives classically made from soybeans or wheat gluten, have to be fortified with vitamn B12. Tofu, yeast spreads, soy milk, and cheese analogs are also often fortified with cyanocobalamin. Moreover, it has been found that vitamin B12 is possibly absorbed better from fortified products than that found naturally in foods (Tucker et al., 2000).

Some fortificant loss is inevitable, the degree of loss being dependent on factors such as the temperature used during food processing or preparation, the moisture content, extrusion temperatures and pressures, the presence of other micronutrients (in the premix and in the fortified food), the nature of the packaging, and the anticipated shelf-life of the fortified product. Vitamin B12 recoveries in bread made from fortified flour range from about 70% to 95% for niacin, and from 75% to 90% for thiamin and pyridoxine. About 70% of any added thiamin, pyridoxine and niacin is retained when enriched flour is used to prepare pasta, even after drying and cooking. On this basis, and assuming that any added B vitamins are 100% absorbed, in flour an overage of approximately 20–30% is thus usually sufficient to provide the desired amount in food products such as breads and cereals. Coated forms of the water-soluble vitamins, such as thiamin and vitamin B6, are available if off-flavors or other problems arise.

2.12 Vitamin H

Vitamin H (biotin) is a heterocyclic compound formed by an imidazolidone ring joined to a tetrahydrothiophene ring with a valeric acid side chain. D(+)-biotin is the only one occurring in nature and binds to and activates four carboxylases in the human body. The vitamin acts as part of enzyme systems involved in building up chemicals containing carbon and oxygen, such as fats and glucose. Infants may be at risk from biotin deficiency, which shows up as a "seborrheic dermatitis" that responds to biotin. Also, some infants have a metabolic disorder requiring extra biotin. There has been some suggestion that "cot deaths" or sudden infant death syndrome (SIDS) may in some cases be due to an inadequate intake of biotin.

Nuts, root vegetables, and eggs are among our best sources of biotin. RDI is set at 100–200 μg. The biotin in human milk averages about 10 μg per 1000 kcal and in infant formula is usually at least 15 μg per 1000 kcal. However, a higher concentration of biotin may be preferable for infant formula because nutrients can be more biologically available to the infant from human milk than from infant formula.

Biotin deficiency can occur while avidin-rich food is consumed, mainly raw eggs, as avidin binds and inactivates biotin. Biotin can be made by gut bacteria and absorbed from the large bowel, so that not all biotin needs to be obtained from food. Antibiotic therapy may reduce the amount of available biotin. Biotin is water soluble, stable at pH 5 to 8, but sensitive to air, oxygen, light, heat, and also to alkaline conditions. Oxidation of the sulfur atom and shortening of the valeric acid side chain result in loss of vitamin activity. D-biotin can be used for food fortification. Genereally, the addition of vitamin B7 is performed together with other vitamins and does not influence the sensory profile and acceptance of biscuits (Tsikritzi et al., 2014) and sorghum-based high protein blended foods (Joseph, 2016). However, eggs are one of the best natural sources of biotin and studies on their fortification by the modification of fodder are still being carried out. The successful enrichment of eggs with biotin was achieved for example by Zang et al. (2011).

2.13 Vitamin C

Vitamin C is a redox system comprised of ascorbic acid and dehydroascorbic acid, which acts as an electron donor. Its main metabolic function is the maintenance of collagen formation, and is also an important antioxidant. Although severe vitamin C deficiency (scurvy) is now relatively rare, the prevalence of milder or marginal deficiency is probably quite high. Vitamin C is widely available in foods of both plant and animal origin, but the best sources are fresh fruits and vegetables, and offal; as germination increases vitamin C content, germinated grains and pulses also contain high levels of vitamin C. However, because vitamin C is unstable when exposed to an alkaline environment or to oxygen, light and heat, losses may be substantial during storage and cooking. Deficiency is usually a result of a low consumption of fresh fruits and vegetables, caused by any one or a combination of factors such as seasonal unavailability, transportation difficulties, and/or unaffordable cost. Displaced populations who rely on cooked, fortified rations and who do not have access to fresh fruits and vegetables are at a high risk for deficiency. For these populations, vitamin C supplementation is recommended. Chronic alcoholics, institutionalized elderly, infants, and people living on restricted diets are also at risk of vitamin C deficiency. Severe vitamin C deficiency (symptoms appear within 3–4 months of a very low, i.e., <2 mg vitamin C daily intake) may lead to follicular hyperkeratosis, haemorrhagic manifestations, swollen joints, swollen bleeding gums and peripheral edema, and even death. From the other side, high consumption of ascorbic acid, due to its reducing and chelating properties, is related to a substantial increase of Fe absorption (Teucher et al., 2004). Ascorbic acid addition to Fe-fortified foods is thus a widely adopted practice throughout the food industry, especially for processed foods. Simultaneous fortification of whole cow milk with ferrous gluconate and ascorbic acid is a common practice in Chile and Mexico, and it has been claimed efficacious in reducing the prevalence of anemia and in improving iron status of small children (Villalpando et al., 2006). However, because of stability issues it is not recommended for staple food and condiments, such as fortified milk powder. To retain vitamin C stability, food, preferably not cooked, must therefore be appropriately packaged, or the ascorbic acid used in an encapsulated form. Chemical forms of vitamin C permitted for fortification include L-ascorbic acid, sodium-L-ascorbate, calcium-L-ascorbate, potassium-L-ascorbate, and L-ascorbyl 6-palmitate. They are often added to oils, fats, soft drinks, and various other foods as a stability enhancer of other added micronutrients, for example vitamin A. The addition of vitamin C to commercially processed foods, such as dry milk, infant formulas, cereal-based complementary foods, chocolate drink powders, and beverages, has been found to be successful in increasing intakes of this nutrient. As sugar helps to protect the ascorbic acid in soft drinks, sugar has been proposed as a possible vehicle for the vitamin.

Fortifying commonly consumed foods and beverages offers a great opportunity of increasing the nutrient intake of young children, thereby improving their nutritional status. Beverages are easily consumed along with meals and so they are good vehicles for delivery of nutritional supplements into the body. The first fortified beverage to appear in the world market was *Aqua Libra,* launched in England in the 1980s. Over the years, many such products have appeared on the market and they address such health problems as aging, stress, and weakness. Therefore, beverages are often fortified with multiple vitamins and minerals for greater nutritional impact, as opposed to fortification with a single micronutrient. On a weight basis, as a percentage of the total dry beverage formulation they are generally in the range between 0.01% and 5%. The choice of nutrients used to fortify beverages is based on a number of factors such as the chemical form of the micronutrient in terms of its bioavailability, the effects on the organoleptic characteristics of the particular beverage, and cost. Ingredient interactions are common, so one way to minimize interactions is to separate vitamins and other ingredients into two individual premixes.

As a beverage becomes fortified by vitamins and minerals or other components, the pH of the beverage rises and therefore the beverage becomes more basic. The ascorbic acid is added to bring the pH of the beverage down and counter the effects of stability of all nutrition components and fortification. As the beverage is more acidic, it becomes more resistant to microbial growth. In most cases, the pH of fruit drinks and juices is below 4.5 and the heat treatment required is pasteurization. Some loss of heat-labile vitamins, thiamin, folic acid, and ascorbic acids occurs as a result of the thermal treatment. The acidity of these drinks causes problems of stability with vitamin A, folic acid, and calcium pantothenate. Carbonation of these beverages, with the resultant exclusion of oxygen, improves the stability of vitamins.

Fortification of fruit juices and beverages with vitamin C is a common practice. Vitamin C is a well-known micronutrient, which is added to food products not only in order to extend shelf life, but also enhance nutritional levels. Mostly, the fortification levels follow recommendations for vitamin C daily intake: 75 (women) and 90 (men) mg/day (Allen et. al., 2006). However, vitamin C is also known to promote anthocyanins degradation (Remini et al., 2015) in pigment-rich juices, that is, cranberry, chokeberry, strawberry, and black currant, thereby affecting the consumer acceptance of the products. Roidoung et al. (2017) suggest that the fortification of vitamin C from 40 to 80 mg/100 mL significantly accelerated color degradation of cranberry juice. Therefore, encapsulation on vitamin C or anthocyanin structure modification has been suggested to improve stability of bioactive compounds.

Precautions included the use of stainless equipment, addition of vitamins at the latest possible stage, avoidance of excessive aeration or even de-aeration, rapid cooling after thermal treatment and the avoidance of readily auto-oxidisable ingredients. Riboflavin and thiamin showed good stability but vitamin C showed about 23% loss.

Additionally, it is not easy to add fat-soluble vitamins such as vitamin E to aqueous foods while retaining their activity. For instance, vitamin E is liposoluble and easily oxidized in the air (Ordoñez et al., 1998), while vitamin C is thermolabile and is degraded after thermal treatments (Lešková et al., 2006). Therefore, it would be very useful to add vitamin C along with other antioxidant vitamins such as α-tocopherol. The addition of these vitamins to aqueous foods using liposomes appears to be a promising solution. Liposomes are microscopic spherical vesicles composed of polar lipids like phospholipids, which enclose liquid compartments within their structure (consisting of lipid bilayers) and enable the encapsulation of both hydrophilic and lipophilic materials (Marsanasco et al., 2011). With respect to vitamin E, it was demonstrated that its absorption and bioavailability are increased when it is encapsulated in liposomes. Also, results showed that liposomes are very useful in protecting vitamins and maintaining their activity in aqueous foods, especially in the case of the thermolabile vitamin C (Marsanasco et al., 2011).

The stability of vitamins is affected by a number of factors, such as temperature, moisture, oxygen, light, pH, minerals (especially iron and copper), vitamin-vitamin interactions, other food components, processing methods, and storage. In order to compare quantitatively the published results, that temperature is the most important factor affecting the degradation. The various forms of vitamin C degrade at different rates and in different forms. From the rate constants, as present (De Ritter et al., 1976), the order of rate constants is ascorbic acid > L-ascorbate 2-monophosphate > L-ascorbate 2-polyphosphate. Approximately the same order can be seen for the potato flakes (Park et al., 1994).

The matrix also affects the rate constants of degradation. For liquid matrices and for comparable temperatures, the rate constants are much higher for the degradation in milk that in fruit juices and drinks. This could be caused by different pH in both matrices. It has been reported that the rate of degradation increases remarkably when pH > 5.7 (Assiry et al., 2006). As for the solid matrices, the rate constants of vitamin C degradation in bread are by 2–3 orders of magnitude higher than those for the bran flakes, cereals, dried apple chips, and potato flakes. Stability of vitamin C in plant products showed that the relative humidity and the quality of packaging could also have some effect on the rate constant .

In addition, Choi et al. (2002) studied retention of ascorbic acid and pigment stability in blood orange juice packed in Tetra Brik Aseptic cartons. Fortified and controlled samples of juices were stored for 7 weeks at 4.5°C, and it was noted that a greater retention at the level of 25% of ascorbic acid was observed. Experiments showed that the most important for stability and protection of vitamin wasbut the storage temperature.

Vitamin C retention in cereal-based products appears to be dependent on time, temperature, and product moisture. Storage time and baking decrease ascorbic acid content; however, encapsulation in soybean oil appears to reduce its losses.

Wang et al. (1995) studied bran flakes fortified with varied forms vitamin C. Bran flakes were stored for 7 months at 25–40°C in moisture about 7%–11%. Loss of ascorbic acid was rapid, that is, 80% after 1 month at 40°C, and a higher moisture (11%) and only 5% after at 25°C and 7% moisture.

Wang et al. (1995) evaluated stability of different forms of vitamin C. Three forms of vitamin C (L-ascorbic acid, L-ascorbate 2-polyphosphate and L-ascorbate 2-mono-phosphate) were added for fortified mashed potatoes and they stored at 25°C. The retention of L-ascorbic acid was 18%, L-ascorbate 2-polyphosphate 84% and L-ascorbate 2-monophosphate 88%. It was concluded that L-ascorbate 2-monophosphate was more stable in stored potatoes (Wang et al., 1995).

Adding vitamin C to meats is difficult because it is not very stable at meat pH and tends to promote lipid oxidation (Decker and Park, 2010). However, sodium ascorbate is routinely applied during meat processing, for example while curing the raw meat before further conversion to smoked products, sausages, and so on. Vitamin C is required in meat processing due to acceleration of color development and prevention of color fading, inhibition of nitrosamine formation, and prevention of lipid and protein oxidation. The use of vitamin C in meat processing has to be strictly controlled due to its prooxidative action in lipids rich environments, especially. Fortification of meat products is usually performed together with α-tocopherol and other nutrients, for example, calcium addition to assure optimum conditions for physico-chemical and sensory parameters, as well as to oxidatively stabilize the product (Serdaroglu and Yildiz, 2004; Mehta et al., 2015).

2.14 Choline

Choline is a β-hydroxyethyltrimethylammonium hydroxide. It is an essential nutrient in the production of phosphatidylcholine, responsible for building a living cell structure and function of all cells, including those building heart, intestines, muscle, and so on. Moreover, acetylcholine is a signal molecule or neurotransmitter responsible for normal action of a nervous system and brain function. The human requirement for dietary choline is 425 mg/day for women and 550 mg/day for men (Young and Garza, 1998). The most common form of choline provided by foods is phophatidylcholine found in egg yolk, beef, liver, fish and seafood, Brussel sprouts, spinach, nuts, and cauliflower. Choline deficiency may led to liver damage, fatigue, and low levels of energy, cognitive function decline and memory loss, learning difficulties, nerve dysfunction and damage, muscle aches and pains, mood swings, and emotional disorders. Choline can be added to prepared foods, beverages, and dietary supplements as a water-soluble salt (choline chloride or choline bitartrate). It is recognized as a GRAS ingredient (21 CFR 182.8250 &8252), and it is stable in high temperature processing and long term storage. Choline (lecithin and/or a choline salt) fortified cereal (US 20040175482 A1) is a good example of a well-balanced ready-to-eat source of choline in daily diet. Further development of extrusion technology can lead to the production of a wide selection of choline-enriched functional cereal-based products (Asomaning et al., 2017).

2.15 Encapsulation

Another approach to food fortification, despite direct applications, is to encapsulate certain vitamins. The primary objective of encapsulation is to extend the shelf life and quality of the product by separating the fortificants from the vehicle components and environment until release is desired. Microencapsulation is a technology wherein small solid, liquid or gas particles are coated with or entrapped within a continuous film of polymeric material. The coated material is called core material, actives, fill, internal phase, or payload and can be encapsulated pure or in combination with other materials. The final products of microencapsulation procedure are small particles (between few μm and few mm) which provide an effective protection of core material regarding the surrounding environment.

Microencapsulation of vitamins (fat and water soluble forms), especially fat soluble, has been proposed as a solution for its chemical instability. Fat-soluble vitamins (A, D, E, K) are hydrophobic compounds and therefore easily become inactive or rapidly degrade in the presence of aqueous systems, and they are poorly soluble in aqueous solvents (Goncalves et al., 2016). The increase of stability and dispersibility of vitamins can be achieved by incorporation of vitamins into carriers with advantageous physical and chemical properties, using suitable encapsulation methods. This strategy may also be beneficial for vitamins in controlled-release experiment promoting the release of this compound at the target site and optimizing the absorption to prevent its ineffective use (Sauvant et al., 2012). The final purpose and its application in food production is to ensure higher bioavailability in the human body. Encapsulation can be also used to mask undesirable flavors and to isolate reactive components to prevent the degradation of micronutrients (Ghosh, 2006). Nowadays nanoencapsulation of vitamins will be much more popular with different techniques and it is expected to be a crucial field of research in the coming years.

Encapsulated vitamins are used for fortified products such as beverages, bread, and cookies. Tomiuk et al. (2012) prepared L-5-methyltetrahydrofolic acid (L-5-MTHF) microcapsules using skim milk as the encapsulating agent for the fortification of bread to increase its bioavailability. Another research group prepared biscuits with encapsulated and unencapsulated 5-methyltetrahy-drofolic acid (5-CH3THF) and studied its stability under different baking conditions. The retention of folic acid content in the biscuits fortified with the encapsulated 5-CH3THF was high (19.1, 8.5, 4.9 at 180, 200, and 220°C, respectively) compared to that in the biscuits fortified with the unencapsulated 5-CH3THF (5.4, 6.7, 4.4 at 180, 200, and 220°C, respectively) (Shrestha et al., 2012).

The literature data indicate that encapsulation is the best way of protecting vitamin C. For the application in solid food systems (cereals, bread, and biscuits), spray-cooling, spray-chilling and fluidized bed appear to be the best ways of encapsulation. In liquid food systems, liposomes represent the best form of encapsulation.

2.16 Monitoring of fortified food products

EU Member States may request notification to their competent authority of the placing on the market in their territory of foods to which vitamins have been added and of foods containing substances listed in Annex III, Parts B and C in accordance with Article 15 of the Regulation.

References

Aaron, G. J., Dror, D. K., and Yang, Z. 2015. Multiple-micronutrient fortified non-dairy beverage interventions reduce the risk of anemia and iron deficiency in school-aged children in low-middle income countries: A systematic review and meta-analysis. *Nutrients* 7:3847–3868.

Allen, L. H., Benoist, B., Dary, O., and Hurrell, R. 2006. *Guideline of Food Fortification with Micronutrients*. Geneva: World Health Organization, Food and Agricultural Organization of the United Nations.

ANZ Food Standards. 2009. Supporting document 1. Technical and nutrition assessment – Application A1104. Voluntary addition of vitamins & minerals to nut- and seed- based beverages. pp. 1-62 (http://www.foodstandards.gov.au/code/applications/Documents/A1104%20Nut%20and%20seed%20beverages%20SD1%20Tech%20and%20nutritn%20assess.pdf)

Arroyave, G., Mejia, L. A., and Aguilar, J. R. 1981. The effect of vitamin A fortification of sugar on the serum vitamin A levels of preschool Guatemalan children: A longitudinal evaluation. *American Journal of Clinical Nutrition* 34:41–49.

Asomaning, J., Zhao, Y. Y., Lewis, E. D. et al. 2017. The development of a choline rich cereal based functional food: Effect of processing and storage. *LWT - Food Science and Technology* 75:447–452.

Assiry, A. M. Sastry, S. K., and Samaranayake, C. P. 2006. Influence of temperature, electrical conductivity, power and pH on ascorbic acid degradation kinetics during ohmic heating using stainless steel electrodes. *Bioelectrochemistry* 68:7–13.

Australian Goverment, National Health and Medical Research Council. Nutrient Reference Values. https://www.nrv.gov.au/

Banville, C., Vuillemard, J. C., and Lacroix, C. 2000. Comparison of different methods for fortifying Cheddar cheese with vitamin D. *International Dairy Journal* 10:375–382.

Bell, J. A., Griinari, J. M., and Kennelly, J. J. 2006. Effect of safflower oil, flaxseed oil, monensin, and vitamin E on concentration of conjugated linoleic acid in bovine milk fat. *Journal of Dairy Science* 89:733–748.

Bender, P. E. 1996. Nutritional effects of food processing. *Journal of Food Technology* 1:261–269.

Bender, D. A. 1989. Vitamin B6 requirements and recommendations. *European Journal of Clinical Nutrition* 43:289–309.

Berendsen, A. A. M., van Lieshout, L. E. L. M., van den Heuvel, E. G. H. M., Matthys, C., Péter, S., and de Groot, L. C. P. G. M. 2016. Conventional foods, followed by dietary supplements and fortified foods, are the key sources of vitamin D, vitamin B6, and selenium intake in Dutch participants of the NU-AGE study. *Nutrition Research* 36:1171–1181.

Boeneke, C. A. and Aryana, K. J. 2008. Effect of folic acid fortification on the characteristics of lemon yogurt. *LWT - Food Science and Technology* 41:1335–1343.

Bolger, Z., Brunton, N. P., Lyng, J. G., and Monahan, F. J. 2016. Quality attributes and retention of vitamin E in reduced salt chicken sausages fortified with vitamin E. *Journal of Food Science and Technology* 53:3948–3959.

Bolger, Z., Brunton, N. P., Lyng, J. G., and Monahan, F. J. 2017. Comminuted meat products—consumption, composition, and approaches to healthier formulations. *Food Reviews International* 33:143–166.

Bou, R., Codony, R., Tres, A., Decker, E. A., and Guardiola, F. 2009. Dietary strategies to improve nutritional value, oxidative stability, and sensory properties of poultry products. *Critical Reviews in Food Science and Nutrition* 49:800–822.

Browning, L. C. and Cowieson, A. J. 2014. Vitamin D fortification of eggs for human health. *Journal of the Science of Food and Agriculture* 94:1389–1396.

Butt, M. S., Arshad, M. U., Alam, M. S., and Nadeem, M. T. 2007. Bioavailability and storage stability of vitamin A fortificant (retinyl acetate) in fortified cookies. *Food Research International* 40:1212–1219.

Caceres, E., Garcia, M. L., and Selgas, M. D. 2008. Conventional and fat-reduced cooked sausages enriched with folic acid. *Fleischwirtschaft International* 23:58–60.

Cashman, K., Duffy, S., Hayes, A. et al. 2015. Biofortification of eggs and pork with vitamin D as a means of increasing dietary supply. *FASEB Journal* 29(Suppl. 1):758–813.

Castellini, C., Dal Bosco, A., and Bernardini, M. 1999. Effect of dietary vitamin E supplementation on the characteristics of refrigerated and frozen rabbit meat. *Italian Journal Food Science* 11:151–159.

Castellini, C., Dal Bosco, A., Bernardini, M., and Cyril, H. W. 1998. Effect ofdietary vitamin E on the oxidative stability of raw and cooked rabbit meat. *Meat Science* 50:153–161.

Choi, M. H., Kim, G. H., and Lee, H. S. 2002. Effects of ascorbic acid retention on juice colour and pigment stability in blood orange (Citrus sinensis) juice during refrigerated storage. *Food Research International* 35:753–759.

Casey J., Whalen P. 2004. Choline-fortified cereal and method. US Patent 20040175482 A1

Combs, G. F. 2012. *The Vitamins: Fundamental Aspects in Nutrition and Health*, 4th ed. Amsterdam: Elsevier.

Corino, C., Pastorelli, G., Pantaleo, L., Oriani, G., and Salvatori, G. 1999. Improvement of color and lipid stability of rabbit meat by dietary supplementation with vitamin E. *Meat Science* 52:285–289.

Cosgrove, M., Flynn, A., and Kiely, M. 2004. Impact of disaggregation of composite foods on estimates of intakes of meat and meat products in Irish adults. *Public Health Nutrition* 8:327–337.

D.03.002, FDR. 2017. Foods to which vitamins, mineral nutrients and amino acids may or must be added. Food and Drug Regulations C.R.C., c. 870 January 31, 2017 Published by the Minister of Justice, http://laws-lois.justice.gc.ca.

Dal Bosco, A. and Castellini, C. 1998. Effet de l'addition de vitamin E dans l'aliment e desconditions de conservation des carcasses sur les caractéristiques physico-chimiques de la viande chez le lapin. *Proceed. 7èmes Journees de la Recherche Cunicole*, Lione, France, pp. 111–114.

Dal Bosco, A., Castellini, C., and Bernardini, M. 2001. Nutritional quality of rabbit meat as affected by cooking procedure and dietary vitamin E. *Journal of Food Science* 66:1047–1051.

Dalle Zotte, A., Cossu, M. E., and Parigi Bini, R. 2000. Effect of the dietary enrichment with animal fat and vitamin E on rabbit meat shelf-life and sensory properties. *Proceedings of the 46th International Congress of Meat Sciences and Technology*, August, Buenos Aires, Argentina, 542–543.

Day, B. P. F. and Gregory, J. F. 1983. Thermal stability of folic acid and 5-methyltetrahydrofolic acid in liquid model food systems. *Journal of Food Science* 48:581–587, 599.

Delles, R. M., Xiong, Y. L., True, A. D., Ao, T., and Dawson, K. A. 2014. Dietary antioxidant supplementation enhances lipid and protein oxidative stability of chicken broiler meat through promotion of antioxidant enzyme activity. *Poultry Science* 93:1561–1570.

De Ritter, E. 1976. Stability characteristics of vitamins in processed foods. *Food Technology* 30: 43-54.

Dhaussy, A. 2014. Vitamin D recommendations, fortification in France, and communication. *Oilseeds and Fats, Crops and Lipids* 21(3):D305. doi:10.1051/ocl/2013063.

Donhowe, E. G., Flores, F. P., Kerr, W. L., Wicker, L., and Kong, F. 2014. Characterization and in vitro bioavailability of b-carotene: Effects of microencapsulation method and food matrix. *LWT - Food Science and Technology* 57:42–48.

Dutra de Oliveira, J. E. D., Desai, I. D., Favaro, R. M. D., and Ferreira, J. F. 1994. Effect of heat treatment during cooking on the biological value of vitamin A fortified soybean oil in humans. *International Journal of Food Science and Nutrition* 45:203–207.

Ebeid, T. A., Zeweil, H. S., Basyony, M. M., Dosoky, W. M., and Badry, H. 2013. Fortification of rabbit diets with vitamin E or selenium affects growth performance, lipid peroxidation, oxidative status and immune response in growing rabbits. *Livestock Science* 155:323–331.

Edelmann, M., Chamlagain, B., Santin, M., Kariluoto, S., and Piironen, V. 2016. Stability of added and in situ-produced vitamin B12 in breadmaking. *Food Chemistry* 204:21–28.

EFSA. Tolerable upper intake levels for vitamins and minerals. 2006. Scientific Committee on Food Scientific Panel on Dietetic Products, Nutrition and Allergies.

FAO, IFAD and WFP. 2015. *The State of Food Insecurity in the World 2015: Meeting the 2015 International Hunger Targets: Taking Stock of Uneven Progress*. Rome: FAO.

Freiser, H. and Jiang, Q. 2009. γ-tocotrienol and γ-tocoperol are primarily metabolized to conjugated 2-(β-carboxyethyl)-6-hydroxy-2,7,8-trimethylchroman and sulfated long-chain carboxychromanols in rats. *Journal of Nutrition* 139:884–889.

Gahruie, H. H., Eskandari, M. E., Mesbahi, G., and Hanifpour, M. A. 2015. Scientific and technical aspects of yogurt fortification: A review. *Food Science and Human Wellness* 4:1–8.

Galan, I., Garcia, M. L., and Selgas, M. D. 2010. Effects of irradiation on hamburgers enriched with folic acid. *Meat Science* 84:437–443.

Galvez, F.C.F., Francisco, F.M.dL., Villarino, B.J., Lustre, A.O., Resurreccion, A.V.A. 2006. Vitamin A fortification of stabilized peanut butter by direct addition. In: Vitamin A fortified peanut butter. Ed. by United States Agency for International Development Peanut Collaborative Research Support Program, Project 04, USA and Philippines, University of Georgia, Griffin, Georgia, USA, No. 5, pp. 81-97.

Gerling, E. M. and Ternes, W. 2014. Stability of a-tocotrienol and atocopherol in salami-type sausages and curing brine depending on nitrite and pH. *Meat Science* 98:657–664.

Ghosh, S. K. 2006. Functional coatings and microencapsulation: A general perspective. In: Ghosh, S. K. (Ed.). *Functional Coating*. Weinheim: Wiley-VCH, pp. 1–26.

Gomes Ribeiro, E. M., Chitchumroonchokchai, C., Jaeger de Carvalho, L. M., and Failla, M. L. 2015. Effect of style of home cooking on retention and bioaccessibility of pro-vitamin A carotenoids in biofortified pumpkin (*Cucurbita moschata* Duch.). *Food Research International* 77:620–626.

Goncalves, A., Estevinho, B. N., and Rocha F. 2016. Microencapsulation of vitamin A: A review. *Trends in Food Science and Technology* 51:76–87.

Gregory, J. I. 1989. Chemical and nutritional aspects of folate research, analytical procedures, methods of folate synthesis, stability and bioavailability of dietary folate. *Advances in Food and Nutrition Research* 33:1–101.

Hennessy, A., Walton, J., and Flynn, A. 2013. The impact of voluntary food fortification on micronutrient intakes and status in European countries: A review. *Proceedings of the Nutrition Society* 72:433–440.

Hoffpauer, D. W. and Bonnette III, R. E. 1998. Enrichment update on folic acid. *Cereal Foods World* 43:365–367.

Holick, M. F. 1999. Vitamin D. In: Shils, M. E., Olson, J. A., Shike, M., and Ross, A. C. (Eds.). *Modern Nutrition in Health and Disease,* 19th ed. Philadelphia, PA: Lippincott Willams & Wilkins, pp. 329–345.

Holmes, R. P. and Kummerow, F. A. 1983. The relationship of adequate and excessive intake of vitamin D to health and disease. *Journal of American Collage of Nutrition* 2:173–199.

Ilic, D. and Ashoor, S. 1988. Stability of vitamins A and C in fortified yogurt. *Journal of Dairy Science* 71:1492–1498.

Jakobsen, J. and Knuthsen, P. 2014. Stability of vitamin D in foodstuffs during cooking. *Food Chemistry* 148:170–175.

Johnson, L.E. 1998. Oils, fats and margarine: overview of technology. In: Micronutrient Initiative, ed. *Food fortification to end micronutrient malnutrition. State of the Art.* Ottawa, Micronutrient Initiative, 22–26

Johnson, M. A. 2007. If high folic acid aggravates vitamin B12 deficiency what should be done about it? *Nutritional Review* 65:451–458.

Joseph, M. V. 2016. Extrusion, physico-chemical characterization and nutritional evaluation of sorghum-based high protein, micronutrient fortified blended foods. PhD dissertation, Kansas State University, Manhattan, Kansas.

Kazmi, S. A., Vieth, R., and Rousseau, D. 2007. Vitamin D3 fortification and quantification in processed dairy products. *International Dairy Journal* 17:753–759.

Kim, Y. J. and Choi, I. H. 2012. Utilization of dried garlic powder and alphatocopherol to improve the shelf-life of emulsion-type sausage during refrigerated storage. *Korean Journal of Food Science and Animal Resources* 32:725–731.

Knapen, M. H. J., Braam, L. A. J. L. M., Teunissen, K. J., Zwijsen, R. M. L., Theuwissen, E., and Vermeer, C. 2015. Yogurt drink fortified with menaquinone-7 improves vitamin K status in a healthy population. *Journal of Nutritional Science* 4:e35, 1–8. doi:10.1017/jns.2015.25.

Kurzer, A. B. 2013. The protective effect of antioxidants on vitamin A stability in nonfat dry milk during thermally accelerated storage. MSc thesis, Brigham Young University, Provo, Utah.

LeBlanc, J. G., Rutten, G., Bruinenberg, P., Sesma, F., de Giori, G. S., and Smid, E. J. 2006. A novel dairy product fermented with Propionibacterium freudenreichii improves the riboflavin status of deficient rats. *Nutrition* 22:645–651.

Leeson, S. and Caston, L. J. 2003. Vitamin enrichment of eggs. *Journal of Applied Poultry Research* 12:24–26.

Lešková, E., Kubíková, J., Kováčiková, E., Košická, M., Porubská, J., and Holčíková, K. 2006. Vitamin losses: Retention during heat treatment and continual changes expressed by mathematical models. *Journal of Food Composition and Analysis* 19:252–276.

Lo Fiego, D., Santoro, P., Macchioni, P. et al. 2004. The effect of dietary supplementation of vitamin C and E on the α-tocopherol content of muscles, liver and kidney, on the stability of lipids, and on certain meat quality parameters. *Meat Science* 67:317–327.

Mahmood, S., Masood, S. B., Faqir, M. A., and Haq, N. 2008. Baking and storage stability of retinyl acetate (vitamin A) fortified cookies. *Pakistan Journal of Nutrition* 7:586–589.

Marsanasco, M., Márquez, A. L., Wagner, J. R., Alonso, S. d. V., and Chiaramoni, N. S. 2011. Liposomes as vehicles for vitamins E and C: An alternative to fortify orange juice and offer vitamin C protection after heat treatment. *Food Research International* 44:3039–3046.

Martin, P. R., Singleton, C. K., and Hiller-Sturmhofel, S. 2003. The role of thiamin deficiency in alcoholic brain disease. *Alcohol Research and Health* 27:134–142.

Martinez-Villaluenga, C., Michalska, A., Frias, J., Piskula, M. K., Vidal-Valverde, C., and Zielinski, H., 2009. Effect of flour extraction rate and baking on thiamin and riboflavin content and antioxidant capacity of traditional rye bread. *Journal of Food Science* 74(1):C49–C55. doi:10.1111/j.1750-3841.2008.01008.x.

Mehansho, H., Hughes, D. L., Nakel, G. M., and Heckert, D. C. 1989. Stable nutritional vitamin and mineral supplemented beverage. US 4992282 A.

Mehta, N., Sharma, B. D., Kumar, R. R., Kumar, P., Malav, O. P., and Kumar Verma, A. 2015. Fortification of low-fat chicken meat patties with calcium, vitamin E and vitamin C. *Nutrition and Food Science* 45:688–702.

Meineri, G., Medana, C., Giancotti, V., Visentin, S., and Peiretti, P. G. 2013. Effect of dietary supplementation of vitamin E in pigs to prevent the formation of carcinogenic substances in meat products. *Journal of Food Composition and Analysis* 30:67–72.

Mercier, Y., Gatellier, P., Viau, M., Remignon, H., and Renerre, M. 1998. Effect of dietary fat and vitamin E on colour stability and on lipid and protein oxidation in turkey meat during storage. *Meat Science* 48:301–318.

Mihhalevski, A., Nisamedtinov, I., Halvin, K., Oseka, A., and Paalme, T. 2013. Stability of B-complex vitamins and dietary fiber during rye sourdough bread production. *Journal of Cereal Science* 57:30–38.

Monahan, F. J., Gray, J. I., Asghar, A. et al. 1994. Influence of diet on lipid oxidation and membrane structure in porcine muscle microsomes. *Journal of Agricultural Food Chemistry* 42:59–63.

Murphy, S. C. and Newcomer, C. 2001. Guideline for vitamin A & D fortification of fluid milk. The Dairy Practices Council® http://phpa.dhmh.maryland.gov/OEHFP/OFPCHS/Milk/Shared%20Documents/DPC053_Vitamin_AD_Fortification_Fluid_Milk.pdf.

Norman, A. W. 1996. Vitamin D. In: Zeigler, E. E. Jr. and Filer, L. J. (Eds.). *Present Knowledge in Nutrition*, 7th ed. Washington, DC: ILSI Press, pp. 120–129.

Ordoñez, J. A., Cambera, M. I., Fernández, L. et al. 1998. *Tecnología de los Alimentos. Componentes de los alimentos y procesos*, 1st ed., Chaps. 3 and 6. Madrid: Síntesis.

Park, H., Seib, P. A., and Chung, O. K. 1994. Stabilities of several forms of vitamin C during making and storing of pup-loaves of white pan bread. *Cereal Chemistry* 71:412–417.

Petrogianni, M., Kanellakis, S., Moschonis, G., and Manios, Y. 2014. Fortification of vitamin A in a phytosterol enriched milk maintains plasma beta-carotene levels. *Journal of Food Science and Technology* 51:196–199.

Regulation (EC) No 1925/2006 of the European Parliament and of the Council of 20 December 2006 on the addition of vitamins and minerals and of certain other substances to foods, http://data.europa.eu/eli/reg/2006/1925/oj.

Reichel, H., Koeffler, H. P., and Norman, A. W. 1989. The role of the vitamin D endocrine system in health and disease. *New England Journal of Medicine* 320:980–991.

Remini, H., Mertz, C., Belbahi, A., Achir, N., Dornier, M., and Madani, K. 2015. Degradation kinetic modelling of ascorbic acid and colour intensity in pasteurised blood orange juice during storage. *Food Chemistry* 173:665–673.

Riccio, F., Mennella, C., and Fogliano, V. 2006. Effect of cooking on the concentration of vitamins B in fortified meat products. *Journal of Pharmaceutical and Biomedical Analysis* 41:1592–1595.

Rohde, C. M., Manatt, M., Clagett-Dame, M., and DeLuca, H. F. 1999. Vitamin A antagonizes the action of vitamin D in rats. *Journal of Nutrition* 129:2246–2250.

Roidoung, S., Dolan, K. D., and Siddiq, M. 2017. Estimation of kinetic parameters of anthocyanins and color degradation in vitamin C fortified cranberry juice during storage. *Food Research International* 94:29–35.

Roman, M. J., Burri, B. J., and Singh, R. P. 2012. Release and bioaccessibility of β-carotene from fortified almond butter during in vitro digestion. *Journal of Agricultural Food Chemistry* 60:9659–9666.

Rosli, W. I. W., Babji, A. S., Aminah, A., Foo, S. P., and Abd Malik, O. 2006. Vitamin E contents of processed meats blended with palm oils. *Journal of Food Lipids* 13:186–198.

Rosli, W. I. W., Babji, A. S., Aminah, A., Foo, S. P., and Abd Malik, O. 2010. Effect of retorting and oven cooking on the nutritional properties of beef frankfurters blended with palm oils. *International Journal of Food Science and Nutrition* 61:519–535.

Sauvant, P., Cansell, M., Sassi, A. H., and Atgie, C. 2012.Vitamin A enrichment: Caution with encapsulation strategies used for food applications. *Food Research International* 46:469–479.

Schellack, G., Harirari, P., and Schellack, N. 2015. B-complex vitamin deficiency and supplementation. *South African Pharmaceutical Journal* 82:28–33.

Selim, N. A., Abdel-Khalek, A. M., Nada, S. A., and El-Medany, S. H. A. 2008. Response of growing rabbits to dietary antioxidant vitamins E and C. 2. Effects on meat quality. *Proceedings of the 9th World Rabbit Congress*, Verona, Italia, pp. 1437–1442.

Serdaroglu, M. and Yildiz, T. G. 2004. Effect of ascorbic acid, rosemary extract and alpha tocopherol/ascorbic acid on some quality characteristics of frozen chicken patties. *Electronic Journal of Polish Agricultural Universities* 7:5.

Shrestha, A. K., Arcot, J., Dhital, S., and Crennan, S. 2012. Effect of biscuit baking conditions on the stability of microencapsulated 5-methyltetrahydrofolic acid and their physical properties. *Food and Nutrition Sciences* 3:1445–1452.

Sloan, A. E. 2000. The top ten functional food trends. *Food Technology* 54:33–62.
Solon, F. S., Klemm, R. D. W., Sanchez, L., Darnton-Hill, I., Craft, N. E., Christian, P., West Jr, K. P. 2000. Efficacy of a vitamin A-fortified wheat-flour bun on the vitamin A status of Filipino schoolchildren. *American Journal of Clinical Nutrition* 72:738–744.
Solon, F. S., Solon, M. S., Mehansho, H. et al. 1996. Evaluation of the effect of vitamin A-fortified margarine on the vitamin A status of preschool Filipino children. *European Journal of Clinical Nutrition* 50:720–723.
Spiro, A. and Buttriss, J. L. 2014. Vitamin D: An overview of vitamin D status and intake in Europe. *Nutrition Bulletin* 39:322–350.
Teucher, B., Olivares, M., and Cori, H. 2004. Enhancers of iron absorption: Ascorbic acid and other organic acids. *International Journal of Vitamins and Nutrition Research* 74:403–419.
Thacher, T. D. and Clarke, B. L. 2011. Vitamin D insufficiency. *Mayo Clinic Proceedings* 86:50–60.
Tiong, S. A., Chandra-Hioe, M. V., and Arcot, J. 2015. Thiamin fortification of bread-making flour: Retention in bread and levels in Australian commercial fortified bread varieties. *Journal of Food Composition and Analysis* 38:27–31.
Tippetts, M., Martini, S., Brothersen, C., and McMahon, D. J. 2012. Fortification of cheese with vitamin D3 using dairy protein emulsions as delivery systems. *Journal of Dairy Science* 95:4768–4774.
Tomiuk, S., Liu, Y., Greeen, T. J., King, M. J., Finglas, P. M., and Kitts, D. D. 2012. Studies on the retention of microen- capsulated L-5-methyltetrahydrofolic acid in baked bread using skim milk powder. *Food Chemistry* 133:249–255.
Tres, A., Bou, R., Codony, R., and Guardiola, F. 2008. Influence of dietary doses of n-3- orn-6 rich vegetable fats and α-tocopheryl acetate supplementation on raw andcooked rabbit meat composition and oxidative stability. *Journal of Agriculture and Food Chemistry* 56:7243–7253.
Tres, A., Bou, R., Codony, R., and Guardiola, F. 2010. Moderately oxidized oils and dietary zinc and α-tocopheryl acetate supplementation, Effects on the oxidative stability of rabbit plasma, liver, and meat. *Journal of Agrcultural Food Chemistry* 58:9112–9119.
Tsikritzi, R., Moynihan, P. J., Gosney, M. A., Allencand, V. J., and Methven, L. 2014. The effect of macro- and micro-nutrientfortification of biscuits on their sensoryproperties and on hedonic liking of olderpeople. *Journal of the Science of Food and Agriculture* 94:2040–2048.
Tucker, K. L., Qiao, N., and Maras, J. E. 2010. Simulation with soy replacement showed that increased soy intake could contribute to improved nutrient intake profiles in the U.S. population. *Journal of Nutrition* 140:2296S–2301S.
Tucker, K. L., Rich, S., Rosenberg, I. et al. 2000. Plasma vitamin B-12 concentrations relate to intake source in the Framingham Offspring study. *American Journal of Clinical Nutrition* 71:514–522.
Uchendu, F. N., Atinmo, T., and Oyewole, O. 2012. Stability of vitamin a in selected Nigerian bread made from commercial fortified wheat flour. *International Journal of Applied Science and Technology* 2:93–98.
U.S. Food and Drug Administration. 1996. Food standards: Amendment of standards of identity for enriched grain products to require addition of folic acidexternal link disclaimer. *Federal Register* 61(44) 8781–8797.
U.S. NA, Institute of Medicine, Food and Nutrition Board. 2010. *Dietary Reference Intakes for Calcium and Vitamin D.* Washington, DC: National Academy Press.

Villalpando, S., Shamah, T., Rivera, J. A., Lara, Y., and Monterrubio, E. 2006. Fortifying milk with ferrous gluconate and zinc oxide in a public nutrition program reduced the prevalence of anemia in toddlers. *Journal of Nutrition* 136:2633–2637.

Wang, X. Y., Seib, P. A., and Ra, K. S. 1995. L-ascorbic acid and its 2-phosphorylated derivatives in select- ed foods: Vitamin C fortification and antioxidant properties. *Journal of Food Science* 60:1295–1300.

Wen, J., Morrissey, P. A., Buckley, D. J., and Sheehy, P. J. 1997. Supranutritional vitamin E supplementation in pigs: Influence on subcellular deposition of α-tocopherol and on oxidative stability by conventional and derivative spectrophotometry. *Meat Science* 47:301–310.

Whitfield, K. C., Karakochuk, C. D., Kroeun, H. et al. 2017. Household consumption of thiamin-fortified fish sauce increases erythrocyte thiamin concentrations among rural Cambodian women and their children younger than 5 years of age: A randomized controlled efficacy trial. *Journal of Pediatrics* 181:242–247.

WHO, FAO, UNICEF, GAIN, MI, & FFI. 2009. Recommendations on wheat and maize flour fortification. Meeting Report: Interim Consensus Statement. World Health Organization, Geneva, http://www.who.int/nutrition/publications/micronutrients/wheat_maize_fort.pdf.

Wien, T. N., Pike, E., Wisloff, T., Staff, A., Smeland, S., and Klemp M. 2012. Cancer risk with folic acid supplements: A systematic review and meta-analysis. *BMJ Open* 2(1):e000653. doi:10.1136/bmjopen-2011-000653.

Yeh, E. B. 2017. The role of vitamin fortification on flavor of fluid milk. MSc thesis, North Carolina State University, Raleigh, NC, https://repository.lib.ncsu.edu/bitstream/handle/1840.20/33470/etd.pdf?sequence=1&isAllowed=y.

Young, V. and Garza, C. 1998. *Dietary Reference Intakes for Thiamin, Riboflavin, Niacin, Vitamin B6, Folate, Vitamin B12, Pantothenic Acid, Biotin, and Choline.* Washington, DC: National Academy Press.

Zang, H., Zhang, K. I., Ding, X. I., Bai, S. I., Hernández, J. M., and Yao, B. 2011. Effects of different dietary vitamin combinations on the egg quality and vitamin deposition in the whole egg of laying hens. *Revista Brasileira de Ciência Avícola* 13:189–196.

Zhang, W., Wang, X. P., Wang, C. Y., and Li, F. C. 2012. Effects of dietary vitamin E supplementation on meat quality, vitamin E contents and oxidative stability of rabbit meat. *Proceedings of the 10th World Rabbit Congress*, Sharm El-Sheikh, Egypt, pp. 871–874.

Zhao, L. L., De, P. Y., Pu, C., Wei, X. D., and Wang, D. M. 2008. Supplementation with selenium and vitamin E improves milk fat depression and fatty acid composition in dairy cows fed fat diet. *Asian-Australian Journal of Animal Science* 21:838–844.

Zsédely, E., Tòth, T., Eiben, Cs., Viràg, Gy., Fàbiàn, J., and Schmidt, J. 2008. Effect of dietaryvegetable oil (sunflower, linseed) and vitamin E supplementation on the fatty acidcomposition, oxidative stability and quality of rabbit meat. *Proceedings of the 9th World Rabbit Congress*, June 10–13, Verona, Italy, pp. 1473–1477.

chapter three

Advances in food fortification with essential minerals

Izabela Michalak

Contents

3.1 Introduction

Fortification of food with essential minerals aims to prevent micro- and macroelemental deficiencies in humans. It is estimated that two thirds of the world population is missing one or more essential minerals (White and Broadley, 2009). Fortification can complement traditional dietary diversification and mineral supplementation. According to FAO/WHO, food fortification is "the addition of one or more essential nutrients to a food, whether or not it is normally contained in the food, for the purpose of preventing or correcting a demonstrated deficiency of one or more nutrients in the population or specific population groups." The most popular food products that undergo fortification (enrichment) are cereals and cereal-based products (e.g., rice, whole cereal grains, breakfast cereals, cornmeal, bread, pasta, flours), milk and milk products (e.g., liquid milk, powdered milk, other dairy products), fats and oils (e.g., margarine, oil), accessory food items (e.g., salt, monosodium glutamate, sugar, sauces), tea and other beverages (fruit juices and drinks), and infant formulas (Clarke, 1996). Nowadays, practically every type of beverage, such as mineral water, energy drink, soy milk, nectar, or juice has a fortified product line (Gerstner, 2003). Food products are mainly fortified with minerals (iron, iodine, zinc, calcium, magnesium, selenium and fluoride), vitamins (vitamin A, vitamin C, vitamin D, vitamin B_9—folate, vitamin B_{12}, and other B vitamins, includiing thiamine, riboflavin, niacin, and vitamin B_6), pigments (β-carotene) (WHO/FAO, 2006), polyunsaturated fatty acids (PUFA) including omega-3 and omega-6 fatty acids, dietary fibers, and probiotics (Jakubowska and Staniewska, 2015).

This chapter highlights the importance of minerals, which are a tool to prevent micronutrient deficiencies, also referred to as "hidden hunger" because these deficiencies are often not clinically visible. People might suffer from them without being aware of a shortage of minerals (Mulualem, 2015). These deficiencies are mainly observed in the developing countries (Smith, 2015). Children (e.g., Serra-Majem, 2011; Gibson et al., 2011; Das et al., 2013; de Barros and Cardoso, 2016) and young women (e.g., Sivakumar et al., 2001; Thuy et al., 2003; Das et al., 2013) are highly vulnerable to mineral deficiencies. Food fortification is an effective, easy, fast, safe, and relatively inexpensive process (Nilson and Piza, 1998; Thuy et al., 2003).

Decisions about which nutrients should be added to food and in what amounts must be guided by the nutritional needs of the population, its consumption profile of the potential fortified food and other existing nutrition programs and their assumptions (Kuong et al., 2016). A crucial issue is the selection of the appropriate fortificant (e.g., mineral salt) for a specific application. The solubility of mineral salt, the content of a given mineral, effect on the taste of the fortified product, bioavailability to humans, animals, and plants, as well as economic considerations should be taken into account (Gerstner, 2003).

Another strategy to prevent micronutrient deficiencies is biofortification which, using the best traditional breeding practices and modern biotechnology (including genetic modification [Nestel et al., 2006]), aims to produce crops with a higher content of micronutrients (Cakmak, 2008; White and Broadley, 2009; Smith, 2015). Biofortified crops can further be used in food production. Such nutrients, sufficiently bioavailable to humans, must be retained during food processing and cooking (Bouis et al., 2011). Biofortificaton is used to enrich crops with minerals that are most commonly lacking in the human diet, for example, iron, zinc, copper, calcium, magnesium, iodine, and selenium (White and Broadley, 2009). The general scheme of different fortification strategies that address mineral malnutrition is presented in Figure 3.1.

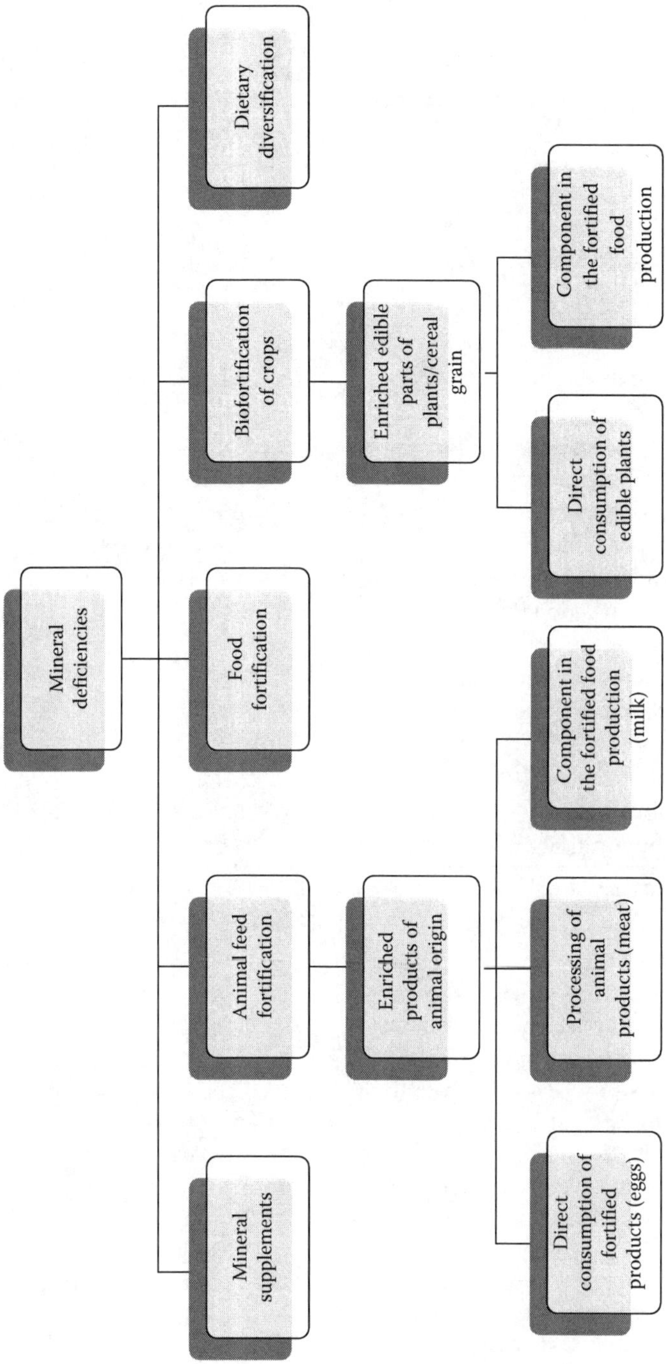

Figure 3.1 Strategies to combat mineral deficiencies in the human diet.

Table 3.1 The number of scientific papers on food fortification/biofortification*

Words in the topic of a scientific paper	Number of papers in years 1945–2017	Number of papers in years 2000–2017
Fortification	9037	7386
Food fortification	3479	3091
Mineral fortification	547	493
Fortification of milk	1152	958
Fortification of milk and minerals	122	106
Fortification of flour	844	740
Fortification of flour and minerals	70	68
Fortification of cereals	588	498
Fortification of cereals and minerals	84	77
Fortification of rice	362	330
Fortification of rice and minerals	44	43
Food fortification and iron	1033	928
Food fortification and zinc	400	382
Food fortification and calcium	343	316
Food fortification and iodine	184	175
Food fortification and magnesium	56	53
Food fortification and selenium	55	52
Food fortification and fluorine	1	-
Biofortification	1255	1255
Biofortification of crops	651	651
Mineral biofortification	262	262
Agronomic biofortification	142	142

* According to the Web of Knowledge; January 2, 2017.

In Table 3.1, the number of scientific papers concerning fortification/biofortification is summarized (according to Web of Knowledge database). Generally, the papers on fortification were written mainly in the last 17 years and on biofortification only in the last 17 years. In the case of vehicles used for fortification, the most often fortified (according to the table) are milk, flour, cereals, and rice. Fourteen percent of the papers on cereal fortification concern enrichment with minerals, 12% in the case of rice, 11% in the case of milk, and 8% for flour. The main minerals that are used for food fortification are iron, zinc, calcium iodine, magnesium, and selenium.

In this chapter, I will deal with the fortification/biofortification of food with such minerals whose deficiencies are a major public health concern in many countries. Special attention will also be paid to the technological advances and the stability of the fortified food.

3.2 *Food fortification technologies*

For most foods, the technology of fortification is quite simple. Water-soluble nutrients can be dissolved in water and then added to liquid foods such as dairy products, fruit juices, and beverages. While fortifying liquid drinks, special attention should be paid to the solubility of the minerals, sedimentation behaviors, and stability of the final formulation. Minerals with low solubility tend to sediment during storage (Gerhart and Schottenheimer, 2013).

Another method of fortification is mixing of the powdered nutrients with foods such as flour (e.g., wheat, maize), corn starch, instant powdered beverages, and dry milk (Nilson and Piza, 1998). The application of micronized mineral salts (for example micronized tricalcium citrate in the fortification of dairy products with calcium [Münchbach and Gerstner, 2010]) is also a good option. For salts significantly smaller than 20 μm, fortification levels can be much higher than in the case of dissolved minerals. In addition, the speed of sedimentation is reduced when the particle size is decreased (Gerhart and Schottenheimer, 2013).

The general overview of fortification technologies (in single-element and multiple systems) is presented in Table 3.2. Kuong et al. (2016) proposed a method for fortified rice production, which involves mixing

Table 3.2 Examples of the technology of food fortification (a) single-element fortification and (b) multiple fortification

Element	Food	Technology of fortification	Reference
	(a) Single-element fortification		
Iron as sodium ferric ethylenediamine-tetracetate (NaFeEDTA)	Fish sauce	Mixing of fish sauce with iron using a water-soluble, highly bioavailable compound NaFeEDTA for 2 hours	Thuy et al. (2003)
Iodine as potassium iodide (KI) and/or potassium iodate (KIO_3)	Salt	*The wet method*: A solution of KIO_3 is dripped or sprayed at a regular rate onto salt passing by on a conveyor belt *The dry method*: KI or KIO_3 powder is sprinkled over dry salt	Zimmerman (2007)

(*Continued*)

***Table* 3.2** (Continued) Examples of the technology of food fortification (a) single-element fortification and (b) multiple fortification

Element	Food	Technology of fortification	Reference
Calcium as soluble salts: calcium chloride·$2H_2O$ tricalcium citrate·$4H_2O$ calcium lactate·$5H_2O$ calcium lactate gluconate *Calcium* as insoluble salts: tricalcium phosphate calcium carbonate	UHT Milk	Standardization of milk – addition of insoluble mineral salt as powder – homogenization (250/50 bar at 55°C) – heat treatment and cooling – addition of soluble mineral salt via ultrafiltrated/ sterile solution – aseptic filling	Gerhart and Schottenheimer (2013)
Magnesium as trimagnesium citrate anhydrous or trimagnesium citrate·$9H_2O$	Yogurt	Fermentation of milk to yogurt – homogenization (75/15 bar) – addition of mineral salts via fruit preparation or compound – heat treatment and cooling – aseptic filling	Gerhart and Schottenheimer (2013)
	(b) Multiple fortification		
Iron as ferrous sulfate heptahydrate ($FeSO_4 \cdot 7H_2O$) *Iodine* as potassium iodide (KI) or potassium iodate (KIO_3)	Iodine and iron-fortified salt	Dry-mixing process in a ribbon blender (produced salt retains the original color of the unfortified salt, the distribution of iodine and iron is uniform)	Ranganathan et al. (1996)
Iron as ferrous fumarate ($C_4H_2FeO_4$) *Selenium* as sodium selenite (Na_2SeO_3) *Zinc* as zinc oxide (ZnO)	Cereal-based infant foods—porridge	Porridge based on maize, beans, bambaranuts and groundnuts	Gibson et al. (2011)

(*Continued*)

Table 3.2 (Continued) Examples of the technology of food fortification (a) single-element fortification and (b) multiple fortification

Element	Food	Technology of fortification	Reference
Calcium as calcium chloride *Magnesium* as magnesium chloride·$6H_2O$	Potato starch	Immersion in 0.5% $CaCl_2$ for the calcium-fortified starch Immersion in 1% $MgCl_2 \cdot 6H_2O$ for the magnesium-fortified starch for 3 hours. The obtained fortified starch was washed twice with distilled water and dried at 20 °C	Noda et al. (2014)
Iron as ferric pyrophosphate *Zinc* as zinc oxide	Rice (the mixing ratio of rice premix to normal rice kernels was 1%)	Techniques for rice premix production: Coating of rice kernels with a mixture of premix (vitamins and minerals) and waxes sprayed on normal rice kernels Cold extrusion of a mixture of rice flour, premix (vitamins and minerals) and a binding agent, such as alginate, <70 °C Hot extrusion of a mixture of rice flour and premix (vitamins and minerals); >70 °C, use of steam	Kuong et al. (2016)

normal with artificially fortified rice kernels (rice premix) at a ratio of 100:1. The rice premix is obtained by the addition of a vitamin-mineral premix either to rice flour or as a coat over normal rice kernels. Some authors indicate that rice grains are not very good vehicles for mineral fortification because it is difficult to fortify them (Thuy et al., 2003). Other food products (e.g., milk, yogurt salt) can be fortified mainly with iron, iodine, calcium, and magnesium.

3.3 Food fortification with minerals

In this section, examples of food fortification with calcium, magnesium, zinc, iron, selenium, iodine, and fluorine are presented.

3.3.1 Food fortification with calcium and magnesium

The function, absorption and excretion, sources, status of the population, and bioavailability of calcium and magnesium are well known and described in the literature (e.g., Abrams and Atkinson, 2003; Gerstner, 2006; Noda et al., 2014). In the case of food fortification with calcium and magnesium, interelemental interaction should be taken into account because they act antagonistically toward each other (Abrams and Atkinson, 2003; Gerstner, 2006).

Regulation of the European Commission No. 1825/2006 approves fortificants containing calcium and magnesium. The former include soluble salts (calcium chloride·$2H_2O$, tricalcium citrate·$4H_2O$, calcium lactate·$5H_2O$, calcium lactate gluconate as calcium lactate and calcium gluconate) and insoluble salts (tricalcium phosphate and calcium carbonate) as well as seaweed calcium, consisting mainly of calcium carbonate (Münchbach and Gerstner, 2010). The latter include soluble salts (magnesium carbonate basic·$5H_2O$, trimagnesium citrate anhydrous, trimagnesium citrate·$9H_2O$, magnesium lactate·$2H_2O$, magnesium sulfate·$7H_2O$), and the insoluble salt trimagnesium phosphate·$5H_2O$. Several scientific studies indicate that organic mineral salts such as citrates, lactates, or gluconates have higher bioavailability than inorganic mineral sources such as oxides, carbonates, and phosphate (Gerhart and Schottenheimer, 2013). That is why trimagnesium citrates (anhydrous and nonahydrate) due to their high solubility as well as bioavailablity have been widely used in food supplements, sports nutrition, baby food, and other dietary products (Gerstner, 2006).

3.3.1.1 Calcium

Calcium is an essential mineral for a variety of physiological and biochemical functions. Since it reduces the risk of cardiovascular diseases and osteoporosis (Heaney et al., 2000; Aguilar et al., 2012), it is added to such dairy products as yogurts, yogurt drinks, fat free milk, milk drinks, and evaporated milk (Münchbach and Gerstner, 2010). Clear beverages (e.g., still mineral water, apple juices), cloudy beverages (e.g., nectars, soy milk, orange, grapefruit, cranberry juices), as well as instant beverages (e.g., instant tea drink, beverage powder) are also commonly fortified with calcium (Gerstner, 2003). Some interesting examples are presented below. Konar et al. (2015) proposed fortification of milk chocolates with calcium in the form of calcium carbonate. Chocolate was chosen as a food vehicle since it is consumed all over the world by all segments of society and by people of all ages. The added calcium, beside calcium enrichment, improved the visual quality and shelf life of the product. Soy milk is another calcium-fortified product that is growing in popularity, particularly among vegetarians (Heaney et al., 2000). The concentration of calcium in such milk can range from 80 to 500 mg/serving, whereas the native soy milk contains only <10 mg Ca/serving. Unfortunately, calcium from soy milk is absorbed at only 75% efficiency as compared to that of cow milk.

3.3.1.2 Magnesium

A diet is usually supplemented with magnesium together with calcium with the advocated weight ratio of 4:1 or lower of calcium to magnesium (Abrams and Atkinson, 2003). Noda et al. (2014) proposed the promising technology of the production of calcium and magnesium fortified potato starches. Starch is widely used in the food production systems. Therefore, fortified starch can enhance the nutritional value of food products based on it. Starch contributes also to the textural properties of foods. Fortified starch (by immersion in aqueous solutions of $CaCl_2$ and $MgCl_2{\cdot}6H_2O$) contained more than six times more calcium (a maximum of 686 mg/kg) and over four times more magnesium (a maximum of 421 mg/kg) than control potato starch.

3.3.2 Food fortification with iron and zinc

Food fortification with iron aims mainly at combating anemia, one of the most widespread public health problems that affects communities in many, especially developing, countries (Rohner et al., 2016). The primary cause of anemia is iron deficiency. The deficiencies of zinc are also very often associated with poor growth and development and impaired immune response). Multiple fortification with iron and zinc requires that interelemental interactions are taken into consideration (Whittaker, 1998; Zlotkin et al., 2003). Whittaker (1998) showed that high iron concentrations can negatively affect zinc absorption in adults when these trace minerals are given in solutions to fasted/famished/starved individuals. When iron and zinc are given in a meal, this effect is not observed.

3.3.2.1 Iron

Dary (2002) presented examples of different iron compounds that can be used as fortificants in food (e.g., ferrous sulfate, ferrous fumarate, ferrous bisglycinate, NaFeEDTA). It was found that the absorption of ferrous bisglycinate and NaFeEDTA is usually two and three times better than that of ferrous fumarate or ferrous sulfate used for flour fortification (Layrisse et al., 2000; Dary, 2002). Examples of fortified food products involve bread prepared from either precooked corn flour or white wheat flour, meal based on corn tortillas and black bean paste, whole-maize porridge, milk formulas, water, and so on. (Dary, 2002). In the case of iron-fortified food, special attention should be paid to the presence of iron inhibitors (e.g., phytate and polyphenols) that can reduce its absorption (Layrisse et al., 2000).

The iron-fortified food is mainly examined in populations where anemia is diagnosed. For more detailed information see, for example, Whittaker (1998), Dary (2002), Gera et al. (2012). For example, Rohner et al. (2016) estimated the iron status of preschool children and women of reproductive age in households consuming fortified wheat flour for at least 4 months. Significantly higher hemoglobin concentrations were found in urban children and women having access to adequately fortified flour products (content of iron ≥ 48 mg/kg). In India, Sivakumar et al. (2001) proposed the fortification of salt with iron (as ferric orthophosphate) as a strategy for the control of anemia caused by iron deficiency (similarly to the fortification of salt with iodine). Salt fulfils the required criteria for a fortificant vehicle. First of all, it is eaten by a large proportion of the target population and the intake is fairly regular through the year (Zimmerman, 2007). Moreover, Sivakumar et al. (2001) developed a formulation for double fortification of salt with iodine and iron. The efficacy of iron fortified salt (1 mg of iron per gram of salt) was tested among 5–15-year-old school children in rural (Hyderabad, New Delhi, Calcutta, India) and in urban areas in Madras (India) and its surroundings over one year. The introduction of iron-fortified salt significantly improved hemoglobin status and, what follows, reduced the occurrences of anemia in both rural and urban communities. Thuy et al. (2003) proposed consumption of fish sauce that contained 10 mg Fe, supplied as sodium ferric ethylenediamine-tetracetate (NaFeEDTA), as an additive to snacks, based on noodles or rice, by women in Vietnam. After 6 months of a 28-day feeding experiment it was observed that the concentrations of hemoglobin and serum ferritin were higher and serum transferrin receptor concentrations were lower in the iron-fortified group than in the control group.

3.3.2.2 Zinc

Zinc deficiency is responsible for many severe health complications, including impairments of physical growth, immune system, and learning ability, combined with increased risk of infections, DNA damage, and cancer development (Cakmak, 2008). Therefore, zinc fortification of food is recommended as an appropriate strategy to enhance population zinc status (Brown et al., 2010). Hess and Brown (2009), Brown et al. (2010), and Das et al. (2013) review zinc fortification trials. The main types of fortified foods, intended for the consumption by zinc-deficient women, newborns, infants, and children, include infant milk formula, bread, porridge, and cereals (wheat flour, maize flour, or rice). Consumption of zinc-fortified food was associated with significant improvement in plasma zinc concentration, which is a functional indicator of zinc status. The same Regulation of the European Commission referred to above approves some soluble zinc salts (zinc citrate·$3H_2O$ [31% of Zn], zinc sulfate·$7H_2O$ [23%], zinc gluconate·xH_2O [13%] and insoluble zinc oxide [80%]) for food fortification. The most commonly used are zinc oxide and zinc sulfate (Whittaker, 1998; Hess and Brown, 2009; Das et al., 2013). Hotz et al. (2005) compared zinc absorption from maize tortilla fortified with zinc sulfate, zinc oxide, zinc oxide+EDTA or sodium–zinc EDTA (3.3 mg of zinc) in women 19–44 years old (Mexico). It was found that inorganic forms of zinc were well absorbed when added as fortificants to a maize-based diet. EDTA did not increase zinc absorption in this diet type. It was also found that high-phytate meals depress zinc absorption from zinc-fortified foods (Hess and Brown, 2009).

Zinc deficiency is also a major contributor to diarrhea in the developing countries (Galetti et al., 2015). Galetti et al. (2015) proposed using filtered water fortified with a low dose of highly bioavailable zinc. The authors conducted a trial in which Beninese school children (N=277) from rural settings received a daily portion of zinc-fortified filtered water delivering 2.8 mg of Zn, non-fortified filtered water, or non-fortified nonfiltered water for 20 weeks. Plasma zinc concentration in the group with fortified water was significantly higher than in the other examined groups. Water is a very good vehicle for fortification, since it is free of absorption inhibitors. The efficacy of water as a carrier of iodine (Elnagar et al., 1997) and iron (de Almeida et al., 2014) was previously shown. Iodine has limited stability in water (< 24 hours) so the regular daily dosing is required (Zimmerman, 2007).

3.3.2.3 *Iron and zinc fortified food*

Zlotkin et al. (2003) examined the effect of sprinkles home-fortified with iron (as ferrous fumarate; $C_4H_2FeO_4$) and zinc (as zinc gluconate; $C_{12}H_{22}O_{14}Zn$) and with iron alone on the concentration of these elements in plasma in anemic infants (6–18 months old) in the Brong Ahafo Region of Ghana for two months. Sachets containing microencapsulated iron (80 mg of elemental iron) and zinc (10 mg of zinc) and ascorbic acid (50 mg) and sachets containing only Fe (80 mg) were added to the child's meal after it was cooked. It was found that the fortified sprinkles were very successful in treating anemia, however the rate of recovery from anemia was higher in the Fe group compared with the Fe-Zn group. On the other hand, sprinkles fortified only with Fe were insufficient to improve zinc status. Herman et al. (2002) proposed to additionally enrich the previously iron-fortified wheat flour, which in Indonesia contains 60 mg Fe/kg, with zinc (as sulfate and oxide). It was found that iron and zinc from prepared dumplings were well absorbed; however, zinc sulfate decreased iron absorption in Indonesian children. The highest iron absorption was in the Fe group (15.9%±6.8%), then in the Fe+ZnO group (14.0%±8.9%), and finally in the Fe+$ZnSO_4$ group (11.5%±4.9%). Therefore, special attention should be paid to the food made from iron fortified flour with zinc, especially with zinc sulfate.

3.3.3 *Food fortification with selenium*

Selenium, an important antioxidant that protects cells from free radicals, can by the same token protect a human body from cancer or cardiovascular diseases (Ježek et al., 2012; Giacosa et al., 2014). Food, especially plant food, is a basic source of selenium in human nutrition (Ježek et al., 2012, Liang et al., 2014). Fortification of crops (edible parts of plants—biofortification, described in the first chapter of this book) with selenium can increase the selenium content in diet (Carvalho et al., 2003; Ježek et al., 2012). Sodium selenite (Na_2SeO_3) was shown to be a suitable form of selenium for foliar application in plant cultivation (e.g., potatoes, tomatoes, lettuce, radish, strawberry, sunflower, oat) (Ježek et al., 2012). Gibson et al. (2011) examined the effect of cereal-based infant food fortified with iron (as ferrous fumarate), selenium (as sodium selenite), and zinc (as zinc oxide) on hemoglobin and biochemical iron, zinc, and selenium status of urban Zambian infants for 12 months. This research focused on selenium because, like zinc, it is an important immune factor and it has been neglected in fortified infant feeding trials so far. It was found that fortified food reduced anemia and improved iron and selenium status but had no effect on serum zinc.

Liang et al. (2014) proposed to drink enriched green tea, which will supplement selenium in organically bound, natural food form (about 80% of the selenium in green tea exists in organic form). Green tea is a popular drink that contains a variety of bioactive compounds, such as polyphenols, polysaccharides, and minerals. The natural selenium level in local soils in which tea is grown influences selenium content in enriched green tea, which can be enlarged by agronomic biofortification. Two methods are applied: either selenium-containing fertilizers are added to the soil or selenate or selenite are sprayed onto tea leaf surface. Foliar fertilization with sodium selenate (Na_2SeO_4) was also applied by Giacosa et al. (2014) in order to obtain fortified rice. This method proved to be very efficient: the selenium content in the fortified rice was 1.64±0.28 μg/g of rice, while in the control rice it was 0.36 ± 0.15 μg/g, with the difference being statistically significant. The trial conducted on Italian women showed that a twenty-day intake of Se-enriched-rice increased the serum selenium levels and erythrocyte glutathione peroxidase activity.

The selenium-fortified plants can also be used as components of animal feed that contain organic selenium, and are therefore readily available to animals. Animal products fortified with selenium (meat, milk, eggs) can cover human demand for this element (Ježek et al., 2012).

3.3.4 Food fortification with iodine

In the case of iodine, universal salt iodization for humans (especially pregnant and/or lactating women and infants) and livestock consumption is recommended (Zimmerman, 2007; Charlton and Skeaff, 2011). Iodine is required by the body for the synthesis of the thyroid hormones tetraiodothyronine (T4) and triiodothyronine (T3). The richest natural food sources of iodine are fish and other seafood because they are able to bioaccumulate this essential nutrient (Charlton and Skeaff, 2011).

Salt is the most common food additive used for iodine fortification, which is usually added as potassium iodide (KI) and potassium iodate (KIO_3). Iodine from iodized salt is well absorbed and iodized salt does not affect the sensory properties of food (Zimmerman, 2007). Beside salt, other foodstuffs and drinks can be used for iodine fortification, for example bread (the application of salt enriched with iodine), sugar, fish sauce, vegetable oil, milk, and water (Zimmerman, 2007).

The fortification of salt with iodine and its effects are well documented (e.g., Zimmerman, 2007; Charlton and Skeaff, 2011; Speeckaert et al., 2011; Leung et al., 2012), therefore, this chapter more attention is paid to other examples. Seal et al. (2007) found that the replacement of regular salt with iodized salt in bread resulted in a significant improvement in iodine status in school children aged 8–11 in Tasmania. After it had been found out that the Australian population had an inadequate iodine intake, in October 2009, in all Australian States and Territories, a mandatory iodine fortification of bread was introduced (Clifton et al., 2013). Clifton et al. (2013) found, however, that pregnant women in South Australia were unlikely to reach recommended iodine levels after consumption of iodine fortified bread without an iodine supplement. Spohrer et al. (2015) proposed to use bouillon cubes and powders produced with iodized salt as cooking ingredients in many recipes. In the study it was shown that iodine was retained in broth and absorbed into rice that was cooked in broth containing bouillon cubes with iodine. Ranganathan et al. (1996) examined the effect of doubly fortified salt (with iron as ferrous sulfate heptahydrate [$FeSO_4{\cdot}7H_2O$] and iodine as potassium iodide [KI] or potassium iodate [KIO_3]) on the level of these elements in pregnant and lactating women in India. It was found that doubly fortified salt effectively controlled iodine deficiency, but a clear impact on reducing anemia was not demonstrated.

3.3.5 Food fortification with fluorine

After a successful implementation of salt iodization, some of the efforts were directed at examining the feasibility of fortifying salt with fluorine together with iodine. Several aspects must be taken into account, for example the minimum levels and maximum limits of fluoride ion in salt and the approved fluoride substances (potassium/sodium fluoride). The content of fluoride in salts available on the European market ranges from 90–250 mg/kg (Götzfried, 2006). Fluoride is beneficial to the health of teeth in that it acts against the acids formed by the oral bacteria growing on tooth surface. The use of fluoride (systemic fluoride—salt, water, or milk fluoridation and use of fluoride-containing toothpastes) are recommended by WHO (Marthaler et al., 2011).

3.4 Stability of fortified food

One of the criteria that must be met by fortified food is the stability of the added nutrients under customary conditions of packing, storage, distribution, and use (Nilson and Piza, 1998). Thuy et al., (2003) evaluated the stability of iron in fish sauce by exposing the fortified sauce in clear and amber bottles to different light conditions (artificial and natural sunlight, fluorescent light, or indirect sunlight and darkness) during different periods of time, ranging from two weeks to one year. Kuong et al. (2016) examined the stability of iron and zinc in fortified rice during storage at two different environments (25±5 °C at a humidity of 60% and 40±5°C at a humidity of 75%) for up to one year. The results showed that losses of these elements in fortified rice were negligible. Therefore addition of zinc and iron to rice could be an effective strategy to improve their status of the population with microelemental deficiencies.

In order to ensure the stability of fortified salts, appropriate humidity should be maintained. Zimmerman (2007) underlined that the stability of iodine in salt depends on salt humidity, acidity, and purity. To reduce losses during storage, iodized salt should be as dry as possible and properly packaged. In the case of salt fortified simultaneously with iron and iodine, the addition of a stabilizer such as sodium hexametaphosphate or encapsulation of one of the nutrients is necessary to preserve the acceptable color and stability of iodine in the doubly fortified salt (Sivakumar et al., 2001).

The stability of biofortified food can also be changed during its processing. Cerretani et al. (2014) evaluated the stability of iodine in biofortified potatoes, which are an ingredient of three Italian typical dishes: dumplings, vegetable pie, and focaccia bread. Good stability of iodine was observed during the baking of focaccia bread, whereas during boiling of dumplings and baking of vegetable pie, significant losses of iodine were detected. However, all dishes preserved good final iodine content.

Another factor crucial to the stability of the mineral in fortified food is its form. In the case of milk fortification with calcium, the organic tricalcium citrate (tetrahydrate form) is recommended because it shows a slight solubility (1 g/L) and has a low effect on the product's pH value and thus a minor effect on product stability, even when applied at higher concentrations (Gerhart and Schottenheimer, 2013).

3.5 *Fortification of animal feeds*

Mineral fortification of animal feed can be useful in increasing the content of micro- and macroelements in animal products. For example, WHO (2014) suggests that dairy products, beside their natural pro-health properties, can also be a good source of minerals (e.g., iodine) if cattle are fed with iodine-enriched feed. Next to iodine-fortified products (salts) available on the market, milk, or other dairy products can constitute supplementation of minerals.

The fortification of animal feed involves the addition of minerals in a highly bioavailable form (organic rather than inorganic). Witkowska et al. (2015) proposed adding soy bean meal enriched with microelements (Cu[II], Fe[II], Zn[II] and Mn[II]) rather than inorganic salts to the diet of goats. It was assumed that microelement bioavailability from enriched biomass will be higher than that from an inorganic source. Fortified milk and cheese obtained in that way can be used in the prevention of micronutrient deficiencies.

Algae enriched with microelements (green macroalga *Enteromorpha* sp. enriched with copper and zinc [Michalak et al., 2015a] and microalga *Spirulina maxima* enriched with copper [Saeid et al., 2013]) were proposed as biological feed additives for pigs. The resultant meat came under examination. In the case of macroalga *Enteromorpha* sp., the content of elements in pork was higher (manganese: 49% [statistically significant difference], iron: 13%, copper: 12%, and zinc by only 4.0%) than in the pork from the control group (pigs fed with inorganic salts as a source of microelements) (Michalak et al., 2015a). For enriched *Spirulina maxima,* the copper content in pork was 8.3% higher than in the control group (Saeid et al., 2013).

Different microelement-enriched biomasses—mixture of green macroalgae *Enteromorpha prolifera* and *Cladophora* sp. (Michalak et al., 2011), microalga *Spirulina maxima* (Saeid et al., 2016) and duckweed *Lemna minor* (Witkowska et al., 2012)—used as feed additives for laying hens were examined. Michalak et al. (2011) reported the effect of algal biomass enriched with Cu(II), Zn(II), Co(II), Mn(II), Cr(III) on their content in eggs (separately yolk and white). It was found that the content of chromium, zinc, and copper in egg white from the experimental groups was 723%, 171%, and 56% higher respectively than in the egg white from the control group. Higher amounts of chromium (by 70%), copper (by 37%), and manganese (by 29%) in yolks were observed for the experimental groups as compared with the control group (elements served as inorganic salts). Saeid et al. (2016) investigated the effect of microalga enriched with Cu(II) and Fe(II) on the microelements content in eggs. Eggs fortified with Fe, Zn, and Mn were obtained. The content of Fe, Zn, and Mn in the egg albumen was higher (by 860%, 113%, and 195% respectively) compared to the control group. The use of duckweed enriched with Cu(II), Zn(II), Co(II),

Mn(II), Cr(III) (*Lemna minor*) as a feed additive for laying hens resulted in the increase in the content of cobalt (by 533%), chromium (by 6.6%), and zinc (by 7.4%) in the egg yolks from the experimental groups compared to that of the control group. Egg white was enriched mainly with copper (increase by 32%) and zinc (increase by 68%) (Witkowska et al., 2012). Consumption of fortified animal products (eggs, meat, milk, cheese) is tentatively suggested rather than of synthetic supplements with microelements, which, however, requires detailed experiments in the future.

This approach can also be used for the treatment of horses and ponies with diagnosed equine metabolic syndrome (EMS). Obesity, insulin resistance, and laminitis are the main components of this clinical syndrome (Frank et al., 2010; Morgan et al., 2015). Dietary management of EMS in obese horses or ponies involves a reduction of the amount of energy provided in the diet to induce weight loss. Another problem is to lower the nonstructural carbohydrate (NSC) content in the diet in order to reduce glycemic and insulinemic responses to meals: hay with a low NSC content should be provided. The forage diet of obese horses and ponies should also be supplemented with minerals (e.g., copper, zinc, selenium) and vitamins (vitamin E, A) (Frank et al., 2010). Potential therapies that aim at building up/lowering insulin resistance which will decrease the risk of developing laminitis include supplementation of horse diet with chromium and magnesium. The supplementation with these elements can improve insulin sensitivity in insulin-resistant horses (Chameroy, 2010). In the work of Chameroy et al. (2011) it was shown that the supplementation of the diet of laminitic obese horses with chromium (as yeast) and magnesium (as oxide/proteinate) did not alter morphometric measurements, blood variables, resting insulin concentrations, or insulin sensitivity. The authors suggested additional research aimed at determination of the appropriate use of chromium and magnesium supplements in horses. The application of biomass enriched via biosorption (e.g., algae) can constitute, pending future research, a rich and highly bioavailable source of these elements to horses.

3.6 *Biofortification of crops*

Biofortification, like mineral fortification described above, is also a food-based method. It aims at developing nutrient-rich versions of staple crops that have already been consumed by poor communities. These two strategies are used at different stages. Micronutrient fortification has been used with great success for decades (e.g., fortified salt), while very few biofortified crops have been released (Nestel et al., 2006). Taking into account the bioavailability of the fortified minerals, some authors suggest that biofortification can be a better strategy than the traditional fortification (Cakmak, 2008; Gerhart and Schottenheimer, 2013; Cerretani et al., 2014), complementing standard food fortification and mineral supplementation programs (Bouis et al., 2011).

Two approaches—conventional breeding and genetic engineering techniques—can be used to biofortify crops such as wheat, rice, pear millet, bean, maize, cassava, and sweet potato with (mainly) zinc and iron (Mulualem, 2015; Cakmak, 2008). Genetic biofortification appears to be the most sustainable and cost-effective technique useful in improving the mineral content in cereal crops, although this is a long-term process. A quick solution is agronomic biofortification in which microelemental or NPK fertilizers with microelements are applied. The foliar or combined soil and foliar application of microelemental fertilizers under field conditions has been shown to be a highly effective strategy to maximize the uptake and accumulation of microelements in grain (Cakmak, 2008). Microelements applied to the soil are mainly in the form of inorganic salts or chelates (Cakmak, 2008; Michalak et al., 2015b).

Some of the examples of agronomic biofortification are presented below. Zanirato and Mayerle (2009) obtained iodine-fortified potatoes, carrots, and onions through foliar fertilization (spray) with aqueous solutions of iodine salt (preferably potassium iodide). Michalak et al. (2015b) proposed using biomass enriched with microelements, via a biosorption process, as a component of traditionally used fertilizers. As shown in this review paper, different types of biomass, including waste biomass from agronomic production (e.g., wheat bran, straw, algae, grass, hazelnut shell, peat, rice husk, sewage sludge, soybean meal, maize cob, sugarcane bagasse) are able to bind metal ions (e.g., Zn(II), Mn(II), Cu(II), Co(II), etc.) from aqueous solutions. Tuhy et al. (2014) showed that the bioavailability of zinc from the enriched biomass of peat, bark, seaweeds, seaweed post-extraction residues, and spent mushroom substrate to garden cress (*Lepidium sativum*; germination tests) was higher as compared with traditional fertilizers such as zinc sulfate and Zn-EDTA. Biofortification of plants in this micronutrient was observed. In the next work, post-extraction residue (after supercritical fluid extraction with carbon dioxide of microalga *Spirulina platensis*) was used as a fertilizer component in field trials on maize. Before field experiments, the biomass was fortified with zinc, copper, and manganese. As a result, biofortified maize was produced. The best results were obtained for *Spirulina* supplied in doses of 150% of the recommended requirements for microelements for the commercial product which is NPK(MgS) fertilizer with micronutrients (Zn, Cu, Mn) added as technical salts. The zinc and manganese content in grain was 11% higher and the copper content was 32% higher compared to the control group (Tuhy et al. 2015). Such biofortified plant products can be consumed directly (e.g., garden cress, carrot, onion) or can constitute an ingredient of prepared meals.

3.7 Conclusions

Food fortification is recognized as an effective technique for improving the micronutrient status of a target population. Fortified food can be obtained not only by the addition of minerals to staple food, but also through the fortification of animal feed and the production of enriched with minerals animal based-products, as well as thorough the biofortification of crops. The challenge for the fortified-product manufacturers is to provide products with the highest mineral content, with good taste and appealing properties. Special attention should also be paid to the form of the fortified mineral (organic or inorganic). The consumption of fortified products is an option for the control of mineral deficiencies that are the cause of many diseases, especially in developing countries.

Acknowledgments

This chapter is financed within the framework of the grant titled: "The effect of bioactive algae enriched by biosorption on the certain minerals such as Cr(III), Mg(II) and Mn(II) on the status of glucose in the course of metabolic syndrome horses. Evaluation *in vitro* and *in vivo*" (2015/18/E/NZ9/00607) attributed by The National Science Center in Poland and a grant titled: "Cultivated plants and natural products as a source of biologically active substances assign to the production of cosmetic and pharmaceutical products as well as diet supplements" (BIOSTRATEG2/298205/9/NCBR/2016) attributed by the National Center for Research and Development in Poland.

References

Abrams, S. A. and Atkinson, S. A. 2003. Calcium, magnesium, phosphorus and vitamin D fortification of complementary foods. *Journal of Nutrition* 133:2994S–2999S.

Aguilar, M. C., Mateos, C., Meseguar, I., and Para, M. 2012. Calcium availability in breakfast cereals: Effect of other food components. *European Food Research and Technology* 235:489–495.

Bouis, H. E., Hotz, C., McClafferty, B., Meenakshi, J. V., and Pfeiffer, W. H. 2011. Biofortification: A new tool to reduce micronutrient malnutrition. *Food and Nutrition Bulletin* 32(1):31–40.

Brown, K. H., Hambidge, K. M., and Ranum, P. 2010. Zinc fortification of cereal flours: Current recommendations and research needs. *Food and Nutrition Bulletin* 31(1):62–74.

Cakmak, I. 2008. Enrichment of cereal grains with zinc: Agronomic or genetic biofortification? *Plant Soil* 302:1–17.

Carvalho, K. M., Gallardo-Williams, M. T., Benson, R. F., and Martin, D. F. 2003. Effects of selenium supplementation of four agricultural crops. *Journal of Agricultural and Food Chemistry* 51(3):704–709.

Cerretani, L., Comandini, P., Fumanelli, D., Scazzina, F., and Chiavaro, E. 2014. Evaluation of iodine content and stability in recipes prepared with biofortified potatoes. *International Journal of Food Sciences and Nutrition* 65(7):797–802.

Chameroy, K. A. 2010. Diagnosis and management of horses with Equine Metabolic Syndrome (EMS). PhD dissertation, University of Tennessee, Knoxville, TN. http://trace.tennessee.edu/utk_graddiss/871 (accessed July 13, 2016).

Chameroy, K. A., Frank, N., Elliott, S. B., and Boston, R. C. 2011. Effects of a supplement containing chromium and magnesium on morphometric measurements, resting glucose, insulin concentrations and insulin sensitivity in laminitic obese horses. *Equine Veterinary Journal* 43:494–499.

Charlton, K. and Skeaff, S. 2011. Iodine fortification: Why, when, what, how, and who? *Current Opinion in Clinical Nutrition and Metabolic Care* 14:618–624.

Clarke, R. 1996. Micronutrient fortification of food: Technology and quality control. In: *Food Fortification: Technology and Quality Control. (FAO Food and Nutrition Paper-60)*, Rome, Italy. http://www.fao.org/docrep/W2840E/w2840e0b.htm#TopOfPage (accessed July 6, 2016).

Clifton, V. L., Hodyl, N. A., Fogarty, P. A. et al. 2013. The impact of iodine supplementation and bread fortification on urinary iodine concentrations in a mildly iodine deficient population of pregnant women in South Australia. *Nutrition Journal* 12:32, http://www.nutritionj.com/content/12/1/32 (accessed July 13, 2016).

Dary, O., 2002. Staple food fortification with iron: A multifactorial decision. *Nutrition Reviews* 60(7):S34–S41.

Das, J. K., Kumar, R., Salam, R. A., and Bhutta, Z. A. 2013. Systematic review of zinc fortification trials. *Annals of Nutrition and Metabolism* 62:44–56.

de Almeida, C. A., De Mello, E. D., Ramos, A. P., Joao, C. A., Joao, C. R., and Dutrade-Oliveira, J. E. 2014. Assessment of drinking water fortification with iron plus ascorbic acid or ascorbic acid alone in daycare centers as a strategy to control iron-deficiency anemia and iron deficiency: A randomized blind clinical study. *Journal of Tropical Pediatrics* 60:40–46.

de Barros, S. F. and Cardoso, M. A. 2016. Adherence to and acceptability of home fortification with vitamins and minerals in children aged 6 to 23 months: A systematic review. *BMC Public Health* 16:299. doi:10.1186/s12889-016-2978-0.

Elnagar, B., Eltom, M., Karlsson, F. A., Bourdoux, P. P, and Gebre-Medhin, M. 1997. Control of iodine deficiency using iodination of water in a goitre endemic area. *International Journal of Food Sciences and Nutrition* 48:119–127.

Frank, N., Geor, R. J., Bailey, S. R., Durham, A. E., and Johnson, P. J. 2010. Equine metabolic syndrome. *Journal of Veterinary Internal Medicine* 24:467–675.

Galetti, V., Kujinga, P., Mitchikpe, C. E. S. et al. 2015. Efficacy of highly bioavailable zinc from fortified water: A randomized controlled trial in rural Beninese children. *American Journal of Clinical Nutrition* 102:1238–1248.

Gera, T., Sachdev, H. S., and Boy, E. 2012. Effect of iron-fortified foods on hematologic and biological outcomes: Systematic review of randomized controlled trials. *American Journal of Clinical Nutrition* 96:309–324.

Gerhart, M. and Schottenheimer, M. 2013. Mineral fortification in dairy. *Wellness Foods Europe Minerals* 5:30–36.

Gerstner, G. 2003. How to fortify beverages with calcium. *Food Marketing & Technology*10:16–19.

Gerstner, G. 2006. Trimagnesium citrates: The new healthy choice for functional foods. *European Journal of Nutraceuticals & Functional Foods* 5:1-4 http://www.jungbunzlauer.com/fileadmin/content/_PDF/Trimagnesium_Citrates_-_the_new_healthy_choice_for_functional_foods_Sep06.pdf (accessed July 12, 2016).

Giacosa, A., Faliva, M. A., Perna, S., Minoia, C., Ronchi, A., and Rondanelli, M. 2014. Selenium fortification of an Italian rice cultivar via foliar fertilization with sodium selenate and its effects on human serum selenium levels and on erythrocyte glutathione peroxidase activity. *Nutrients* 6:1251–1261.

Gibson, R. S., Kafwembe, E., Mwanza, S. et al. 2011. Micronutrient-fortified food enhances iron and selenium status of Zambian infants but has limited efficacy on zinc. *Journal of Nutrition* 141(5):935–943.

Götzfried, F. 2006. Legal aspects of fluoride in salt, particularly within the EU. *Schweiz Monatsschr Zahnmed* 4:371–375.

Heaney, R. P., Dowell, M. S., Rafferty, K., and Bierman, J. 2000. Bioavailability of the calcium in fortified soy imitation milk, with some observations on method. *American Journal of Clinical Nutrition* 71:1166–1169.

Herman, S., Griffin, I. J., Suwarti, S. et al. 2002. Cofortification of iron-fortified flour with zinc sulfate, but not zinc oxide, decreases iron absorption in Indonesian children. *American Journal of Clinical Nutrition* 76:813–817.

Hess, S. Y. and Brown, K. H. 2009. Impact of zinc fortification on zinc nutrition. *Food and Nutrition Bulletin* 30(1):S79–S107.

Hotz, C., DeHaene, J., Woodhouse, L. R., Villalpando, S., Rivera, J. A., and King, J. C. 2005. Zinc absorption from zinc oxide, zinc sulfate, zinc oxide + EDTA, or sodium-zinc EDTA does not differ when added as fortificants to maize tortillas. *Journal of Nutrition* 135:1102–1105.

Jakubowska, D. and Staniewska, K. 2015. Information on food fortification with bioactive compounds in observation and consumer studies. *Polish Journal of Natural Sciences* 30(3):307–318.

Ježek, P., Škarpa, P., Lošák, T. Hlšek, J., Jůzl, M., and Elzner, P. 2012. Selenium–an important antioxidant in crops biofortification. In: El-Missiry, M. A. (Ed.). *Antioxidant Enzyme*. InTech Croatia, doi:10.5772/50356. http://www.intechopen.com/books/antioxidant-enzyme/selenium-an-important-antioxidant-in-crops-biofortification (accessed July 14, 2016).

Konar, N., Poyrazoglu, E. S., and Artik, N. 2015. Influence of calcium fortification on physical and rheological properties of sucrose-free prebiotic milk chocolates containing inulin and maltitol. *Journal of Food Science and Technology* 52(4):2033–2042.

Kuong, K., Laillou, A., Chea, C., Chamnan, C., Berger, J., and Wieringa, F. T. 2016. Stability of vitamin A, iron and zinc in fortified rice during storage and its impact on future national standards and programs – case study in Cambodia. *Nutrients* 8(51):1–9.

Layrisse, M., Garcia-Casal, M. N., Solano, L. et al. 2000. Iron bioavailability in humans from breakfast enriched with iron bis-glycine chelate, phytates and polyphenols. *Journal of Nutrition* 130:2195–2199.

Leung, A. M., Braverman, L. E., and Pearce, E. N. 2012. History of U.S. iodine fortification and supplementation. *Nutrients* 4:1740–1746.

Liang, J., Puligundla, P., Ko, S., and Wan, X. C. 2014. A review on selenium-enriched green tea: Fortification methods, biological activities and application prospect. *Sains Malaysiana* 43(11):1685–1692.

Marthaler, T. M., Gillespie, G. M., and Goetzfried, F. 2011. Salt fluoridation in Europe and in Latin America – with potential worldwide. *Kali und Steinsalz Heft* 3:12–25.

Michalak, I., Chojnacka, K., Dobrzański, Z. et al. 2011. Effect of macroalgae enriched with microelements on egg quality parameters and mineral content of eggs, eggshell, blood, feathers and droppings. *Journal of Animal Physiology and Animal Nutrition* 95:374–387.

Michalak, I., Chojnacka, K., and Korniewicz, D. 2015a. New feed supplement from macroalgae as the dietary source of microelements for pigs. *Open Chemistry* 13:1341–1352.

Michalak, I., Witek-Krowiak, A., Chojnacka, K., and Bhatnagar, A. 2015b. Advances in biosorption of microelements – the starting point for the production of new agrochemicals. *Reviews in Inorganic Chemistry* 35(3):115–133.

Morgan, R., Keen, J., and McGowan, C. 2015. Equine metabolic syndrome. *Veterinary Record* 8:173–179.

Mulualem, T. 2015. Application of bio-fortification through plant breeding to improve the value of staple crops. *Biomedicine and Biotechnology* 3(1):11–19.

Münchbach, M. and Gerstner, G. 2010. Calcium fortification in dairy products. *Food Marketing & Technology* 2:4–8.

Nestel, P., Bouis, H. E., Meenakshi, J. V., and Pfeiffer, W. 2006. Biofortification of staple food crops. *Journal of Nutrition* 136(4):1064–1067.

Nilson, A. and Piza, J. 1998. Food fortification: A tool for fighting hidden hunger. *Food and Nutrition Bulletin* 19(1):49–60.

Noda, T., Takigawa, S., Matsuura-Endo, C., Ishiguro, K., Nagasawa, K., and Jinno, M. 2014. Preparation of calcium- and magnesium-fortified potato starches with altered pasting properties. *Molecules* 19:14556–14566.

Ranganathan, S., Reddy, V., and Ramamoorthy, P. 1996. Large scale production of salt fortified with iodine and iron. *Food and Nutrition Bulletin* 17:73–78.

Rohner, F., Raso, G., Aké-Tano, S. O. P., Tschannen, A. B., Mascie-Taylor, C. G. N., and Northrop-Clewes, C. A. 2016. The effects of an oil and wheat flour fortification program on pre-school children and women of reproductive age living in Côte d'Ivoire, a Malaria-Endemic Area. *Nutrients* 8(148):1–11.

Saeid, A., Chojnacka, K., Korczyński, M., Korniewicz, D., and Dobrzański, Z. 2013. Biomass of *Spirulina maxima* enriched by biosorption process as a new feed supplement for swine. *Journal of Applied Phycology* 25:667–675.

Saeid, A., Chojnacka, K., Opaliński, S., Korczyński, M. 2016. Biomass of *Spirulina maxima* enriched by biosorption process as a new feed supplement for laying hens. *Algal Research* 19:342–347. doi:10.1016/j.algal.2016.02.008.

Seal, J. A., Doyle, Z., Burgess, J. R., Taylor, R., and Cameron, A. R. 2007. Iodine status of Tasmanians following voluntary fortification of bread with iodine. *Medical Journal of Australia* 186:69–71.

Serra-Majem, L. 2011. Vitamin and mineral intakes in European children. Is food fortification needed? *Public Health Nutrition* 4(1A):101–107.

Sivakumar, B., Brahmam, G. N. V., Madhavan, N. K. et al. 2001. Prospects of fortification of salt with iron and iodine. *British Journal of Nutrition* 85:S167–S173.

Smith, G. 2015. Micronutrient fortification of food: Issues for Asia. *Journal of Nutritional Science and Vitaminology* 61:183–185.

Speeckaert, M. M., Speeckaert, R., Wierckx, K., Delangheand, J. R., and Kaufman, J. M. 2011. Value and pitfalls in iodine fortification and supplementation in the 21st century. *British Journal of Nutrition* 106:964–973.

Spohrer, R., Knowles, J., Jallier, V. et al. 2015. Estimation of population iodine intake from iodized salt consumed through bouillon seasoning in Senegal. *Annals of the New York Academy of Sciences* 1357:43–52.

Thuy, P. V., Berger, J., Davidsson, L. et al. 2003. Regular consumption of NaFeEDTA-fortified fish sauce improves iron status and reduces the prevalence of anemia in anemic Vietnamese women. *American Journal of Clinical Nutrition* 78:284–290.

Tuhy, Ł., Samoraj, M., Michalak, I., and Chojnacka, K. 2014. The application of biosorption for production of micronutrient fertilizers based on waste biomass. *Applied Biochemistry and Biotechnology* 174:1376–1392.

Tuhy, Ł., Samoraj, M., Witkowska, Z., and Chojnacka, K. 2015. Biofortification of maize with micronutrients by *Spirulina*. *Open Chemistry* 13:1119–1126.

White, P. J. and Broadley, M. R. 2009. Biofortification of crops with seven mineral elements often lacking in human diets – iron, zinc, copper, calcium, magnesium, selenium and iodine. *New Phytologist* 182:49–84.

Whittaker, P. 1998. Iron and zinc fortification in humans. *American Journal of Clinical Nutrition* 68:442S–446S.

WHO. 2014. Guideline: Fortification of food-grade salt with iodine for the prevention and control of iodine deficiency disorders. Geneva: World Health Organization, http://www.ncbi.nlm.nih.gov/books/NBK254243/pdf/Bookshelf_NBK254243.pdf (accessed July 7, 2016).

WHO/FAO. 2006. *Guidelines on Food Fortification with Micronutrients*. Allen, L., de Benoist, B., Dary, O., and Hurrell, R. (Eds.) Geneva, World Heath Organization http://www.who.int/nutrition/publications/guide_food_fortification_micronutrients.pdf (accessed July 6, 2016).

Witkowska, Z., Michalak, I., Korczyński, M. et al. 2015. Biofortification of milk and cheese with microelements by dietary feed bio-preparations. *Journal of Food Science and Technology* 52(10):6484–6492.

Witkowska, Z., Saeid, A., Chojnacka, K. et al. 2012. New biological dietary feed supplement for laying hens with microelements based on duckweed (*Lemna minor*). *American Journal of Agricultural and Biological Sciences* 7:482–493.

Zanirato, V. M. and Mayerle, M. 2009. Method for enriching crops with iodine, and crops thus obtained. International Patent PCT/EP2009/050142.

Zimmerman, M. B. 2007. Key barriers to global iodine deficiency disorder control: A summary. A2Z Technical Brief. http://www.a2zproject.org/pdf/GapAnalysis-Iodine-Final.pdf (accessed July 7, 2016).

Zlotkin, S., Arthur, P., Schauer, C., Antwi, K. Y., Yeung, G., and Piekarz, A. 2003. Home-fortification with iron and zinc sprinkles or iron sprinkles alone successfully treats anemia in infants and young children. *Journal of Nutrition* 133:1075–1080.

chapter four

Advances in food fortification with essential fatty acids

Bogusława Łęska and Grażyna Czyżak-Runowska

Contents

The conception of healthy food has been evolving with time all over the world. Currently, consumers are increasingly making better food choices that provide health benefits. Functional food generally contains one or more functional ingredients that provide a health benefit in addition to the energetic and nutritional aspects that every food must supply (Plaza et al., 2010). Functional food ingredients have biological benefits beyond normal nutrition and have the potential to improve human health. These ingredients are available as dietary supplements or may be incorporated into food products. According to a FAO/WHO definition, fortification is the practice of deliberately increasing the content of an essential micronutrient in a food, so as to improve the nutritional quality of the food supply and provide a public health benefit with minimal risk to health (Allen et al., 2006).

Frequently, food fortification uses the addition of vitamins and minerals, dietary fiber, or unsaturated fatty acids (Table 4.1). Thanks to enriched food products, it is possible to prevent nutrient deficiencies naturally present in minor amounts. Good examples are salt iodization or water fluoridation. Food fortification is also used to balance the nutrient profile, substituting conformed to natural products in terms of nutritional value. In this way, margarine and other dairy products with reduced fat content have been enriched with vitamins A and D or EFA. Besides the direct fortification, that is, during the technological process, it is also possible to

Table 4.1 Types of selected unsaturated fatty acids

Fatty acid (common name)	Chain length (number of carbons)	Type of fatty acid (based on position of first double bond)	Degree of saturation (number of double bonds)
Oleic acid	18	n-9	1
Linoleic acid	18	n–6	2
γ-Linolenic acid	18	n–6	3
α-Linolenic acid	18	n–3	3
Stearidonic acid	18	n–3	4
Arachidonic acid	20	n–6	3
Eicosatetraenoic acid	20	n–3	4
Eicosapentaenoic acid	20	n–3	5
Docosahexaenoic acid	22	n–3	6

indirectly process fortification, such as through the addition of ingredients rich in n-3 fatty acids to animal feed. So, in this way we get fortified meat, milk, or eggs (Woods and Fearon, 2009; Kalogeropoulos et al., 2010; Ganesan et al., 2014).

The chemicals (bioactive compounds) used in the fortification of products must meet several criteria:

- Be bioavailable and cause no danger to life or human health
- Have no effect on the taste, odor, or color of food
- Content scarce ingredient or ingredients in the product must be stable, uniform, and precisely defined
- Enhance the effect was noticeable to the human body

Fortified foods should contain not less than 15% of the recommended daily requirement of the ingredient in 100 g (or 100 mL) of the product, while the maximum amount does not exceed 50% of the recommended daily intake. This level of enrichment is recommended to replenish the nutrients lost during the manufacturing process and the retention period (Baines et al., 2011; Lai et al., 2017). The saturated fatty acids (SFA) contain only single bonds between carbon atoms. Monounsaturated fatty acids have one double bond, whereas polyunsaturated fatty acids (PUFA) contain more than one double bond and depending on the position of the first double bond are divided into two groups: n–3 and n–6. To the most valuable of the n–3 PUFA belong docosahexaenoic (DHA), eicosapentaenoic acids (EPA), and α-linolenic acids (ALA), while n-6 PUFA belong linoleic acid (LA), γ-linolenic acid (GLA), and arachidonic (AA). Until recently it was published that in the absence of appropriate enzymes mammals cannot synthesize *de novo* two of polyunsaturated fatty acids, ALA and LA, hence they have been called essential unsaturated fatty acids (EFA). Nowadays it is known that the term "EFA," used for ALA and LA, are inadequate. In fact, it has been found that ALA and LA can occur in humans from hexadecatrienoic acid C16:3 and C16:2 hexadecadienoic acid. Moreover, most of the effects of EFAs result from their transformation into eicosanoids (Markiewicz-Kęszycka et al., 2013).

Polyunsaturated fatty acids (PUFA) are an important component of membrane phospholipids. They affect the membrane fluidity, transport, and binding of calcium ions and they are precursors of eicosanoids—prostaglandins, prostacyclins, leukotrienes, and thromboxanes (Neijat et al., 2016). Fatty acids (n–3) are delivered to the cells and then in cell membranes can replace n–6 fatty acids or saturated fatty acids. A suitable number of them may decrease the pro-inflammatory factors in the cell, of which the precursors are, *inter alia*, n–6 fatty acids present in increased proportions. By inhibiting the development of inflammation, n–3 fatty acids reduce the excessive blood clotting and reduce fibrinogen levels. In addition, they have effects on regulation of gene expression associated with the process and pro-inflammatory activity of a protein transcription (Gharami et al., 2015; Khan and He, 2017). The results of epidemiological studies show the beneficial effects of n–3 fatty acids, in particular long chain (LC n–3 PUFA), are not only in the prevention of cardiovascular diseases, but also neurological disorders, certain types of cancer, metabolic diseases, type 2 diabetes, as well as allergic diseases (Gogus and Smith, 2010; Bermúdez-Aguirre and Barbosa-Cánovas, 2011; McNamara, 2016).

Because of the specific health benefits posed by the consumption of polyunsaturated fatty acids, the reasonable care of their constant presence in the daily diet is extremely important. The key to selecting individual food products in the diet is to provide an optimum ratio of fatty acids to n–6 and n–3. The analysis of diet in societies of industrial countries, recognizes in them a shortage of long-chain n–3 polyunsaturated fatty acids in ratio to an excess of n–6 fatty acids. It is considered an unfavorable ratio of n–6 / n–3, which is rather estimated at 15–17:1 (Simopoulos, 2008), than the 1–4: 1 ration recommended by nutritionists. This ratio can be improved by increasing the intake of foods rich in n–3 fatty acids. The main representative of this type of fatty acids is α-linolenic acid (ALA), of which the primary source in the diet are plants or vegetable-origin products, mainly vegetable oils (rapeseed oil, linseed oil, soybean oil, walnut oil), and other products such as walnuts, almonds, chia seeds, soya bean, rape seeds, and flax, as well as algae. ALA in the human organism may be subject to some degree of conversion to docosahexaenoic acid (DHA). However, according to results of studies (Burdge and Calder, 2005), the amount of DHA created in this way is not sufficient to maintain the appropriate level in the human body. Therefore, the best way to deliver LC n–3 PUFA, such as EPA and DHA, to the human organism is adequate diet including oily sea fish (salmon, herring, mackerel, sole, cod) and seafood. The daily requirements for these acids have not been clearly defined for each age group and depend on the country and the recommending institutions (Aranceta and Pérez-Rodrigo, 2012). The American Heart Association (AHA) recommends consumption of about 500 mg of EPA and DHA per day as a prophylactic to reduce risk and 1 g per day for treatment of existing cardiovascular disease (Gebauer et al., 2006). This strategy was confirmed in a paper (Harris et al., 2009), according to which at least 0.5 g/d of n–3 PUFAs EPA and DHA are recommended for daily consumption, while preferred intake levels are 2–3-fold higher (Trumbo et al., 2002).

The problem of deficiency of n–3 PUFA in the diet has also been noticed by food manufacturers. Essential fatty acids (EFAs) are key strategic ingredients currently being actively considered in the fortification of food by several food and beverage companies to impart known health benefits and added value in their food products. On the world market, food products can be found in foods enriched with n–3 fatty acids from different categories including dairy products and fats, as well as drinks and cereal products. The most fortified products include full-fat milk, skim milk, yogurt, cheese, margarine, and mixed spreads. Breads, cereals, cereal bars, cookies, salty snacks, and ready meals have been also enriched with n–3 PUFA. In recent years, a plethora of n–3-fortified food products have arrived on the market, ranging from meat, eggs, and dairy products to cereals, cereal bars, and infant formula.

ALA is usually added for the purpose of fortification of food products. Mainly this acid is produced from linseed oil. The other fatty acids (DHA and EPA), which are derived from fish, have also been used in the fortification of food with fatty acids. The frequent use of linseed oil in food fortification is primarily dictated by the more desirable features of a sensory and organoleptic substance compared to fatty acids derived from fish. These features may be particularly problematic in the case of cereal products, or in spreadable fats. However, manufacturers continue to be quite willing to use the fatty acids EPA and DHA fortification of cheese and meat products. Increasing consumer awareness of the health benefits of the essential fatty acids, particularly n–3, is generating a wealth of opportunities for their use in functional foods. The creation of functional foods increasingly uses nanotechnology. Its use in food processing makes it possible to obtain a product enriched with different functional substances (vitamins, antioxidants, fatty acids) which are necessary for the proper functioning of the organism and to better protect food products against harmful environmental factors (Ozimek et al., 2010).

4.1 Application of encapsulation in functional food

Substances introduced into foods are rarely used in pure form. Typically, they are deposited on the media, which is the primary factor limiting the efficacy of functional ingredients in food products. Thus, nanocapsules, micelles, liposomes, emulsions, microspheres, and the biopolymer matrices appear to be good solutions for the provision of various food ingredients (Ozimek et al., 2010). Liposomes have been widely used in food sectors both in research and industry; it has become feasible to use liposomes to deliver functional components such as nutraceuticals, antimicrobials, and flavors to foods because of having a number of benefits, for example the possibility of large-scale production using natural ingredients and entrapment and release of water-soluble, lipid-soluble, and amphiphilic materials as well as target ability (Gallardo et al., 2013; Lin et al., 2015; Cui et al., 2016).

Fish oil has been chosen as a preferred source of long chain n–3 fatty acids due to their proven positive role in infant development and mental illnesses, and their effects against inflammation, platelet aggregation, hypertension, and hyperlipidemia. A good vegetable alternative n–3 source is linseed oil, also known as flaxseed oil, which contains more than 50% of ALA (Gallardo et al., 2013).

Lipids are considered a good product for n–3 fatty acid fortification and nutritional improvement, because of their acceptability among all age groups, longer shelf life, and better taste. But lipid oxidation could lead to the problem of off flavor development in foods and reducing the nutritional and economic value of food products. Synthetic antioxidants such as butylated hydroxy (BHA) and butylated hydroxy toluene (BHT) are widely used as food additives but their safety has been questioned (Mildner-Szkudlarz et al., 2009), which stimulates the search for and evaluation of natural compounds with antioxidant properties. Many naturally occurring compounds from herbs and spices have been extensively studied for their antioxidant activity (Martinez et al., 2013). Among them, rosemary extract (RE) is widely used in food systems (Babuskin et al., 2015). Unfortunately, n–3 PUFA oxidizes easily due to their high melting of unsaturation, the method which comprises the formation of flavor compounds (Kolanowski et al., 2007). Microencapsulation was performed as a key technology delay or inhibitor of oxidation, masking undesirable odors and flavors in the final product. The conversion process oil free flowing powder that can be easily handled and used for nutrients or food fortification. Microencapsulation can be defined as a process in which the fine selected material, namely a core surrounded by a layer of microencapsulation. This coating wall can be made of a wide variety of food-grade materials and protects the entrapped core by providing a physical barrier against environmental conditions. The most popular microencapsulation technique used in the food industry is spray drying, due to the low cost and available equipment (Ozimek et al., 2010). The method comprises spraying the emulsion on the carrier and drying at a high temperature, which causes rapid evaporation of the water. Microencapsulated fish oil has been obtained largely by spray-drying, a product referred to as dried microencapsulated fish oil (DMFO). Many different wall materials have been used, such as skim milk powder or mixtures of Na/Ca caseinate with lactose, mixtures of proteins and carbohydrates, sugar beet pectin, cellulose derivatives (methylcellulose and hydroxypropyl methylcellulose) (Kolanowski et al., 2007), and maltodextrin in combination with branched cyclodextrin and casein (Gallardo et al., 2013). This chapter reviews a short list of various characteristic products present in the diet of the average consumer, together with the methods of enrichment of PUFA.

4.2 Milk and dairy products

Milk and dairy products are consumed all over the world and form an important part of the human diet at any age. Currently the world production of milk is determined by 5 species of animals: cattle, buffalo, goats, sheep, and camels. The global production is dominated by cow's milk, which accounts for 85% of world production, the second is buffalo milk (11%), followed by goat (2.3%), sheep (1.4%) and camel (0.2%) (Gerosa and Skoet, 2012).

Increased interest has recently been seen in continental Europe in more marginal milk animal species, such as mares, whose composition is similar to human milk (Uniacke-Lowe, 2011). The milk from these animals contains far less fat than breast milk, and milk of ruminants is a valuable source of bioactive compounds, including PUFAs (Park et al., 2007; Markiewicz-Kęszycka et al., 2014). Fat is the most variable component of milk, both quantitatively and qualitatively. Its content and the concentration of individual fatty acids is associated with a species of animal, breed, stage of lactation, genetic factors, and nutrition (Tsiplakou et al., 2006; Schwendel et al., 2015; Toral et al., 2015). The greatest amount of fat is observed in the milk of buffalo and sheep, least in the milk of mares (Claeys et al., 2014). Cow's milk contains an average of 3.5% fat, less than the milk of other ruminants, and its contents can vary over a wide range of 2.5%–8.1% (Kennelly, 1996; Butler et al., 2011). Milk fat is its main source of energy and has a high digestibility (97%–99%) and high nutritional value (Barłowska and Litwińczuk, 2009). This type of fat is present in natural form as an emulsion, that is fat-dispersed beads. A high degree of dispersion of the emulsion means it can be absorbed without prior hydrolysis in the gastrointestinal tract. The size of fatty acid beads in cow's milk ranges from 0.1 to 20 μm with an average diameter of about 4.0 μm. In the milk over 400 different fatty acids can be distinguished, of which the majority

(> 98%) are bound in the form of triacylglycerols. The variation in mammary fatty acid secretion and lipogenic responses to changes in diet composition between ruminants reflect inherent interspecies differences in ruminal lipid metabolism and mammary-specific regulation of cellular processes and key lipogenic enzymes involved in the synthesis of milk-fat triacylglycerides (Shingfield et al., 2010).

Among the PUFAs present in cow's milk, the content of ALA is about 10 mg/g of fat, while EPA and DHA are present in small amounts, approximately 0.9 and 1 mg/g of fat, respectively (Ganesan et al., 2014). Particularly noteworthy is conjugated linoleic acid (CLA). Its presence in the milk of ruminants is associated with the processes of isomerization and biohydrogenation of unsaturated fatty acids by rumen bacteria as well as the Δ^9—desaturase activity in the mammary gland (Liu et al., 2016). The main substrates for the synthesis of isomers of CLA in the rumen are linoleic acid and α- linolenic acid. In cow's milk their concentration ranges between 0.56%–0.74% of the total fatty acid content, depending on how the maintenance and the time of year (Butler et al., 2011). More than 20 isomers of CLA have been found in milk. The most important ones exhibit the highest biological activity, C18: 2 c9 t11 (rumenic acid) and C18: 2 t10 c12, which dominate the c9 t11 (75%–90% of linoleic acid conjugated diene) (Lock and Bauman, 2004).

The studies by Pestana et al. (2009) showed that the highest amount of CLA is in high fat dairy products made from cows' milk, particularly in ripened cheeses and to a lesser extent in butter. Isomers of CLA, seen in numerous clinical trials, have immunity-enhancing and anticarcinogenic properties, prevent obesity, atherosclerosis, lower hypertension, and support the treatment of diabetes and osteoporosis (Khanal, 2004). The *cis*-PUFAs are also present in milk in small amounts (<1 mg/g of fat), isomers of fatty acids with 20 or 22 carbon atoms in the molecule. However, so far no evidence has been found that any of them are characterized by pro-health properties (Ganesan et al., 2014).

It is noteworthy that small amounts of *trans*-PUFAs (approximately 15 mg/g of fat) are also present in milk, which are the result of incomplete biohydrogenation of unsaturated fatty acids in the rumen. The impact of these isomers on human health is ambiguous, although recent studies have shown that natural transisomers present in the milk of ruminants is distinguished by comprehensive health-oriented action (Kowalska and Cichosz, 2013). Given the small total content of n–3 PUFA in cow's milk (0.33 mg/100 mL) (Ganesan et al., 2014), it requires enrichment in essential fatty acids.

For many years, studies have been conducted on how to improve the fatty acid profile of the milk of ruminants, using different feeding systems and techniques of managing herds (Lock and Bauman, 2004; Kuczyńska et al., 2013). Among feeding systems the one known as the best in terms of fatty acid profile is feeding and grazing that involves feeding rich in herbage (Butler et al., 2011). With such a system, conducted feed a cow is to increase the CLA content of the milk up to 500%, compared to milk from cows fed in system TMR (total mixed ration) (Dhiman et al., 1999). Fat from the milk of cows fed herbage is characterized by a preferred fatty acid ratio of n–6/n–3 (approximately 2:1) compared to conserved fed, approximately. 4:1 (Haug et al., 2007). Milk sourced from organic farms compared to conventional farms is characterized by a higher content of CLA (Bloksma et al., 2008), Schwendel et al., 2015).

The most common strategy to enhance n–3 PUFA in meat and milk is dietary supplementation with linseeds, linseed oil, marine oil, or marine algae (Dhiman et al., 1999; Chilliard et al., 2002; Andrade and Schmidely, 2006; Tsiplakou and Zervas, 2013; Razzaghi et al., 2016; Cabiddu et al., 2017). The content of n–3 acids in selected oils and marine products is shown in Tables 4.2 and 4.3. It is noteworthy that algae is rich in EPA and to a lesser extent DHA, while vegetable oils are a rich source of LA and ALA, especially linseed oil (approx. 60% ALA).

Their use in the supplementation of different diets has positive effects and increases the level of CLA in milk. Vegetable oil may be added to the feed alone or combined with fish oil, which can significantly increase the proportion of n–3 LC PUFA in the raw material and products. Also the form of grain processing plant oil added to the feed (grain ground, roasted, or flaked) affects the levels of n–3 fatty acids in the milk of animals fed on them (Dhiman et al., 1999; Neveu et al., 2014).

The new sources of fats used in animal nutrition are lupine, naked oats, camelina, hemp, and chia seed (Woods and Fearon, 2009; Gaffney et al., 2014). Suitable feeding of cows makes the milk and dairy products prepared from milk, such as cheese and fermented beverages, discover a number of new bioactive compounds of fatty acids (Bonanno et al., 2013; Pikul et al., 2014; Bodkowski et al., 2016). In order to protect polyunsaturated fatty acids contained in the feed prior to biohydrogenation in the rumen, a protein envelope is used, fixed with formaldehyde or calcium salts of fatty acids (Chilliard et al., 2000; Kupczyński et al., 2012). Fish oil in protected form added to feed contributes more to increased content of EPA and DHA in milk than the addition of unprotected oil (Castañeda-Gutiérrez et al., 2007). However, many studies have shown that the transfer of n–3 fatty acids from food into milk fat is low, even with the increased supply of polyunsaturated fatty acids in protected form (Palmquist and Griinari, 2006; Castañeda-Gutiérrez et al., 2007).

The addition of n–3 PUFAs during the technological process fortifies a wide range of dairy products such as milk, yogurt, buttermilk, cheese, margarine, mixed spreads, ice cream, and foods for infants and young children during the process (Cox et al., 2011; Dal Bello et al., 2015; Gahruie et al., 2015). Fortification of dairy products with fatty acids is recovered as in the case of animal feed, mainly vegetable oils (usually linseed oil) and marine raw

Table 4.2 Plant sources and terrestrial animal sources of dietary lipids containing PUFAs

Source	Linoleic	ALA	EPA	DHA
Plant sources				
Castor oil	4	-	-	-
Coconut oil	1.4		-	-
Corn oil	52	1	-	-
Cottonseed oil	50.5	-	-	-
Linseed oil	14.2	59.8	-	-
Olive oil	18.9	0.8	-	-
Palm oil	11	0.4	-	-
Peanut oil	41.1	0.3	-	-
Rapeseed oil (high erucic)	14	10	-	-
Rapeseed oil (low erucic)	26	10	-	-
Safflower oil (high oleic)	15.8	-	-	-
Safflower oil (high linoleic)	75.3	-	-	-
Sesame oil	45	0.6	-	-
Soybean oil	53	7.5	-	-
Sunflower oil	68.5	0.1	-	-
Terrestrial animal sources				
Human milk fat	7	1	0.1	0.2
Cow milk fat	2	1	-	-
Lard	11.4	1	-	-
Beef	3.7	0.18	-	-
Sheep	1.6	0.2	-	-
Lamb	8.1	1.6	-	-
Chicken breast	18.7	1.1	-	-
Chicken leg	23.5	1	-	-
Turkey	21.3	1.2	-	-
Pork	9.7	0.7	-	-
Chicken eggs	11.1	0.3	-	-

Source: Ganesan, B. et al., *Critical Reviews in Food Science and Nutrition*, 54, 98–114, 2014 *American Journal of Clinical Nutrition* –

materials (fish, algae). Caution should be used in their dosages, especially of fish oil, because of possible deterioration of flavor and reducing the shelf life of the product as a result of oxidation of fats (Dal Bello et al., 2015). In order to mask the flavor of fish oil in the final product, a highly specialized

Table 4.3 Marine animal and algal sources containing PUFAs

Source	Linoleic	ALA	EPA	DHA
Marine animal sources				
Cod liver oil	22.6	-	7	7
Sardine oil	1	-	17	13
Cod	1	-	11	3.5
Sardine	1.3	0.9	16.9	12.9
Herring	2.9	1.1	8.8	10.8
Anchovy	1	-	18	11
Sand Eel	<2	1.1	10.6	8.2
Krill	3.3	1.1	17.4	12.4
Mussels	-	-	10.2	13.4
Oyster	2	3.3	11.2	9.7
Shrimp	1.6	0.8	14.9	12.8
Scallop	0.1	1.2	26	24.1
King crab	3.2	3.3	21.5	10.2
Clam	-	-	10	15
Squid	0.7	0.1	14.6	20.4
Mullet	1.9	0.8	16.5	5.8
Hake	2.2	0.5	6.8	31
Sepia	1.2	0.3	20	20.9
Perch	5.5	0.2	5.6	8.1
Tropical halibut	-	-	2.5	32.3
Shark liver oil	4.1	-	4.3	30
Seal oil	10.3	-	4.7	5.1
Algal sources[2]				
Chlorella officinale	-	2.5	32	-
Chlorella minutissima	-	-	44	-
Phaeodactylum tricornutum	-	-	26	11
Gonyaulox caterella	-	1.3	11.2	34
Crypthecodinium cohnii	-	-	-	P
Schizochytrium	-	-	P	P
Phaeophyceae	-	-	P	-
Phytophthora cinnamomi				

Source: Ganesan, B. et al., *Critical Reviews in Food Science and Nutrition*, 54, 98–114, 2014.

p – can produce PUFAs but not quantified

technology is used to provide a protective barrier, for example by an encapsulation system (Martini et al., 2009; Ghorbanzade et al., 2017).

4.3 Meat and meat products

Meat and meat products are popular in the human diet due to their high nutritional value (Li et al., 2005; Williams, 2007). Until recently they were regarded as the main source of dietary fat, especially saturated fat. Recently carried out, intensive research on the modification of the fatty acid profile in muscle, or fat, contributed to a significant reduction in body fat, particularly in pigs, and improvement in the nutritional quality indicators (Givens and Gibbs, 2006; Janiszewski et al., 2016). The content of lipids in meat depends mainly on the species, sex, age, weight, feeding system, felling technology, the location of muscle tissue in the carcass, and the rest (depending on species, origin, feeding system, and the cut) (Enser et al., 1996; Raes et al., 2004; Łyczyński et al., 2006; Aranceta and Pérez-Rodrigo, 2012; Horcada et al., 2016).

Meat is a naturally poor source of n–3 PUFA, and therefore its fortification is necessary, mainly through appropriate feeding. Diet modification significantly improves the fatty acid profile, particularly in monogastric animals (pigs, poultry) (Cortinas et al., 2004; Mitchaothai et al., 2007; Konieczka et al., 2016) and to a lesser extent in ruminants (such as cattle, sheep, and goats) (Andrés et al., 2014; Abuelfatah et al., 2016; Boughalmi and Arab, 2016; Bravo-Lamas et al., 2016), due to differences in the digestive processes (digestive process). As feed additives in animal nutrition, vegetable oils, fish oils, or fish meal were used and from new sources as well: chia seed, marine algae, camelina, and lupine. Studies (Bourre, 2005) demonstrated that feeding animals with extracts of linseed and rapeseed grains increased the ALA 10-fold in chicken meat, 6-fold in pork, and less than 2-fold in beef. By comparison, feeding animals with fish extracts or algae has raised the level of DHA 7-fold in chicken and less than 2-fold in beef. Rymer and Givens (2006) demonstrated that the inclusion of ALA in poultry feed does not increase EPA and DHA, suggesting either that birds cannot convert ALA to the long-chain fatty acids or that synthesized PUFAs are not deposited in edible tissues.

Although it is difficult to change the ration of meat enriched in PUFA (due to hydrogenation in the rumen) for ruminants, many authors have noted favorable changes in the fatty acid profile. Díaz et al. (2017) generated in the meat light lambs adding microalgae supplementation feed very suitable indicators nutritional quality (PUFA/SFA, n–6/n–3). The research of French et al. (2000) showed almost 3-fold increase of CLA in muscle longissimus dorsi in beef steers and in animals fed with fresh grass compared to animals fed with the addition of the concentrate. The way the transfer of fatty acids from feed to animal tissues takes place has been detailed in a number of review papers (Wood et al., 2008; Woods and Fearon, 2009; Corino et al., 2014).

The analysis of meat carried out by Williams (2007) in animal species indicates a low fat content in meat, and a good ratio of n–6/n–3, which preferably presented in the meat of ruminants (2.0–2.6). However, in pork and poultry without the skin, this ratio is slightly higher than recommended by nutritionists at 7.5 and 8, respectively. The predominant fatty acid in the muscle tissue of pigs, cattle, sheep, and poultry is linoleic acid C18: 2 n–6 (the greatest quantity of its content is observed in poultry meat) and the acid present to a lesser extent is α-linolenic acid C18: 3 n–3 (ALA) (Table 4.2, Ganesan et al., 2014). Particularly noteworthy is the meat of ruminants (beef, lamb, mutton, goat meat). Its uniqueness is related to the CLA content and, in particular isomers (c9 t11 and t9 c12) (Wood et al., 2004; Daley et al., 2010), to which a variety of health benefits are attributed. It should also be emphasized that the thermal processing of meat (cooking, baking, grilling) at temperatures > 60° C leads to the loss of free PUFA (Gerber et al., 2009).

The choice of feed additives (vegetable oils, fish oils) is very important. Pay attention to the level of their dosage, so that diet modification does not worsen the sensory characteristics of raw material (taste and odor), technological suitability of the meat, and its durability. Adequate protection against oxidation processes is necessary; current trends tend to look for natural antioxidants derived mainly from plant sources (Corino et al., 2014; Babuskin et al., 2015).

Encapsulation technology is an effective way, originally developed to improve the oxidation stability and bioavailability of n–3 fatty acids that were added to the meat products. Kitessa et al. (2001) showed a 3-fold increase in the content of EPA in lamb meat after addition into feed of fat in protected form.

4.4 Fish and seafood

The marine world represents a relatively untapped source of functional ingredients that can be applied to numerous aspects of food processing, storage, and fortification. Due to the wide range of environments they survive in, marine organisms have developed unique properties and bioactive compounds that, in some cases, are unparalleled by their terrestrial counterparts. The numerous marine-based compounds have been identified as having diverse biological activities, with some reported to interfere with the pathogenesis of diseases. Fish and seafood are a rich source of PUFA, especially of n–3 fatty acids: eicosapentaenoic acid (EPA) and docosahexaenoic acid (DHA). This applies above all oily sea fish, inhabiting the cold waters, such as herring, anchovies, walleye pollock, capelin, sand eel, krill, and sardine (Huynh and Kitts, 2009; Turchini et al., 2009). The fat (oil) obtained from the fish comprises from 0.2% to 15% of the total fatty acid content. In contrast, much smaller quantities of these acids are present in shellfish (crustaceans), such as shrimp, scallop, crabs, and clams and ranges from 0.1% to 2.5% of the total fatty acid content (Ganesan et al., 2014).

The content of n–3 PUFA in fish depends on many factors, including the species, fish physiological condition, the season, place of fish, feed, and varieties (Grigorakis, 2007; Guler et al., 2008; Lee et al., 2016). The content of PUFA in marine products is shown in Table 4.3 (Ganesan et al., 2014). The chart shows that the fish from the Mediterranean Sea (squid, mullet, hake, and sepia) contain comparably higher amounts of EPA and DHA (15%–30%) than Australian and tropical fish (perch and tropical halibut), 20%–30% fatty acids as EPA and DHA. The fish harvested from the cold northern seas are characterized by higher content of EPA, while the fish caught in the south seas by higher content of DHA (Kolanowski et al., 2007).

Fish living in the wild are also characterized by a higher content of n–3 and n–6, as compared to reduced amounts in fish artificially breeding (Usydus et al., 2011). In contrast, long-chain fatty acid content, defined as the sum of EPA and DHA, is more abundant in farmed fish, than in fish living in the wild (Table 4.4, Gebauer et al., 2006). Fish beyond the preferred ratio of n–6/n–3 are of high nutritional value and a good source of protein (18%–25%), including low-cholesterol (15–25 mg/100 g) (Ganesan et al., 2014). The recommended dose (1 g) of EPA and DHA was contained in about 25 g of Baltic salmon, about 100 grams of Baltic herring, about 55 g of trout farmed in Poland, and in more than 4000 g of sutchi catfish (Usydus et al., 2011).

Table 4.4 Total PUFA, LA, ALA, EPA, and DHA contents of 85 g (3 oz) cooked wild and farm-raised fish of various species

Fish species	Total PUFA	LA	ALA	EPA	DHA	EPA +DHA
Catfish, channel						
Wild	0.541	0.121	*0.082*	*0.085*	*0.116*	*0.201*
Farm	*1.183*	*0.875*	0.07	0.042	0.109	0.151
Trout, rainbow						
Wild	1.556	0.245	*0.159*	*0.398*	0.442	0.84
Farm	*1.981*	*0.807*	0.07	0.284	*0.697*	*0.981*
Salmon, coho						
Wild	1.082	0.048	0.047	0.341	0.559	0.9
Farm	*1.669*	*0.317*	*0.065*	*0.347*	*0.740*	*1.087*
Salmon, Atlantic						
Wild	2.768	0.187	*0.321*	0.349	1.215	1.564
Farm	*3.762*	*0.566*	0.096	*0.587*	*1.238*	*1.825*

Source: Gebauer et al., *American Journal of Clinical Nutrition* 83:1526–1535, 2006.

Higher amounts for each species are italicized.

Oils extracted from fish and later applied as additives to feed for livestock in suitable proportions significantly raise the nutritional value in animal raw materials such as milk, eggs, meat, or fat, adding to their bioactive and health-promoting components (fatty acids and lipid-soluble vitamins). However, research conducted recently on the safety of fish consumption, increasingly points to risks associated with the presence of toxic compounds of mercury and pesticides (Diez, 2009; Anishchenko et al., 2017). Taking into account the so-called "fishy" sea products, there is a limit to their application to many food products (Gallardo et al., 2013).

Marine algae are an alternative to fish oil as a dietary source of n–3 long-chain PUFA, eicosapentaenoic acid (EPA), and docosahexaenoic acid (DHA). The n–3 to n–6 ratio of macroalgae closely matches preferred ratios, which may add to their efficacy as a dietary supplement or as part of a balanced diet (Lunn and Theobald, 2006). Moreover, they contain many essential fatty acids. Red and brown algae, for instance, are particularly rich in the n–3 fatty acids, EPA and α-linolenic acid, and the n–6 fatty acids, AA and linoleic acid, as well as relatively high levels of oleic and palmitic acids (Dawczynski et al., 2007). In contrast, green seaweeds, such as *Ulva pertusa*, are characterized by the presence of hexadecatetraenoic (n–3), oleic and palmitic acids (Lordan et al., 2011). The n–3 fatty acid, octadecatetraenoic acid, is abundant in *Laminaria* sp. and *Undaria pinnatifida* while hexadecatetraenoic acid is prominent in *Ulva* sp. (Sánchez-Machado et al., 2004). In addition to fatty acids, the unsaponifiable fraction of macroalgae contains carotenoids (such as β-carotene, lutein, and violaxanthin in red and green seaweeds, fucoxanthin in brown seaweeds), tocopherols, sterols (such as fucosterol in brown seaweeds), and terpenoids (Lordan et al., 2011).

It is interesting to note that microalgae are the original source of DHA in the marine food chain, dried marine algae having also been included in animal feeds to improve the DHA level of foods of animal origin. The effect of supplementing a basal dairy, cow diet of marine algae (Schizochytrium sp.) has been extensively described by Woods (Woods and Fearon, 2009). They also reported lower content of EPA and DHA in the phospholipid fraction of lamb meat when linseed or PLS (protected linseed) were supplied compared with diets containing fish oil or marine algae. The combination of marine algae with either fish oil or PLS in lambs' diet increased DHA transfer by almost 2.5 times over lambs offered fish oil alone. Other algae containing fatty acids and used in animal feed are described in Table 4.3. Identification and acquisition of nutrients for potential functional properties of marine products is possible with advances in biotechnology.

Fish oils have many dietary benefits, but due to their strong odors and rapid deterioration, their application in food formulations is limited. For these reasons, nano-liposome was used to nano-encapsulate fish oil in this study and encapsulated fish oil was utilized in fortifying yogurt. This study demonstrated that nano-liposome encapsulation resulted in a significant reduction in acidity, syneresis, and proxide value while increasing DHA and EPA stability (Ghorbanzade et al., 2017). Another good example would be adding nanocapsules containing n–3 fatty acids to bread, enriching the daily diet with this essential component. The use of capsules filled with tuna oil provides adequate daily supply of a fatty acid, and bread fortified by encapsulation has no fishy off-taste or smell (Wang et al., 2015).

4.5 Conclusion

The improper eating habits of people are undoubtedly one of the reasons for the increased risk of diet-related diseases. In recent years, research on the exact composition of nutritional supplements are intended to establish a link between the occurrence of various diseases and nutrition. These studies are increasingly common. The significant impact on the nutritional value of food products is the type contained in their fatty acids. Epidemiological studies indicate that in the context of improving health and reducing the risk of various diseases of civilization, it is advantageous to increase the intake of polyunsaturated fatty acids (PUFA) relative to saturated fatty acids (SFA).

This review suggests that the benefits of n–3 PUFA's to human health are widely known. The consumption of n–3 PUFA via incorporation into foods is ultimately the most effective mechanism of providing them to the average consumer. Increasing the n–3 PUFA content of animal feedstuffs can be a promising and sustainable way to improve the nutritional value of meat without forcing consumers to change their eating habits. Consuming of fortified food products, enriched with the unsaturated fatty acids n–3 PUFAs, especially the long-chain fatty acids EPA and DHA, instead of changes in eating habits while maintaining physical activity, can have a significant impact on the improvement of human health.

References

Abuelfatah, K., Zuki, A. B. Z., Goh, Y. M., and Sazili, A. Q. 2016. Effects of enriching goat meat with n–3 polyunsaturated fatty acids on meat quality and stability. *Small Ruminant Research* 136:36–42.

Allen, L., de Benoist, B., Dary, O., and Hurrell, R. 2006. *Guidelines on Food Fortification with Micronutrients*. Geneva, Switzerland: FAO/WHO.

Andrés, S., Morán, L., Aldai, N. et al. 2014. Effects of linseed and quercetin added to the diet of fattening lambs on the fatty acid profile and lipid antioxidant status of meat samples. *Meat Science* 97:156–163.

Anishchenko, O. V., Sushchik, N. N., Makhutova, O. N. et al. 2017. Benefit-risk ratio of canned pacific saury (Cololabis saira) intake: Essential fatty acids vs. heavy metals. *Food and Chemical Toxicology* 101:8–14.

Aranceta, J. and Pérez-Rodrigo, C. 2012. Recommended dietary reference intakes, Nutritional goals and dietary guidelines for fat and fatty acids: A systematic review. *British Journal of Nutrition* 107(S2):8–22.

Babuskin, S., Radhakrishnan, K., Babu, P. A. S. et al. 2015. Effects of Rosemary extracts on oxidative stability of chikkis fortified with microalgae biomass. *Journal of Food Science and Technology* 52:3784–3793.
Baines, J., Cunningham, J., Leemhuis, Ch., Hambridge, T., and Mackerras, D. 2011. Risk assessment to underpin food regulatory decisions: An example of public health nutritional epidemiology. *Nutrients* 3:164–185.
Barłowska, J., and Z. Litwińczuk. 2009. Nutritional and Pro-health properties of milk fat. *Mleka. Review. Medycyna Weterynaryjna (Polish)* 65:171–174.
Bermúdez-Aguirre, D. and Barbosa-Cánovas, G. V. 2011. Quality of selected cheeses fortified with vegetable and animal sources of omega-3. *LWT - Food Science and Technology* 44:1577–1584.
Bloksma, J., Adriaansen-Tennekes, R., Huber, M. et al. 2008. Comparison of organic and conventional raw milk quality in the Netherlands. *Biological Agriculture and Horticulture* 26:69–83.
Bodkowski, R., Czyż, K., Kupczyński, R., Patkowska-Sokoła, B., Nowakowski, P., and Wiliczkiewicz, A. 2016. Lipid complex effect on fatty acid profile and chemical composition of cow milk and cheese. *Journal of Dairy Science* 99:57–67.
Bonanno, A., Tornambè, G., Bellina, V. et al. 2013. Effect of farming system and cheesemaking technology on the physicochemical characteristics, fatty acid profile, and sensory properties of Caciocavallo Palermitano cheese. *Journal of Dairy Science* 96:710–724.
Boughalmi, A. and Araba, A. 2016. Effect of feeding management from grass to concentrate feed on growth, carcass characteristics, meat quality and fatty acid profile of Timahdite lamb breed. *Small Ruminant Research* 144:158–163.
Bourre, J. M. 2005. Effect of increasing the omega-3 fatty acid in the diets of animals on the animal products consumed by humans. *Medicine Sciences (Paris)* 21:773–779.
Bravo-Lamas, L., Barron, L. J. R., Kramer, J. K. G., Etaio, I., and Aldai, N. 2016. Characterization of the fatty acid composition of lamb commercially available in northern Spain: Emphasis on the trans-18:1 and CLA content and profile. *Meat Science* 117:108–116.
Burdge, G. C. and Calder, P. C. 2005. Conversion of α-linolenic acid to longer-chain polyunsaturated fatty acids in human adults - Review. *Reproduction Nutrition Development* 45:581–597.
Butler, G., Stergiadis, S., Seal, C., Eyre, M., and Leifert, C. 2011. Fat composition of organic and conventional retail milk in northeast England. *Journal of Dairy Science* 94:24–36.
Cabiddu, A., Addis, M., Fiori, M., Spada, S., Decandia, M., and Molle, G. 2017. Pros and cons of the supplementation with oilseed enriched concentrates on milk fatty acid profile of dairy sheep grazing Mediterranean pastures. *Small Ruminant Research* 147:63–72.
Castañeda-Gutiérrez, E., de Veth, M. J., Lock, A. L., Dwyer, D. A., Murphy, K. D., and Bauman, D. E. 2007. Effect of supplementation with calcium salts of fish oil on N–3 satty acids in milk fat. *Journal of Dairy Science* 90:4149–4156.
Chilliard, Y., Ferlay, A., Loor, J., Rouel, J., and Martin, B. 2002. Trans and conjugated fatty acids in milk from cows and goats consuming pasture or receiving vegetable oils or seeds. *Italian Journal of Animal Science* 1:243–254.
Chilliard, Y., Ferlay,A., Mansbridge, R., and Doreau, M. 2000. Ruminant milk fat plasticity: Nutritional control of saturated, polyunsaturated, trans and conjugated fatty acids. *Annales de Zootechnie* 49:181–205.

Claeys, W. L., Verraes, C., Cardoen, S. et al. 2014. Consumption of raw or heated milk from different species: An evaluation of the nutritional and potential health benefits. *Food Control* 42:188–201.

Cortinas, L., Villaverde, C., Galobart, J., Baucells, M. D., Codony, R., and Barroeta, A. C. 2004. Fatty acid content in chicken thigh and breast as affected by dietary polyunsaturation level. *Poultry Science* 83:1155–1164.

Corino, C., Rossi, R., Cannata, S., and Ratti, S. 2014. Effect of dietary linseed on the nutritional value and quality of pork and pork products: Systematic review and meta-analysis. *Meat Science* 98:679–688.

Cox, D. N., Evans, G., and Lease, H. J. 2011. The influence of product attributes, consumer attitudes and characteristics on the acceptance of: (1) Novel bread and milk, and dietary supplements and (2) Fish and novel meats as dietary vehicles of long chain omega 3 fatty acids. *Food Quality and Preference* 22:205–212.

Cui, H., Li, W., Li, Ch., Vittayapadung, S., and Lin, L. 2016. Liposome containing cinnamon oil with antibacterial activity against methicillin-resistant Staphylococcus aureus biofilm. *Biofouling* 32:215–225.

Dal Bello, B., Torri, L., Piochi, M., and Zeppa, G. 2015. Healthy yogurt fortified with N–3 fatty acids from vegetable sources. *Journal of Dairy Science* 98:8375–8385.

Daley, C. A., Abbott, A., Doyle, P. S., Nader, G. A., and Larson, S. 2010. A review of fatty acid profiles and antioxidant content in grass-fed and grain-fed beef. *Nutrition Journal* 9:10.

Dawczynski, Ch., Schubert, R., and Jahreis,G. 2007. Amino acids, fatty acids, and dietary fibre in edible seaweed products. *Food Chemistry* 103:891–899.

Dhiman, T. R., Helmink, E. D., McMahon, D. J., Fife, R. L., and Pariza, M. W. 1999. Conjugated linoleic acid content of milk from cows fed different diets. *Journal of Dairy Science* 82:412–419.

Díaz, M. T., Pérez, C., Sánchez, C. I. et al. 2017. Feeding microalgae increases omega 3 fatty acids of fat deposits and muscles in light lambs. *Journal of Food Composition and Analysis* 56:115–123.

Diez, S. 2009. Human health effects of methylmercury exposure. *Reviews of Environmental Contamination and Toxicology* 198:111–132.

Enser, M., Hallett, K., Hewitt, B., Fursey, G. A. J., and Wood, J. D. 1996. Fatty acid content and composition of english beef, lamb and pork at retail. *Meat Science* 42:443–456.

French, P., Stanton, C., Lawless, F. et al. 2000. Fatty acid composition, including conjugated linoleic acid, of intramuscular fat from steers offered grazed grass, grass silage, or concentrate-based diets. *Journal of Animal Science* 78:2849–2855.

Gaffney, M., O'Rourke, R., and Murphy, R. 2014. Manipulation of fatty acid and antioxidant profiles of the microalgae Schizochytrium sp. through flaxseed oil supplementation. *Algal Research* 6:195–200.

Gahruie, H. H., Eskandari, M. H., Mesbahi, G., and Hanifpour, M. A. 2015. Scientific and technical aspects of yogurt fortification: A review. *Food Science and Human Wellness* 4:1–8.

Gallardo, G., Guida, L., Martinez, V. et al. 2013. Microencapsulation of linseed oil by spray drying for functional food application. *Food Research International* 52:473–482.

Ganesan, B., Brothersen, C., and McMahon, D. J. 2014. Fortification of foods with omega-3 polyunsaturated fatty acids. *Critical Reviews in Food Science and Nutrition* 54:98–114.

Gebauer, S. K., Psota, T. L., Harris, W. S., and Kris-Etherton, P. M. 2006. n–3 fatty acid dietary recommendations and food sources to achieve essentiality and cardiovascular benefits. *American Journal of Clinical Nutrition* 83:1526–1535.

Gerber, N., M. R. L Scheeder, and Wenk, C. 2009. The influence of cooking and fat trimming on the actual nutrient intake from meat. *Meat Science* 81:148–154.

Gerosa, S., and Skoet, J. 2012. Milk availability: Trends in production and demand and medium-term outlook. *ESA Working Paper* 12:1–40.

Gharami, K., Das, M., and Das, S. 2015. Essential role of docosahexaenoic acid towards development of a smarter brain. *Neurochemistry International* 89:51–62.

Ghorbanzade, T., Jafari, S. M., Akhavan, S., and Hadavi, R. 2017. Nano-encapsulation of fish oil in nano-liposomes and its application in fortification of yogurt. *Food Chemistry* 216:146–152.

Givens, D. I. and Gibbs, R. A. 2006. Very long chain n–3 polyunsaturated fatty acids in the food chain in the UK and the potential of animal-derived foods to increase intake. *Nutrition Bulletin* 31(2):104–110.

Gogus, U., and Smith, Ch. 2010. n–3 omega fatty acids: A review of current knowledge. *International Journal of Food Science and Technology* 45:417–436.

Grigorakis, K. 2007. Compositional and organoleptic quality of farmed and wild gilthead sea bream (Sparus aurata) and sea bass (Dicentrarchus labrax) and factors affecting it: A review. *Aquaculture* 272:55–75.

Guler, G. O., Kiztanir, B., Aktumsek, A., Citil, O. B., and Ozparlak, H. 2008. Determination of the seasonal changes on total fatty acid composition and n–3/n–6 ratios of carp (Cyprinus Carpio L.) muscle lipids in beysehir lake (Turkey). *Food Chemistry* 108:689–694.

Haug, A., Høstmark, A. T., and Harstad, O. M. 2007. Bovine milk in human nutrition-a review. *Lipids in Health and Disease* 6:25.

Harris, W. S., Mozaffarian, D., Lefevre, M. et al. 2009. Towards establishing dietary reference intakes for eicosapentaenoic and docosahexaenoic acids. *Journal of Nutrition* 139:804–819.

Horcada, A., Polvillo, O., Juárez, M., Avilés, C., Martínez, A. L., and Peña, F. 2016. Influence of feeding system (concentrate and total mixed ration) on fatty acid profiles of beef from three lean cattle breeds. *Journal of Food Composition and Analysis* 49:110–116.

Huynh, M. D. and Kitts, D. D. 2009. Evaluating nutritional quality of pacific fish species from fatty acid signatures. *Food Chemistry* 114:912–918.

Janiszewski, P., Grześkowiak, E., Lisiak, D. et al. 2016. The influence of thermal processing on the fatty acid profile of pork and lamb meat fed diet with increased levels of unsaturated fatty acids. *Meat Science* 111:161–167.

Kalogeropoulos, N., Chiou, A., Gavala, E., Christea, M., and Andrikopoulos, N. K. 2010. Nutritional evaluation and bioactive microconstituents (carotenoids, tocopherols, sterols and squalene) of raw and roasted chicken fed on DHA-rich microalgae. *Food Research International* 43:2006–2013.

Kennelly, J. J. 1996. Producing milk with 2.5% fat–the biology and health implications for dairy cows. *Animal Feed Science and Technology* 60:161–180.

Khan, M. Z., and He, L. 2017. The role of polyunsaturated fatty acids and GPR40 receptor in brain. *Neuropharmacology* 113:639–651.

Khanal, R. C. 2004. Potential health benefits of conjugated linoleic acid (CLA): A review. *Asian Australasian Journal of Animal Science* 17:1315–1328.

Kitessa, S. M., Gulati, S. K., Ashes, J. R., Scott, T. W., and Fleck, E. 2001. Effect of feeding tuna oil supplement protected against hydrogenation in the rumen on growth and n–3 fatty acid content of lamb fat and muscle. *Australian Journal of Agricultural Research* 52:433–437.

Kolanowski, W., Jaworska, D., Laufenberg, G., and Weißbrodtm, J. 2007. Evaluation of sensory quality of instant foods fortified with omega-3 PUFA by addition of fish oil powder. *European Food Research and Technology* 225:715–721.

Konieczka, P., Czauderna, M., and Smulikowska, S. 2016. The enrichment of chicken meat with omega-3 fatty acids by dietary fish oil or its mixture with rapeseed or flaxseed—Effect of feeding duration. *Animal Feed Science and Technology* 223:42–52.

Kowalska, M. and Cichosz, G. 2013. Dairy products–The best source of CLA. *Bromatologia i Chemia Toksykologiczna (Polish)* 46:1–12.

Kuczyńska, B., Nałęcz-Tarwacka, T., and Puppel, K. 2013. Bioactive components as an indicator of the health beneficial quality of the milk. *Medycyna Rodzinna (Polish)* 1:11–18.

Kupczyński, R., Kuczaj, M., Szołtysik, M., and Stefaniak, T. 2012. Influence of fish oil, palm oil and glycerol on milk fatty acid composition and metabolism in cows during early lactation. *Archiv Tierzucht* 55:540–551.

Lai, W. T., Khong, N. M. H., Lim, S. S. et al. 2017. A review: Modified agricultural by-products for the development and fortification of food products and nutraceuticals. *Trends in Food Science & Technology* 59:148–160.

Lee, S., Hung, S. S. O., Fangue, N. A. et al. 2016. Effects of feed restriction on the upper temperature tolerance and heat shock response in juvenile green and white sturgeon. *Comparative Biochemistry and Physiology Part A: Molecular & Integrative Physiology* 198:87–95.

Li, D., Siriamornpun, S., Wahlqvist, M. L., Mann, N. J., and Sinclair, A. J. 2005. Lean meat and heart health. *Asia Pacific Journal of Clinical Nutrition* 14:113–119.

Lin, L., Cui, H., Zhou, H. et al. 2015. Nanoliposomes containing Eucalyptus citriodora as antibiotic with specific antimicrobial activity. *Chemical Communications* 51(13):2653–2655.

Liu, S., Zhang, R., Kang, R., Meng, J., and Ao, Ch. 2016. Milk fatty acids profiles and milk production from dairy cows fed different forage quality diets. *Animal Nutrition* 2:329–333.

Lock, A. L. and Bauman, D. E. 2004. Modifying milk fat composition of dairy cows to enhance fatty acids beneficial to human health. *Lipids* 39:1197–1206.

Lordan, S., Ross, R. P., and Stanton, C. 2011. Marine bioactives as functional food ingredients: Potential to reduce the incidence of chronic diseases. *Marine Drugs* 9:1056–1100.

Lunn, J., and Theobald, H. 2006. The health effects of dietary unsaturated fatty acids. *Nutrition Bulletin* 31:178–224.

Łyczyński, A., Pospiech, E., Rzosińska, E. et al. 2006. Quality of porcine meat in relation to pig genotype and intramuscular fat content. *Animal Science Papers and Reports* 24:195–204.

Markiewicz-Kęszycka, M., Czyżak-Runowska, G., Lipińska, P., and Wójtowski, J. 2013. Fatty acid profile of milk—A review. *Bulletin of the Veterinary Institute in Pulawy* 57:135–139.

Markiewicz-Kęszycka, M., Wójtowski, J., Czyżak-Runowska, G. et al. 2014. Concentration of selected fatty acids, fat-soluble vitamins and β-carotene in late lactation mares' milk. *International Dairy Journal* 38:31–36.

Martinez, M. L., Penci, M. C., Ixtaina, V., Ribotta, P. D., and Maestri, D. 2013. Effect of natural and synthetic antioxidants on the oxidative stability of walnut oil under different storage conditions. *LWT - Food Science and Technology* 51:44–50.

Martini, S., Thurgood, J. E., Brothersen, C., Ward, R., and McMahon, D. J. 2009. Fortification of reduced-fat Cheddar cheese with N–3 fatty acids: Effect on off-flavor generation. *Journal of Dairy Science* 92:1876–1884.

McNamara, R. K. 2016. Role of omega-3 fatty acids in the etiology treatment, and prevention of depression: Current status and future directions. *Journal of Nutrition & Intermediary Metabolism* 5:96–106.

Mildner-Szkudlarz, S., Zawirska-Wojtasiak, R., Obuchowski, W., and Gośliński, M. 2009. Evaluation of antioxidant activity of green tea extract and its effect on the biscuits lipid fraction oxidative stability. *Journal of Food Science* 74:362–370.

Mitchaothai, J., Yuangklang, C., Wittayakun, S. et al. 2007. Effect of dietary fat type on meat quality and fatty acid composition of various tissues in growing-finishing swine. *Meat Science* 76:95–101.

Neijat, M., Ojekudo, O., and House, J. D. 2016. Effect of flaxseed oil and microalgae DHA on the production performance, fatty acids and total lipids of egg yolk and plasma in laying hens. *Prostaglandins Leukotrienes and Essential Fatty Acids* 115 :77–88.

Neveu, C., Baurhoo, B., and Mustafa, A. 2014. Effect of feeding extruded flaxseed with different grains on the performance of dairy cows and milk fatty acid profile. *Journal of Dairy Science* 97:1543–1551.

Ozimek, L., Pospiech, E., Narine, S. 2010. Nanotechnologies in food and meat processing. *Acta Scientarum Polonorum Technologia Alimentaria* 9:401–412.

Palmquist, D. L. and Griinari, J. M. 2006. Milk fatty acid composition in response to reciprocal combinations of sunflower and fish oils in the diet. *Animal Feed Science and Technology* 131:358–369.

Park, Y. W., Juárez, M., Ramos, M., and Haenlein, G. F. W. 2007. Physico-chemical characteristics of goat and sheep milk. *Small Ruminant Research* 68:88–113.

Pestana, J. M., Martins, S. I. V., Alfaia, C. M. M. et al. 2009. Content and distribution of conjugated linoleic acid isomers in bovine milk, cheese and butter from azores. *Dairy Science & Technology* 89:193–200.

Pikul, J., Wójtowski, J., Danków, R. et al. 2014. The effect of false flax (Camelina sativa) cake dietary supplementation in dairy goats on fatty acid profile of kefir. *Small Ruminant Research* 122:44–49.

Plaza, M., Santoyo, S., Jaime, L. et al. 2010. Screening for bioactive compounds from algae'. *Journal of Pharmaceutical and Biomedical Analysis* 51:450–455.

Raes, K., De Smet, S., and Demeyer, D. 2004. Effect of dietary fatty acids on incorporation of long chain polyunsaturated fatty acids and conjugated linoleic acid in lamb, beef and pork meat: A review. *Animal Feed Science and Technology* 113:199–221.

Razzaghi, A., Valizadeh, R., Naserian, A. A., Mesgaran, M. D., Carpenter, A. J., and Ghaffari, M. H. 2016. Effect of dietary sugar concentration and sunflower seed supplementation on lactation performance, ruminal fermentation, milk fatty acid profile, and blood metabolites of dairy cows. *Journal of Dairy Science* 99:3539–3548.

Rymer, C., and Givens, D. I. 2006. Effect of species and genotype on the efficiency of enrichment of poultry meat with n–3 polyunsaturated fatty acids. *Lipids* 41:445–451.

Sánchez-Machado, D. I., López-Cervantes, J., López-Hernández, J., and Paseiro-Losada, P. 2004. Fatty acids, total lipid, protein and ash contents of processed edible seaweeds. *Food Chemistry* 85:439–444.

Schwendel, B. H., Wester, T. J., Morel, P. C. et al. 2015. Invited review: Organic and conventionally produced milk-an evaluation of factors influencing milk composition. *American Dairy Science Association* 98:721–746.

Shingfield, K. J., Bernard, L., Leroux, C., and Chilliard, Y. 2010. Role of trans fatty acids in the nutritional regulation of mammary lipogenesis in ruminants. *Animal* 4:1140–1166.

Simopoulos, A. P. 2008. The importance of the omega-6/omega-3 fatty acid ratio in cardiovascular disease and other chronic diseases. *Experimental Biology and Medicine* 233:674–688.

Toral, P. G., Chilliard, Y., Rouel, J., Leskinen, H., Shingfield, K. J., and Bernard, L. 2015. Comparison of the nutritional regulation of milk fat secretion and composition in cows and goats. *Journal of Dairy Science* 98:7277–7297.

Tsiplakou, E., Mountzouris, K. C., and Zervas, G. 2006. Concentration of conjugated linoleic acid in grazing sheep and goat milk fat. *Livestock Science* 103:74–84.

Tsiplakou, E., and Zervas, G. 2013. The effect of fish and soybean oil inclusion in goat diet on their milk and plasma fatty acid profile. *Livestock Science* 155:236–243.

Trumbo, P., Schlicker, S., Yates, A. A., and Poods, M. 2002. Dietary reference intakes for energy, carbohydrate, fiber, fat, fatty acids, cholesterol, protein and amino acids. *Journal of the American Dietetic Association* 102:1621–1630.

Turchini, G. M., Torstensen, B. E., and Ng, W.-K. 2009. Fish oil replacement in finfish nutrition. *Reviews in Aquaculture* 1:10–57.

Uniacke-Lowe, T. 2011. Studies on equine milk and comparative studies on equine and bovine milk systems. PhD Thesis, University College Cork, Cork, Ireland.

Usydus, Z., Szlinder-Richert, J., Adamczyk, M., and Szatkowska, U. 2011. Marine and farmed fish in the polish market: Comparison of the nutritional value. *Food Chemistry* 126:78–84.

Wang, B., Vongsvivut, J., Adhikari, B., and Barrow, C. J. 2015. Microencapsulation of tuna oil fortified with the multiple lipophilic ingredients vitamins A, D3, E, K2, curcumin and coenzyme Q10. *Journal of Functional Foods* 19:893–901.

Williams, P. G. 2007. Nutritional composition of red meat. *Dietitians Association of Australia* 64(S4):1–6.

Wood, J. D., Enser, M., Fisher, A. V. et al. 2008. Fat deposition, fatty acid composition and meat quality: A review. *Meat Science* 78:343–358.

Wood, J. D., Richardson, R. I., Nute, G. R. et al. 2004. Effects of fatty acids on meat quality: A review. *Meat Science* 66:21–32.

Woods, V. B. and Fearon, A. M. 2009. Dietary sources of unsaturated fatty acids for animals and their transfer into meat, milk and eggs: A review. *Livestock Science* 126:1–20.

chapter five

Advances in food fortification with essential amino acids

Ankit Goyal, Beenu Tanwar, Ami Patel, Nihir Shah, and Manvesh Sihag

Contents

"Health comes from the farm, not the pharmacy."

5.1 Introduction

The relationship between diet and health is a progressive domain of research. A well-balanced diet should not only supply energy but also the essential amino acids; vitamins and trace elements, particularly the uncommon sulfur (S-) rich amino acids; lysine and methionine; vitamins A, C, D, and E; B vitamins; folic acid; and the ionic elements iodine (I), iron (Fe), zinc (Zn), and selenium (Se). Chronic deficiency of these nutrients can lead to developmental disturbances of the fetus, restrictions of cognitive perception in children, lethargy, blindness, and acute immunological malfunctions (WHO, 2002). Since these symptoms are not evidently linked with an inadequate diet, this malnutrition is also designated as *hidden hunger.* The global significance of hidden hunger first caught the eye of the nutrition community in the mid-1980, when protein-energy malnutrition became known as the culprit of the world's nutrition problems (Allen, 2000). Yet today, this global distress affects one in nine people on earth (FAO, 2011). Deficiency in essential amino acids and trace elements is most widespread in developing countries. Proteins are important constituents of the human diet, since they are a principal source of nitrogen and essential amino acids. The nutritional quality of food protein is determined by calculating the amino acid score of a protein, which in turn is calculated by comparing the amounts of individual essential amino acids with the pattern of the requirement for each per unit of its protein. People from developing countries, whose foods are mostly derived from the major cereal and legume crops, suffer from particular deficiencies in the essential amino acids, Lysine and Methionine, respectively (Galili et al., 2005; Wenefrida et al., 2009). Lysine and Methionine belong to the Aspartate family pathway responsible for the synthesis of two other essential amino acids, Threonine and Isoleucine (Galili et al., 2005) and deficiency thereby reduces the nutritional values of crop plants to 50%–75%, compared to those of a diet possessing balanced levels of essential amino acids. This deficiency of essential amino acids can result in nonspecific signs of protein deficiencies in humans, such as lowered resistance to diseases, decreased blood proteins, and retarded mental and physical development in young children, a syndrome referred to as protein-energy malnutrition (PEM). The World Health Organization (WHO) estimates that around 30% of the populations in the developing world suffer from this syndrome (WHO, 2002). According to FAO (2005) about 30% of these populations are poor and have no possibility of growing any crop plants. The poor, in particular, cannot afford a balanced diet, and this group represents a large proportion of the population of large cities. Since the vegetarian diet is usually deficient in essential amino acids, it must be complemented in some way to improve its amino acid pattern (Young and Pellet, 1990). Unfortunately, due to low production of legumes (Hussain et al., 2004), its price has soared just like that of animal protein, beyond the reach of the most vulnerable groups. Hence, there is a need to re-explore the possible value of increasing the amino acid content of staple foods.

Various extensive programs are underway to enrich the nutrient content of plants both to improve health and to prevent disease. There are many interventions that tackle hidden hunger, reduce or eliminate protein deficiency, and improve nutrition, including vitamin and mineral supplementation, to promote dietary diversification and home food production. Yet food fortification—adding a small amount of nutrient/micronutrients to a staple food or condiment—has been shown to be one of the safest and most cost-effective approaches to tackle this global challenge (Bhagwat et al., 2014; Goyal et al., 2015). Various nutrients such as iodine, iron, zinc, calcium, omega-3 fatty acids Vitamin A, B-group vitamins, and

Vitamin D have been successfully incorporated in combinations that did not affect the appearance, taste, texture, or flavor of the food (Goyal et al., 2016; Goyal et al., 2017). Thus, food fortification is designed to build up essential amino acid and micronutrient stores in people over time and without risk, so it is a benign and resourceful way of improving nutrition without making people modify their cooking and eating habits.

A number of methods for fortifying food have been suggested, some of which have potential, while others were unsuccessful either owing to the chemical properties of the substances, hostile conditions for their delivery, or financial reasons (Garcia-Casal et al., 2003). Several researchers are working on increasing the levels of the micronutrients and amino acids in crops by conventional plant breeding, by adding the suitable mineral or inorganic complex to fertilizer, or through biotechnology, in addition to the traditional goals of disease resistance, yield, drought tolerance, and so on; but the challenge is to get consumer recognition and acceptance for bio-fortified crops, thereby increasing the intake of the target nutrients (Hirschi, 2009).

However, the practices of fortification and/or supplementation of essential amino acids performed in cereal and legume's flour, animal feed, and other food products, result in better consumer acceptability, improved nutritional quality in terms of Net protein utilization (NPU), biological value (BV) and chemical score. This chapter focuses on the fortification/supplementation studies of amino acids undertaken to improve nutritional content of animal feeds and food along with their toxicity and regulations.

5.2 Global market

According to a report published by Grand View Research, Inc. in 2015, the global amino acid market is expected to reach $35.4 billion by 2022. Increased meat consumption and thus feed formulation is expected to remain a key factor in an enormous rise of amino acid market globally. Essential amino acids such as lysine, methionine, leucine, threonine, and tryptophan are mainly produced for feed formulations and live-stock production. Increased awareness of health has led to the development of dietary supplements, nutraceuticals, and functional foods, which are the driving factors and have thus influenced positively the growth of this market. For example, aspartame, an artificial sweetener, commonly used in food and beverages, is prepared from L-aspartic acid and phenylalanine. Due to its flavor-enhancing effects, L-glutamic acid has become the leading amino acid in total amino acids production. Owing to their enormous functional potential, the amino acids market is expected to reach 10,117.5 kilotons by 2022 from 6,582.0 kilo tons in 2014, growing at a CAGR (compound annual growth rate) of 5.6% from 2015 to 2022 (Grand View Research, 2015).

5.3 Physiological roles of amino acids in various animal models

Amino acids are the building blocks of proteins and the precursors of various important low-molecular weight substances (nitrogen oxide, thyroid hormones, polyamines, creatine, glutathione, serotonin, heme, melanin, etc.). A wide range of literature is available indicating the physiological roles of individual amino acids in different animal models. Consumption of a suboptimal diet leads to a deficiency of essential amino acids, which adversely affects the optimal growth and development of the body. Apart from the nutrition, some amino acids (such as glycine, proline) act as major constituents of structural proteins (collagen and elastin). Though glycine is considered to be a nonessential amino acid, the chronic deficiency of glycine may cause impaired growth, weak immune response, and other adverse effects on health and metabolism. It is interesting to note that in case of birds, dietary glycine is essential for fetal and neonatal development, as fetus and neonatal cannot synthesize sufficient glycine to support optimal growth (Jackson et al., 2002). Wu (2013) reviewed the physiological function of essential as well as non-essential amino acids comprehensively in various animal and human models. Starting from general nutrition, amino acids regulate gene expression, cell signaling, intestinal microbial growth, immune functions, anti-oxidative response, neurological development, protein synthesis, DNA and protein methylation, growth of small intestine and skeletal muscles, nutrient transport and metabolism, and so on. (Wu, 2013). Some of the functions of amino acids are shown in Figure 5.1.

5.4 Fortification of amino acids

It is well known that lysine and methionine are essential and limiting amino acids in cereals crops and legumes, respectively. Several researchers have worked on increasing the levels of these amino acids in crops by breeding or genetic manipulation; but this approach could not be accepted by a large population. Later on, the practices of fortification and/or supplementation of essential amino acids were performed in cereal and legume's flour, animal feed, and other food products, resulting in better consumer acceptability, improved nutritional quality in terms of net protein utilization (NPU), biological value (BV), and chemical score. Fortification of amino acids is discussed here in the next two major sections.

5.4.1 Fortification of amino acids in foods

A wide range of literature is available on the supplementation of amino acids in animal feed, but it is limited in case of foods intended for human

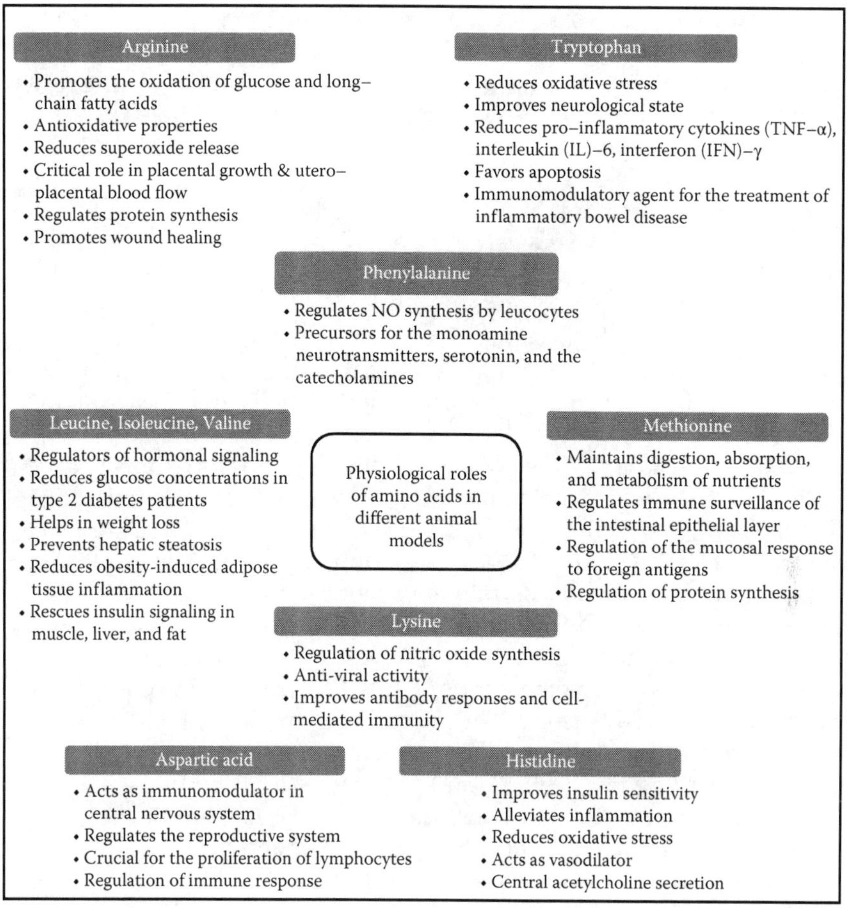

Figure 5.1 Physiological roles of amino acids in different animal models.

consumption. Fortification of amino acids was done not only to enhance the protein's quality, but also to reduce the acrylamide formation in baked products. It is well known that asparagine reacts with reducing sugars in dough and forms acrylamide (a carcinogen) at baking temperature. Claeys et al. (2005) reported a significant reduction in acrylamide content on supplementation of cysteine into dough. Cysteine or other amino acids (other than asparagine) compete with asparagine for the reaction with reducing sugars and thus reduce the acrylamide formation (Wedzicha et al., 2005). Similar effects were reported by Mustafa et al. (2009) and Rydberg et al., (2003), who studied the effect of addition of glycine on acrylamide content in yeast-leavened wheat bread. However, Fink et al. (2006) observed contrary results with no significant reduction in acrylamide content on addition of glycine in dough.

Several authors worked on the supplementation of amino acid in legume and wheat flour and observed a significant improvement in nutritional quality of final product. De Oliveira et al. (1973) suggested improved protein quality when manioc flour (cassava flour) was supplemented with 0.2%–0.4% methionine. Similarly, when Hegsted (1971) added 0.2% L-lysine-HCl in white flour, net utilizable protein increased from 3.2% to 5.3%. By this approach, protein quality of plant origin foods can be enhanced up to the levels of meat, fish and/or egg proteins. Fomon et al. (1973) used the same approach and fortified methionine at the level of 0.5% of soybean flour in infant formula, which was judged equivalent in proteins value to the proteins of milk, meat and eggs.

The protein of wheat, the most common cereal consumed all over the world (in the form of bread), is limiting in lysine and threonine. Various epidemiological and animal studies have shown that lysine fortification in bread and other wheat products significantly improved the normal growth and development in various animals (Rosenberg and Rohdenburg, 1952; Stillings et al., 1971; Jansen et al., 1964). In a study conducted by Fleming and Sosulski (1977), nutritive value of bread fortified with legume protein concentrate and lysine was analyzed in terms of net protein retention (NPR) and protein efficiency ratio (PER) of animals. Results indicated the highest growth rate in rats fed on casein diet irrespective of lysine supplementation; while the group fed on lysine-fortified bread was rated second. The animals grown on control wheat flour bread showed the minimum NPR values. In another study, directed by Geervani and Eggum (1989), BV and NPU were significantly increased on the addition of lysine at the level of 0.6g/100g of five minor varieties of millets (Kodo, Little, Barnyard, French and Italian). In this study, lysine supplementation improved the range of BV from 45.7-64.1 to 76.1-90.3 and NPU from 41.1-51.0 to 62.7-83.3. Similarly, Ifon et al., (1980) found that soy proteins fortification significantly improved nutritive value of millet porridge in terms of NPU, PER, BV, and NPR. In developing countries, wheat provides a major portion of protein and caloric intake of the population. By considering this factor, Hussain et al., (2004) investigated the effect of lysine fortification in wheat flour and studied the selected indices of nutritional status of predominantly cereal (wheat)-eating families. A double-blind study was performed on two groups having a total of 80 families (40 families per group). One group received lysine fortified flour and other group was control, consumed flour without added lysine. Though weight and height increased in both groups during the study, in the lysine group, significantly higher values were observed in children. A similar trend was observed in haemoglobin values of women. There was no significant change in Hb value of control (9.6 mg/dl). However, a significant change from 8.8 to 9.6 mg/dl was observed in Hb of women, who received the lysine fortified flour.

Several researchers associated lysine with the psychobehavioral and logical response, colonic health, and thus quality of life (Smriga et al., 2002; Smriga and Torii, 2003; Srinongkote et al., 2003; Smriga et al., 2004). Smriga et al. (2002) demonstrated that dietary L-lysine deficiency caused interference with the normal release of serotonin neurotransmitter, which further enhanced the footshock stress-induced anxiety. On the basis of results, it was concluded that severe deficiency of dietary lysine changed psychobehavioral responses to stress and increased fecal excretion in rats. Stress-induced anxiety has been reported to have a positive and strong correlation with irritable bowel syndrome (Lydiard, 1992). In continuation with the previous work, Smriga et al. (2004) investigated a similar effect in family members of the Syrian community. It was a 3-month randomized double-blind study, in which the effect of lysine fortification in wheat on stress-induced anxiety and stress-responses was investigated. Results suggested that some stress responses can be improved by lysine fortification in humans also. In a study conducted by Srinongkote et al. (2003), pigs received a diet rich in lysine and arginine. It was observed that Lys and Arg diet significantly inhibited stress-induced increase in locomotion without affecting body weight, and concluded that the combination of the same may improve pig welfare during exposure to environmental stress. Several recent studies have been shown on the effects of fortification/supplementation of essential amino acids in diet in Table 5.1.

5.4.2 Fortification of amino acids in animal feed

Animal proteins are the major ingredients of animal feed due to better quality, higher digestibility, and enhanced bioavailability. Animal proteins, such as whey protein concentrates, fish meal, and so on, constitute all essential amino acids and thus improve nutritional status and feed digestibility. However, due to higher price and variable availability of animal proteins, cost of animal feed increases greatly and affects the overall cost of animal production. This cost can be reduced using fortification of essential amino acids in animal feed, which not only improve the quality of animal feed, but also reduce the overall cost of feed and animal production. In this regard, Zhao et al. (2014) conducted a study as to whether amino acids (Lys, Thr, Trp, Met, Val, and Ile) could replace fish meal and whey protein concentrate in diet, and investigated the effect of fortification on growth, immune status, and gut health of weanling pigs. It was concluded that fortification of six amino acids could successfully replace the fish meal and whey protein concentrate without any significant effects on growth performance, immune functions, or gut health of pigs.

Methionine is the most common essential amino acid supplemented in animal feed. Generally, corn and soybeans are the major feed ingredients for calorie and protein requirements of non-ruminants. When corn

Table 5.1 Recent clinical studies showing the effects of dietary supplementation of amino acids in animal/human models

Amino acid involved	Experiment	Model system	Significant findings	Reference
L-lysine	L-lysine was supplemented at 1.35% in zein basal diet for 3 weeks	Weaned piglets	Dietary supplementation of lysine significantly increased villus height, crypt depth in jejunum ($P<0.05$), and enhanced the expression of amino acid transporters to modulate absorption of protein and other amino acids.	He et al. (2013)
L-Tryptophan	L-Tryptophan @ 110 mg/kg.bodywt.day was administered in a porcine model of dextran sodium sulfate (DSS)-induced colitis (irritable bowel syndrome)	Piglets	L-Tryptophan reduced the expression of pro-inflammatory cytokines, TNF-α, interleukin-6, interferon (IFN)- γ; and increased the expression of apoptosis initiators caspase-8. Overall, it enhanced the recovery rate of DSS-induced colitis.	Kim et al. (2010)
L-Arginine	L-arginine @ 155 mmolArg-HCl/kg body weight was supplemented to underfed ewe.	Ewes	L-arginine supplemented underfed ewe showed no significant difference in birth weight of lambs than that of control. Arg supplementation prevented fetal growth restriction and provided scope to ameliorate Intrauterine growth restriction (IUGR) in humans.	Lassala et al. (2010)
L-Arginine	L-Arginine was mixed with the basal diet based on corn and soybean at the levels of 0, 0.5 and 1%, at the beginning when the body wt. was ~60kg.	Pigs	No significant effect on growth performance or carcass traits. Arg supplementation decreased drip loss at postmortem and increased intramuscular fat. 1% Arg enhanced antioxidant capacity and glutathione peroxidase activity in serum. Overall, it improved meat quality and attenuated oxidative stress.	Ma et al. (2010)

(*Continued*)

Table 5.1 (Continued) Recent clinical studies showing the effects of dietary supplementation of amino acids in animal models/human

Amino acid involved	Experiment	Model system	Significant findings	Reference
L-Arginine	Digestible L-Arginine was administered @ 0.96, 1.16, 1.36, 1.56, and 1.76% levels with basal diet based on corn and soybean for 9 weeks.	Broiler breeder hens	Animals received 1.36% Arg supplemented diet showed highest laying rate and total-antioxidant capacity; and lowest methane dicarboxylic aldehyde content. It was concluded that 1.36% digestible Arg (1972 mg/d) was optimal to satisfy nutritional needs during late laying periods for hens.	Duan et al. (2015)
D-Aspartic acid	Sodium D-aspartate (40 mM) was orally administered for 12-16 days with basic diet.	Rats	Animals possessing high levels of D-Asp in hippocampus were found much faster in searching of hidden platform of Morris water maze system; suggesting its important role in modulation of learning and memory.	Topo et al. (2010)
L-Tryptophan	Fish fed basic diet supplemented with 0.7 (control), 1.7, 3.1, 4.0, 5.2, and 6.1 g/kg diet for 8 weeks.	Fish	Tryptophan supplementation significantly ($P < 0.05$) increased % weight gain, feed intake and feed efficiency and decreased plasma ammonia content. Collectively, Trp improved growth performance, intestinal immune response, barrier functions and antioxidant status.	Wen et al. (2014)
D-Aspartic acid	Dose of Na-D-aspartate (10 ml of 2.0 M sdium D-aspartate) was given to patients affected by oligo-asthenozoospermia and asthenozoospermia for 90 days.	Humans	Significant increase in concentration and motility of spermatozoa. 1.6–2.0 fold increase in sperm concentration in sub-fertile patients. Spermatozoa motility increased from 15.5% to 23.19% after D-aspartate treatment.	D'Aniello et al. (2012)

(Continued)

Table 5.1 (Continued) Recent clinical studies showing the effects of dietary supplementation of amino acids in animal models/human

Amino acid involved	Experiment	Model system	Significant findings	Reference
Glycine, Glutamine, Valine, and Isoleucine	Suboptimal basal diet (low crude-protein diet) was supplemented with Glycine, Glutamine, Valine and Isoleucine, individually and in combination.	Broilers	Gly and Glu addition improved body weight gain and feed conversion ratio. Supplementation of Ile, Glu, and Gly increased breast meat yield compared with broilers received diets supplemented with only Val.	Berres et al. (2010)
Leucine	Leucine (4g/meal; 3 meals/d) was supplemented to normal meals of older individuals for 2 weeks	Humans	Leucine supplementation improved postabsorptive muscles fraction synthesis rate and response to the meal. However, no significant change in fat free mass was observed. It was concluded that leucine supplementation may improve muscle protein synthesis in response to low protein diet in older adults.	Casperson et al. (2012)
L-Methionine	Basal diet supplemented with Met (0.12%) was fed for 14 days to weaning piglets of 28 days of age	Piglets	Higher average daily gain and improved feed efficiency was observed in Met supplemented group. Content of sulfur containing amino acids, Glu, Gln, and taurine were found to be higher in plasma of Met supplemented group. As compared to control, Met-group exhibited improved villus structure.	Chen et al. (2014)

(maize) makes up a major portion of the animal's diet, feed becomes deficient in lysine and threonine. On the other hand, when soybean makes up a substantial portion of the diet, feed does not provide a sufficient amount of methionine and cysteine. In such cases, fortification of limiting amino acids provides a better approach to improve nutritional as well as protein quality of animal feed. Though fortification of essential amino acids is a common practice in animal feed, in contrast nonessential amino acids' supplementation could not provide significant improvement. For example, Awad et al. (2015) studied the individual nonessential amino acids (NEAA) fortification of a low-protein diet for broilers under specific conditions and observed that no individual NEAA fortification was able to compensate the depressed growth. Here, it is interesting to note that when the same authors (Awad et al., 2014) conducted a similar experiment except the amino acids were fortified in combinations (Gly, Glu, Pro, Ala, and Asp) unlike in the previous study; they observed that combination of NEAAs could overcome depressed growth and performance in broilers. In another study conducted by Han et al. (1992), the effect of amino acid fortification in a low-protein diet based on corn and soybean meal (CS) in chicks was investigated. When the low-protein (16%) CS diet was fortified with Met, Lys, Arg, Val, and Thr individually, weight gain and feed efficiency substantially increased, similar to that of positive control fed with 23% CS diet.

5.5 Biofortification of essential amino acids

The term biofortification is widely employed in agriculture crops that may be described as the development of nutrient-dense staple crops using the best conventional breeding practices and modern biotechnology, without affecting their normal agronomic performance and important consumer-preferred traits (Anon, 2014). People from underdeveloped countries cannot afford supplemented or diversified foods, hence research and development of protein or amino acid enriched biologically fortified crops should be a vital alternate to solve this problem. Biofortification differs from regular fortification, rather than incorporating nutrients into the foods when they are being processed it focuses on building plant foods more nutritious as the plants are growing. Plant scientists are working on biofortifying major staple crops including wheat and potato, rice (Asia), maize (Latin America), cassava (Africa) with iron, vitamins such as folic acid, and essential amino acids such as lysine. Some recent studies are discussed in Table 5.2. These investigations offered a a significant solution to the amino acid deficiencies in staple crops, while at the same time addressing concerns about food safety and physiological abnormalities in biofortified agriculture crops.

Table 5.2 Studies on biofortification of essential amino acids in different agriculture crops

Crop with cultivar	Transferred gene(s)	Promoter used	Major finding(s)	Reference
Rice (Oryza sativa L.)	Aspartate kinase and dihydrodipicolinate synthase	Endosperm-specific GLUTELIN1 promoter (GT1)	Increase in total free amino acids and a slight increase in total protein content; the growth of HFL transgenic rice was normal, except for a slight difference in plant height and grain color	Yang et al. (2016)
Rice (Oryza sativa L.)	Lysine-rich protein gene (LRP) from Psophocarpustetragonolobus (L.) DC	Endosperm-specific GLUTELIN1 promoter (GT1)	Lys content was significantly increased in seeds of transgenic rice; furthermore, Lys content in the hybrid of the transgenic plants also had an approximate 20% increase compared to hybrid control	Liu et al. (2016)
Rice (Oryza sativa L.)	Lysine-rich histone proteins, RLRH1 and RLRH2	Glutelin promoter	Lysine content in the transgenic rice seeds was enhanced by up to 35%,	Wang et al. (2015)
Oryza sativa L., Japonica cv. Wuxiangjing 9	E. coli AK, DHPS and RNAi of LKR/SDH	CaMV 35S promoter, rice endosperm specific glutelinGt1 promoter	Increased lysine levels up to ~12-fold in leaves and ~60-fold in seeds	Long et al. (2013)
Oryza sativa L. cv. Taipei 309	E. coli serineacetyltransferase	Ubiquitin promoter	Enhanced cysteine, glutathione, and methionine levels in crop	Nguyen et al. (2012)

(*Continued*)

Table 5.2 (Continued) Studies on biofortification of essential amino acids in different agriculture crops

Crop with cultivar	Transferred gene(s)	Promoter used	Major finding(s)	Reference
Mtr1	Rice Mtr1 mutant gene (mtr1-D)	Maize ubiquitin promoter	Increased Phenylalanine and Tryptophan levels	Yamada et al. (2008)
Oryza sativa L. cv. Nipponbare	Rice OASA1D	Maize ubiquitin promoter	Doubled the amount of free Tryptophan as compared to wild plants	Wakasa et al. (2006)
Oryza sativa L. cv. Taipei	Sunflower Seed Albumin	1Dx5 and Bx17 wheat High molecular weight glutelin promoter	Enhanced cysteine content; grains observed little change in total sulfur amino acid content	Hagan et al. (2003)
Oryza sativa L., japonica cv. TNG67	Sesame 2S Albumin precursor polypeptide	Glutelin promoter	Observed 29%-76% rise in methionine and 31%-75% rise in cysteine levels	Lee et al. (2003)
Japonica variety Nagdongbyeo	Maize Dihydrodipicolinate synthase	CaMV 35S and the rice glutelin GluB-1 promoter	Increased free lysine in seeds	Lee et al. (2001)
Oryza sativa cv. Nipponbare	Rice OASA1 and OASA2 (encodes Anthranilate synthase)	Maize Ubi1 promoter	Mutation of OASA1 resulted in accumulation of Tryptophan	Tozawa et al. (2001)

5.6 FDA regulations, GRAS status, and toxicity

L-lysine and its monohydrochloride form- L-lysine monohydrochloride, are approved as food additives by the FDA (21CFR 172.320) and can be used directly to fortify foods for enhanced nutrition and normal consumption. As per this regulation, the amount of L-lysine should not exceed 6.4% of the total protein in final food product (GRAS, 2011). This amount includes the L-lysine added for nutritive purpose and natural lysine (free and combined as protein) already present in food product. As the daily reference value of protein is 50 g/d (for adult), the amount of L-lysine must not exceed 3200 mg/day. Lysine can be present in other forms also such as Maillard reaction products, which could be absorbed, but its utilization for protein synthesis is precluded. According to the report published by FDA, neither L-lysine nor its degradation products cause any toxicological hazards or safety concerns, when used at intended levels (GRAS, 2011). Dubow et al. (1958) investigated the tolerance level in most sensitive population, i.e., infants to L-lysine supplementation. In this study, 4–11 month old infants (n=6) received whole cow milk supplemented with L-lysine monohydrochloride at the levels of 60, 120, 240, 480, 720, 960 and 1080 mg per 8 ounces of milk. If milk protein concentration is taken into consideration, the highest amount of supplementation increased L-lysine content to 17.7% versus 7.4% for control milk. Results showed that all supplemented milk samples were well tolerated. Though lysine levels in plasma varied, but urinary lysine levels were roughly proportional to the supplementation amount. No signs of cystinuria were observed in any of the infants. In another study, Sackler and Sophian (1957a, 1957b, 1958) investigated the effect of supplementation of a single dose of 5 g L-lysine hydrochloride with basic diet of bread and water. A similar experiment was performed with arginine monohydrochloride. It was reported that both the amino acids were well tolerated. Recently, Wass et al. (2011) studied the effect of L-lysine (6 g/d) supplementation for schizophrenia patients (n=10) for 8 weeks. In this study, it was reported that L-lysine treatment significantly increased the blood concentration in lysine-supplemented patients and was well tolerated without any adverse side effects. As per the literature discussed in an FDA report (GRAS, 2011), oral LD_{50} of 10 g/kg body weight for lysine suggests a very low order of toxicity.

Other amino acids such as L-arginine and L-valine are also approved by FDA and are GRAS recognized when fortified to a certain prescribed level. However, a recent study suggested that when high concentration of branched-chain amino acids (BCAA) (2.5 mM Valine, 2.5 mM Leucine, 2.5 mM Isoleucine) were administered to cortical or hippocampal neuronal cell cultures of Wistar rat embryos, it significantly increased excitotoxicity and showed neurotoxicity to certain brain areas, specifically cortical neurons (Contrusciere et al., 2010). In another study, elevated plasma levels of BCAA promoted the oxidative stress and pro-inflammatory status (Zhenyukh et al., 2017; Hoffmann et al., 2006; Mescka et al., 2015; Gleeson, 2005). Pencharz et al. (2012) and Rasmussen et al. (2016) studied the safety levels of L-leucine in adult men and elderly men, respectively, and concluded that safe upper limit of leucine intake in humans is $<550\ mg{\cdot}kg^{-1}\cdot d^{-1}$ or <39 g/d.

5.7 Conclusion

It can be concluded that amino acids play a critical role in normal growth and development of the animals. Beginning from the nutrition and building of muscles, amino acids perform a vast variety of functions such as regulate gene expression, immune response, absorption and transport of nutrients, hormonal secretion, release of signaling molecules, and so on. A large population depends on cereals and legumes for their daily needs, which are deficient in lysine and sulfur-containing amino acids, respectively. Therefore, fortification could be a better approach to supplement limiting amino acids in normal diet; so that the adverse effects on health and metabolism could be controlled.

References

Allen, L.H. 2000. *Ending hidden hunger: The history of micronutrient deficiency control*. Washington, DC: Background Analysis for the World Bank-UNICEF Nutrition Assessment Project World Bank.

Anon, 2014. *Biofortification through biotechnology to combat malnutrition*. Available from: https://croplife.org/news/biofortification-through-biotechnology-to-combat-malnutrition/last accessed on February 02, 2017.

Awad, E.A., Zulkifli, I., Farjam, A.S. and Chwen, L.T. 2014. Amino acids fortification of low-protein diet for broilers under tropical climate. 2. Nonessential amino acids and increasing essential amino acids. *Italian Journal of Animal Science* 13(3):631–636.

Awad, E.A., Zulkifli, I., Soleimani, A.F. and Loh, T.C. 2015. Individual non-essential amino acids fortification of a low-protein diet for broilers under the hot and humid tropical climate. *Poultry Science* 94(11):2772–2777.

Berres, J., Vieira, S.L., Dozier, W.A., Cortes, M.E.M., De Barros, R., Nogueira, E.T. and Kutschenko, M., 2010. Broiler responses to reduced-protein diets supplemented with valine, isoleucine, glycine, and glutamic acid. *The Journal of Applied Poultry Research* 19(1):68–79.

Bhagwat, S., Gulati, D., Sachdeva, R. and Sankar, R. 2014. Food fortification as a complementary strategy for the elimination of micronutrient deficiencies: Case studies of large scale food fortification in two Indian States. *Asia Pacific Journal of Clinical Nutrition* 23(S1):s4–s11.

Casperson, S.L., Sheffield-Moore, M., Hewlings, S.J. and Paddon-Jones, D. 2012. Leucine supplementation chronically improves muscle protein synthesis in older adults consuming the RDA for protein. *Clinical Nutrition* 31(4):512–519.

Chen, Y., Li, D., Dai, Z., et al. 2014. L-Methionine supplementation maintains the integrity and barrier function of the small-intestinal mucosa in post-weaning piglets. *Amino Acids* 46(4):1131–1142.

Claeys, W. L., De Vleeschouwer, K., and Hendrickx, M. E. 2005. Effect of amino acids on acrylamide formation and elimination kinetics. *Biotechnology Progress* 21:1525–1530.

Contrusciere, V., Paradisi, S., Matteucci, A. and Malchiodi-Albedi, F. 2010. Branched-chain amino acids induce neurotoxicity in rat cortical cultures. *Neurotoxicity Research* 17(4):392–398.

D'Aniello, G., Ronsini, S., Notari, T., et al. 2012. D-Aspartate, a key element for the improvement of sperm quality. *Advances in Sexual Medicine* 2:47–53.

De Oliveira, D.J.E., Salata, E.B. and Campos, J. 1973. Manioc flour as a methionine carrier to balance common bean-based diets. *Journal of Food Science* 38(1):116–118.

Duan, X., Li, F., Mou, S., Feng, J., Liu, P. and Xu, L. 2015. Effects of dietary L-arginine on laying performance and anti-oxidant capacity of broiler breeder hens, eggs, and offspring during the late laying period. *Poultry Science* 94(12):2938–2943.

Dubow, E., Maher, A., Gish, D. and Erk, V. 1958. Lysine tolerance in infants. *The Journal of Pediatrics* 52(1):30–37.

FAO. 2005. Agriculture Organization of the United Nations, Economic and Social Department, 2005. The State of Food Insecurity in the World 2005: Eradicating World Hunger-Key to Achieving the Millennium Development Goals. *Food & Agriculture Organization*. Viale delle Terme di Caracalla, Rome, Italy. Available from: ftp://ftp.fao.org/docrep/fao/008/a0200e/a0200e.pdf

FAO. 2011. Quinoa: An ancient crop to contribute to world food security. In: A. Bojanic (Ed). *Regional Office for Latin America and the Caribbean*, Rome, Italy: Food and Agriculture Organization: pp. 63.

Fink, M., Andersson, R., Rosen, J., and Aman, P. 2006. Effect of added asparagine and glycine on acrylamide content in yeast-leavened bread. *Cereal* 83:218–222.

Fleming, S.E. and Sosulski, F.W., 1977. Nutritive value of bread fortified with concentrated plant proteins and lysine. *Cereal Chemistry* 54(6):1238–1248.

Fomon, S.J., Thomas, L.N., Filer, L.J., Anderson, T.A. and Bergmann, K.E. 1973. Requirements for protein and essential amino acids in early infancy: Studies with a Soy-Isolate Formula. *Acta Paediatrica* 62(1):33–45.

Galili, G., Amir, R., Hoefgen, R. and Hesse, H. 2005. Improving the levels of essential amino acids and sulfur metabolites in plants. *Biological Chemistry* 386(9):817–831.

Garcia-Casal, M.N., Layrisse, M., Pena-Rosas, J.P., Ramirez, J., Leets, I. and Matus, P. 2003. Iron absorption from elemental iron-fortified corn flakes in humans. *Role of vitamins A and C. Nutrition Research* 23(4):451–463.

Geervani, P. and Eggum, B.O. 1989. Effect of heating and fortification with lysine on protein quality of minor millets. *Plant Foods for Human Nutrition* 39(4):349–357.

Gleeson, M. 2005. *Interrelationship between physical activity and branched-chain amino acids, American Society for Nutrition* 135:1591S–1595SS.

Goyal, A., Sharma, V., Sihag, M.K. et al. 2015. Development and physico-chemical characterization of microencapsulated flaxseed oil powder: A functional ingredient for omega-3 fortification. Powder Technology 286:527–537.

Goyal, A., Sharma, V., Sihag, M. K., Singh, A. K., Arora, S. and Sabikhi, L. 2016. Fortification of dahi (Indian yoghurt) with omega-3 fatty acids using microencapsulated flaxseed oil microcapsules. Journal of Food Science and Technology 53(5):2422–2433.

Goyal, A., Sharma, V., Sihag, M. K., Singh, A. K., Arora, S. and Sabikhi, L. 2017. Oxidative stability of alpha-linolenic acid (ω-3) in flaxseed oil microcapsules fortified market milk. International Journal of Dairy Technology 70(2):188–196.

Grand View Research, 2015. Available from http://www.grandviewresearch.com/press-release/global-amino-acids-market Last accessed: February 7, 2017.

GRAS, 2011. Available from: http://www.fda.gov/downloads/Food/IngredientsPackagingLabeling/GRAS/NoticeInventory/ucm299316.pdf Last accessed: February 7, 2017.

Hagan, N. D., Upadhyaya, N., Tabe, L. M., and Higgins, T. J. V. 2003. The redistribution of protein sulfur in transgenic rice expressing a gene for a foreign, sulfur-rich protein. *The Plant Journal* 34:1–11.

Han, Y., Suzuki, H., Parsons, C.M. and Baker, D.H., 1992. Amino acid fortification of a low-protein corn and soybean meal diet for chicks. *Poultry Science* 71(7):1168–1178.

He, L., Yang, H., Hou, Y. et al. 2013. Effects of dietary L-lysine intake on the intestinal mucosa and expression of CAT genes in weaned piglets. *Amino Acids* 45(2):383–391.

Hegsted, D. M. 1971. In: Scrimshaw, N. S. and Altschul, A. M. (Eds.) *Amino Acid Fortification of Protein Foods,* Cambridge, Massachusetts: MIT Preff; pp. 175

Hirschi, K.D. 2009. Nutrient biofortification of food crops. *Annual Review of Nutrition* 29:401–421.

Hoffmann, B., Helbling, C., Schadewaldt, P., Wendel, U. 2006. Impact of longitudinal plasma leucine levels on the intellectual outcome in patients with classic MSUD. *Pediatric Research* 59:17–20.

Hussain, T., Abbas, S., Khan, M.A. and Scrimshaw, N.S. 2004. Lysine fortification of wheat flour improves selected indices of the nutritional status of predominantly cereal-eating families in Pakistan. *Food and Nutrition Bulletin* 25(2):114–122.

Ifon, E.T. 1980. Biological evaluation of the nutritive value of the millet porridge-a traditional Nigerian weaning food-before and after fortification with soya proteins. *Nutrition Reports International* 22(1): 109–116.

Jackson, A.A., Marchand, M.C. and Langley-Evans, S.C. 2002. Increased systolic blood pressure in rats induced by a maternal low-protein diet is reversed by dietary supplementation with glycine. *Clinical Science* 103(6):633–639.

Jansen, G.R., Ehle, S.R. and Hause, N.L. 1964. Studies of the nutritive loss of supplemental lysine in baking. 1. Loss in a standard white bread containing 4% nonfat dry milk. *Food Technology* 18:367–371.

Kim, C.J., Kovacs-Nolan, J.A., Yang, C., Archbold, T., Fan, M.Z. and Mine, Y. 2010. L-Tryptophan exhibits therapeutic function in a porcine model of dextran sodium sulfate (DSS)-induced colitis. *The Journal of Nutritional Biochemistry* 21(6):468–475.

Lassala, A., Bazer, F.W., Cudd, T.A. et al. 2010. Parenteral administration of L-arginine prevents fetal growth restriction in undernourished ewes. *The Journal of Nutrition* 140(7):1242–1248.

Lee, S. I., Kim, H. U., Lee, Y. H. et al. 2001. Constitutive and seed-specific expression of a maize lysine-feedback-insensitive dihydrodipicolinate synthase gene leads to increased free lysine levels in rice seeds. *Molecular Breeding* 8:75–84.

Lee, T. T., Wang, M. M., Hou, R. C. et al. 2003. Enhanced methionine and cysteine levels in transgenic rice seeds by the accumulation of sesame 2S albumin. *Bioscience, Biotechnology, and Biochemistry* 67:1699–1705.

Liu, X., Zhang, C., Wang, X. et al. 2016. Development of high-lysine rice via endosperm-specific expression of a foreign Lysine rich protein gene. *BMC Plant Biology* 16(1):147.

Long, X., Liu, Q., Chan, M., Wang, Q., and Sun, S.S. 2013. Metabolic engineering and profiling of rice with increased lysine. *Plant Biotechnology Journal* 11(4):490–501.

Lydiard, R.B. 1992. Anxiety and the irritable bowel syndrome. *Psychiatric Annals* 22(12):612–618.

Ma, X., Lin, Y., Jiang, Z. et al. 2010. Dietary arginine supplementation enhances antioxidative capacity and improves meat quality of finishing pigs. *Amino Acids* 38(1):95–102.

Mescka, C.P., Guerreiro, G., Donida, B. et al. 2015. Investigation of inflammatory profile in MSUD patients: Benefit of L-carnitine supplementation. *Metabolic Brain Disease* 30:1167–1174.

Mustafa, A., Fink, M., Kamal-Eldin, A., Rose´n, J., Andersson, R., and Aman, P. 2009. Interaction effects of fermentation time and added asparagine and glycine on acrylamide content in yeast-leavened bread. *Food Chemistry* 112:767–774.

Nguyen, H. C., Hoefgen, R., and Hesse, H. 2012. Improving the nutritive value of rice seeds: Elevation of cysteine and methionine contents in rice plants by ectopic expression of a bacterial serine acetyltransferase. *Journal of Experimental Botany* 63:5991–6001.

Pencharz, P.B., Elango, R. and Ball, R.O. 2012. Determination of the tolerable upper intake level of leucine in adult men. *The Journal of Nutrition* 142(12):2220S–2224S.

Rasmussen, B., Gilbert, E., Turki, A., Madden, K. and Elango, R. 2016. Determination of the safety of leucine supplementation in healthy elderly men. *Amino Acids* 48(7):1707–1716.

Rosenberg, H.R. and Rohdenburg, E.L. 1952. The fortification of bread with lysine. II. The nutritional value of fortified bread. *Archives of Biochemistry and Biophysics* 37(2):461–468.

Rydberg, P., Eriksson, S., Tareke, E., Karlsson, P., Ehrenberg, L., and Tornqvist, M. (2003). Investigations of factors that influence the acrylamide content of heated foodstuffs. *Journal of Agricultural and Food Chemistry* 51:7012–7018.

Sackler, A.M., Sophian, L.H. 1957a. Gastric secretagogue effect of lysine monohydrochloride. *Science* 126:255–256.

Sackler, A.M., Sophian, L.H. 1957b. The effect of the ingestion of amino acid on gastric secretion with particular reference to L-lysine monohydrochloride. *Journal of Clinical Pathology* 28:258–263.

Sackler, A.M., Sophian, L.H. 1958. The effects of amino acid ingestion on gastric secretion: comparison of lysine and arginine. *Journal of Laboratory and Clinical Medicine* 52:43–47.

Smriga, M., Ghosh, S., Mouneimne, Y., Pellett, P.L. and Scrimshaw, N.S. 2004. Lysine fortification reduces anxiety and lessens stress in family members in economically weak communities in Northwest Syria. Proceedings of the National Academy of Sciences of the United States of America 101(22):8285–8288.

Smriga, M., Kameishi, M., Uneyama, H. and Torii, K., 2002. Dietary L-lysine deficiency increases stress-induced anxiety and fecal excretion in rats. *The Journal of Nutrition* 132(12):3744–3746.

Smriga, M. and Torii, K. 2003. Prolonged treatment with L-lysine and L-arginine reduces stress-induced anxiety in an elevated plus maze. *Nutritional Neuroscience* 6(2):125–128.

Srinongkote, S., Smriga, M., Nakagawa, K. and Toride, Y. 2003. A diet fortified with L-lysine and L-arginine reduces plasma cortisol and blocks anxiogenic response to transportation in pigs. *Nutritional Neuroscience* 6(5): 283–289.

Stillings, B.R., Sidwell, V.D. and Hammerle, O.A. 1971. Nutritive quality of wheat flour and bread supplemented with either fish protein concentrate or lysine. *Cereal Chemistry* 48(3):292–302.

Topo, E., Soricelli, A., Di Maio, A., D'Aniello, E., Di Fiore, M.M. and D'Aniello, A. 2010. Evidence for the involvement of D-aspartic acid in learning and memory of rat. *Amino acids* 38(5):1561–1569.

Tozawa, Y., Hasegawa, H., Terakawa, T., and Wakasa, K. 2001. Characterization of rice anthranilate synthase α-subunit genes OASA1 and OASA2. Tryptophan accumulation in transgenic rice expressing a feedback-insensitive mutant of OASA1. *Plant Physiology* 126:1493–1506.

Wakasa, K., Hasegawa, H., Nemoto, H., et al. 2006. High-level tryptophan accumulation in seeds of transgenic rice and its limited effects on agronomic traits and seed metabolite profile. *Journal of Experimental Botany* 57:3069–3078.

Wass, C., Klamer, D., Katsarogiannis, E. et al. 2011. L-lysine as adjunctive treatment in patients with schizophrenia: a single-blinded, randomized, crossover pilot study. *BMC Medicine* 9:40:1–8.

Wedzicha, B. L., Mottram, D. S., Elmore, J. S., Koutsidis, G., and Dodson, A. T. 2005. Kinetic models as a route to control acrylamide formation in food. *Advances in Experimental Medicine and Biology* 561:235–253.

Wen, H., Feng, L., Jiang, W. et al. 2014. Dietary tryptophan modulates intestinal immune response, barrier function, antioxidant status and gene expression of TOR and Nrf2 in young grass carp (Ctenopharyngodon idella). *Fish & Shellfish Immunology* 40(1):275–287.

Wenefrida, I., Utomo, H.S., Blanche, S.B. and Linscombe, S.D., 2009. Enhancing essential amino acids and health benefit components in grain crops for improved nutritional values. *Recent Patents on DNA & Gene Sequences* 3(3):219–225.

WHO, 2002. *The World Health Report 2002: Reducing Risks, Promoting Healthy Life.* World Health Organization. Geneva, Switzerland. Available from: http://www.who.int/whr/2002/en/whr02_en.pdf?ua=1

Wu, G., 2013. Functional amino acids in nutrition and health. *Amino Acids* 45(3):407–411.

Yamada, T., Matsuda, F., Kasai, K. et al. 2008. Mutation of a rice gene encoding a phenylalanine biosynthetic enzyme results in accumulation of phenylalanine and tryptophan. *Plant Cell* 20:1316–1329.

Yang, Q.Q., Zhang, C.Q., Chan, M.L. et al. 2016. Biofortification of rice with the essential amino acid lysine: Molecular characterization, nutritional evaluation, and field performance. *Journal of Experimental Botany* 67(14):4285–4296.

Young, V.R. and Pellett, P.L. 1990. Current concepts concerning indispensable amino acid needs in adults and their implications for international nutrition planning. *Food and Nutrition Bulletin* 12(4):289–300.

Zhao, Y., Weaver, A.C., Fellner, V., Payne, R.L. and Kim, S.W. 2014. Amino acid fortified diets for weanling pigs replacing fish meal and whey protein concentrate: Effects on growth, immune status, and gut health. *Journal of Animal Science and Biotechnology* 5(57):1–10.

Zhenyukh, O., Civantos, E., Ruiz-Ortega, M. et al. 2017. High concentration of branched-chain amino acids promotes oxidative stress, inflammation and migration of human peripheral blood mononuclear cells via mTORC1 activation. *Free Radical Biology and Medicine* 104:165–177.

chapter six

Advances in food fortification with phytonutrients

D. Suresh Kumar

Contents

6.1 *Medicine in ancient Greece*

Mankind has always been interested in food. Food is one of the most important elements guiding the rise of human civilization. During its journey through the ages, human civilization realized that food may possess the ability to prevent diseases and even to cure them. Twenty-five hundred years ago the Greek physician Hippocrates proclaimed "Food is thy medicine and medicine thy food" (Wildman, 2000). Ancient Greek medicine firmly advocated the view that a good diet was one that ensured good health. Scribonius Largus, a contemporary of emperor Claudius (A.D. 41–54) summed up the stages of medical care as diet first, then drugs, and finally surgery (Grant, 2000).

The boundary between food and drug was very thin in Hippocratic medicine. Hippocratic authors often referred to both drugs and foods while describing treatments. For example, the following description can be found in the *Hippocratic Corpus*, which is a collection of nearly 60 early ancient Greek medical works closely associated with Hippocrates and his teachings: "In this case (a black disease) it is necessary to purge with medicaments (*pharmaka*) (that purge) from below and from above, and after that to drink ass's milk, and use foods (*sitia*) that are as emollient and cold as possible: shore-fish, cartilaginous fish, beet, colocynth, and minced meat" (Jouanna, 1983).

In ancient Greece many drugs were used as primary items of diet, a good example being garlic. It was used in such quantities that during the period after the death of Alexander the Great in 323 B.C. there were attempts at specialized cultivation of garlic in Ptolemaic Egypt (Crawford, 1973). In addition to its use as a dietary ingredient it was often recommended by physicians as a food to be used by patients after a treatment. The author of the Hippocratic treatise *Nature of Woman* advised a woman treated for "displacement of the womb" to consume the following foods: "And let her eat a lot of garlic, both raw and boiled, and drink its juice as a soup, and let her make use of emollient foods" (Potter, 2012; Totelin, 2015).

By the end of the fifth century B.C. dietetics had become an established discipline, mainly through the teachings of Hippocrates. Many modern scholars see ancient dietetics as superior to pharmacotherapy or surgery. Foucault (1984) argued that the body is passive when it undergoes drug or surgical treatments, while the soul actively learns when dietetic treatment is employed (Temkin, 1953; Sassi, 2001).

Advances in nutritional science and pharmacology highlight the importance of the quality of food that one consumes. Recent research has provided striking evidence for the influence of dietary factors on specific molecular mechanisms which maintain mental function. Many gut hormones that can enter the brain influence cognitive ability. Additionally, well-established regulators of synaptic plasticity can function as metabolic modulators, responding to peripheral signals like food intake (Gómez-Pinilla, 2008).

Recent studies also show that food can influence psychic activity. The British Cheese Board conducted in 2005 a study on the effects of eating cheese on dreams. The study carried out with 200 volunteers provided evidence that different types of cheese can induce different types of dreams. For example, eating Stilton cheese many a time led to crazy or vivid dreams and subjects eating cheddar cheese often dreamed of celebrities (Anonymous, 2016a). Nielsen and Powell (2015) conducted a study on the perception of food-dependent dreaming. Three-hundred and ninety-six students took part in this study. Both disturbing dreams and vivid dreams were reported by the subjects. Poorer sleep, binge-eating, eating of dairy products, and eating for emotional reasons were associated with reports of disturbing dreams. In contrast, reports of vivid dreams were associated with better sleep, a healthier diet and longer times between meals.

6.2 Indian systems of medicine

6.2.1 Ayurveda

Ayurveda, the traditional medical system of India is based on the basic axiom that diseases spring from disturbance of three factors *vāta, pitta,* and *kapha,* collectively known as *tridōṣa*. The state of health follows when the *tridōṣa* are in steady state. Very similar to the view held by Hippocrates, Ayurveda maintains that both food and herbs influence health. Indian cuisine is largely based on principles of Ayurveda. Thus we come across numerous foods that are made with herbs or vegetables having medicinal properties. Asafoetida (*Ferula asafoetida*), black pepper (*Piper nigrum*), coriander (*Coriandrum sativum*), cumin seeds (*Cuminum cyminum*), curry leaves (*Murraya koenigii*), bitter gourd (*Momordica charantia*), drumstick (*Moringa oleifera*), fenugreek (*Trigonella foenum-graecum*), ginger (*Zingiber officinale*), mustard (*Brassica juncea*), inflorescence and pseudostem of banana (*Musa paradisiaca*), onion (*Allium cepa*), and turmeric (*Curcuma longa*) used in the preparation of these foodstuffs have medicinal properties. They are digestive stimulants, antidiabetic agents, cardioprotectants, litholytics, antioxidants, and antimutagenics (Srinivasan, 2011). Ayurveda also recommends the consumption of powders of herbs mixed with common food ingredients such as milk, butter, buttermilk, yogurt, sesame oil, and honey for curing specific diseases (Kumar 2016a). These are the ayurvedic equivalents of modern-day functional foods or nutraceuticals.

6.2.2 *Unani*

Unani, which is an amalgam of Greco-Arabic medicine and Ayurveda (Verma and Keswani, 1974) also employs medicated food in the treatment of diseases. To improve patient compliance, *Unani* physicians started administering medicaments through three matrices: *halwa*, *sharbat*, and *murabba*. A *halwa* is prepared by bringing to thick consistency a mixture of flour, milk, clarified butter, sugar, and herbs. Examples are *Halwa-i-Badam*, *Halwa-i-Murgh* and *Halwa-i-Ghaikwar*. A *sharbat* is a sweet beverage containing sugar, citric acid, and extracts of herbs. The common examples are *Sharbat Alu Balu*, *Sharbat Afsantin*, and *Sharbat Sandal*. Being sweet or less bitter in taste both *halwa* and *sharbat* are easily accepted by patients. *Murabba* are fruit pickles usually made out of rhizomes of *Zingiber officinale*, and fresh fruits of *Emblica officinalis*, *Ananas sativus*, *Aegle marmelos*, *Benincasa cerifera*, and *Terminalia chebula* (Kumar, 2016a).

6.3 Chinese medicine

Huang-Di-Nei-Jing, an ancient (100 B.C.) and standard text of traditional Chinese medicine, preferred the use of food to drugs in the treatment of diseases. This view has shaped the value of Chinese alimentotherapy. In contemporary China around 77 traditional foodstuffs are known to have medicinal properties. These food items are prepared from many fungi, herbs, and in some cases animals (Jiang et al. 2011). Two medicinal foods popular in China are soy beans and *XiangGu*.

The functional property of soy beans is made use of in nonfermented and fermented soy products. Soy milk, tofu, and soy sprouts are the nonfermerted soy food, while the fermented ones include soy sauce, *sufu, douchi, miso, tempeh, onchom,* and *natto* (Jiang et al. 2011).

During the ripening of *sufu* isoflavones such as genistein and daidzein increase nearly 20 times. These isoflavones have a preventive effect on the development of cancers of the breast, intestines, liver, bladder, skin, and stomach (Adlercreutz et al. 1992; Wei et al. 1993). *Sufu* extract is also found to have considerable angiotensin I–converting enzyme inhibitory activity (Ni et al. 1997; Wang et al. 2003). The insoluble fraction of *sufu* exhibits hypocholesterolemic activity (Zhang et al. 1998).

Fermented soy foods such as *natto* and *tempeh* have stronger antioxidant activity than the unfermented ones (Ren et al. 2006; Wang et al. 2004). During the manufacturing of *sofu* many ingredients such as red kojic rice (angkak) are added. These also have functional property (Wang et al. 1997).

XiangGu (*Lentinus edodes*) is a nonpathogenic fungus found growing on many underutilized logs of trees. Its meaty texture and woody taste make it a pleasant ingredient of food (Wu, 2002; Wu and Chen, 2002). *XiangGu* is mostly used as a flavoring for stews, gravies, stuffing, dips, and spreads (Jiang et al. 2011). *XiangGu* contains 18 amino acids and a unique one among them, eritadenine, seems to be responsible for the hypocholesterolemic property of the fungus (Bai, 2007).

Research carried out during the last two decades confirms the functional nature of *XiangGu*. The polysaccharides present have immune stimulating properties. Lentinan, a β-glucan inhibits tumorigenesis by activating the immune system and inducing gene expression of immunomodulatory cytokines (Liu et al. 2002). Results of experiments conducted by Duan et al. (1997) show that the extract of *XiangGu* can repair genetic damage induced by radiation. *XiangGu* also possesses antiviral (Chihara, 1993; Zhang et al. 2006), antimicrobial (Masatomo et al. 1999), cholesterol-lowering (Fulushima et al. 2001), and hepatoprotective (Lin and Huang, 1987) activities.

6.4 The concept of functional foods

The concept of functional foods was born in Japan when faced with escalating health care costs. As a result of the systematic and large-scale research on chemical compounds derived from natural products, the concept of Foods for Specific Health Use (FOSHU) was born in 1991 (Kubomara, 1998). These foods are intended to improve the lives of people and the manufacturer is permitted to display the specific health claims on the container. Japan is the only country that has legally defined functional foods. The Japanese functional food market is now one of the most advanced in the world (Henry, 2010). Functional foods are also known as nutraceuticals, designer foods, farmafoods, pharmafoods, medifoods, vitafoods, dietary supplements, fortified foods, or foodaceuticals (Roberfroid, 2008). The term *functional food* first appeared in an article in 1993 in *Nature* (Swinbanks and O'Brien, 1993). The term *nutraceutical* was first coined by Stephen DeFelice at a biomedical management course held in Villa Olmo, Como, Italy (DeFelice, 1992).

The adoption of the Alma Ata Declaration by World Health Organization in 1978 (Anonymous, 1978), and growing evidence on the positive effects of phytonutrients on health, have popularized the use of herbal medicinal products in the developed world (Pietta, 2000; Buttriss, 2012). Simultaneously, fortification of food and beverages with phytonutrients has also advanced. The trend for fortified foods continues to gain momentum, as the educated consumer looks at herbs and food for solving their health problems (Borzalleca, 1994).

6.5 *Fortification of food and beverages*

A wide variety of foods and beverages can be fortified with phytonutrients. Fortification is achieved by adding the phytonutrient in question (fortificant or additive) to the food matrix. Bread, biscuits, soups, sausages, cheese, mayonnaise, margarine, sauces, yogurt, pickles, chutneys, confectioneries, jams, jellies, and marmalades can be fortified in this manner. The first step in this long process is the extraction of the phytonutrients.

6.5.1 *Extraction of phytonutrients*

A high quality extract is manufactured using a high-quality herb, an appropriate solvent and equipment, good manufacturing technology and robust analytical methods. Information on medicinal herbs is available in compendia of Ayurveda, *Unani*, Siddha medicine and W.H.O. monographs (Kumar, 2016b). Initial samples of the herb are procured from reliable suppliers and the quality of the herb established using standard methods. Thereafter, raw material specifications for the herb are prepared, the herb cleaned and comminuted, and the extraction process optimized using response surface methodology. On completion of the optimization process, pilot scale extraction is carried out. Extracts obtained by solvent extraction frequently undergo a process of enrichment to enhance the content of the active ingredient. After preparation of the specifications of the extract, its costing, assessment of stability and safety of the extract, its commercial manufacture is undertaken. However, before that the critical control points that can contribute to the variability of the final extract are identified. After formulation and finishing the extract is packed in appropriate containers (Kumar, 2016b). The major steps in the manufacture of the extract and its application in food fortification are presented in Figure 6.1.

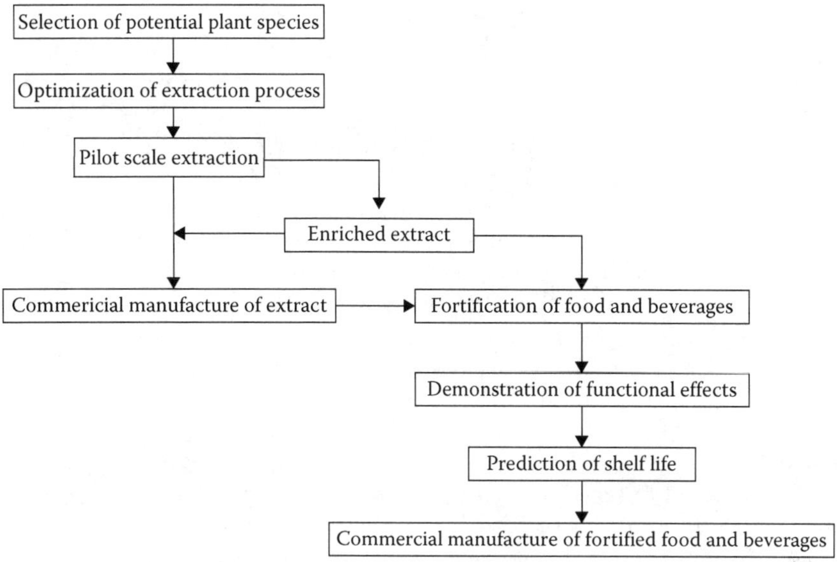

Figure 6.1 Scheme showing the major steps in food fortification with phytonutrients.

6.5.2 *Technical aspects of food fortification*

6.5.2.1 *Maintaining good taste*

Analysis of mass market response shows that though the lay public wants to consume healthy foods, it is always the taste of the fortified food that determines its repeated purchase. A consumer understands good taste in the light of attributes such as mouth feel, taste, and smell. Therefore, formulating fortified food is a really challenging task. The phytonutrients added to the food matrix may interact with other components of the food and alter its flavor. In addition to that, there is the problem of geo-cultural sensory preferences. The best way to control taste in fortified food and beverages is to select appropriate ingredients that can minimize or modify the unpleasant tastes generated during the formulation of these food and beverages (Wright et al. 2001; Chaudhari and Fanion, 2008).

6.5.2.2 *Taste challenges*

At one time, food manufacturers used to formulate healthier products by adding one or two ingredients that allowed them to promote a simple consumer message. They chose ingredients that could be easily incorporated into their product line and avoided working with ingredients that were difficult to process or were known for bad taste and aroma. Polyunsaturated fatty acids and choline are examples of ingredients that bestow nutrient value but whose smell and taste are unacceptable to many consumers. Some vitamins, such as B_1, can impart a bitter taste and sulfurous egg aroma, and minerals such as zinc, copper, and iron can give a metallic taste (Chaudhari and Fanion, 2008).

In recent years, consumer interest in fortified food has compelled manufacturers to change their old strategy. They now strive to find ways to make the difficult ingredients work. Moreover, today's consumer is looking for more complex products that are formulated to deliver a health benefit suitable to their gender, age, or to address specific health conditions such as cardiovascular and digestive problems. This means overcoming the issues of formulating and processing multiple ingredients. This necessitates finding effective means to make the functional ingredients work in the type of products consumers look forward to (Chaudhari and Fanion, 2008).

When a food formulator works with multiple functional ingredients, the core challenge facing him is the complexity of the food matrix. A food product consists of many different ingredients which when present together create a wholesome and balanced nutritional system. Many of these ingredients are multifunctional. Therefore, removing or adding new functional food ingredients may disrupt the balance of the product. Adding common nutrients in demand may affect the taste, consistency, or texture that constitute perceived product quality (Chaudhari and Fanion, 2008).

Unwanted interactions between the various components of complex foods and beverages increase the risk of deterioration of their quality. Prominent among them is moisture transfer between components with different water activity. Other interactions that can spoil the sensory quality of a product include migration of color, fats, oxygen, and other flavoring substances. These changes further challenge taste and stability of the product (Chaudhari and Fanion, 2008).

6.5.2.3 Off-flavors

Different elements in a food matrix can generate off-flavors individually. Nevertheless, some off-flavors may be generated from interaction of compounds in food during formulation or packaging. Reactions may also be stimulated by the manufacturing process (Spinnler, 2003).

Packaging used to protect the food from contamination and spoilage can also be at times a source of taints or atypical taste or odor caused by the presence of some chemicals. Plastics, plastic laminates, glass, paper board, paper plastic laminates, metal composites, metals, regenerated cellulose films, printing inks, varnishes, adhesives, and additives can be the cause of off-flavors and taints. Mostly aldehydes and ketones are responsible for taints (Lord, 2003).

Microbiological spoilage of food can be a cause of off-flavors. Since 1980, a great number of spoilage organisms and their metabolites have been identified as the cause of off-flavors in foods (Whitfield, 2003).

Oxidative rancidity can also be a source of off-flavors. Though carbohydrates and protein components of food can generate off-flavors, it is mainly the lipid part of food that gives rise to off-flavors. One simple way to prevent rancidity is to store the food in a good container and at a low temperature. Use of antioxidants such as TBHQ continues to be the most preferred method to prevent rancidity (Hamilton, 2003). However, natural antioxidants such as tocopherols, tocotrienols, flavonoids, green tea catcechins, and carnosic acid derivatives are also becoming popular (Yanishlieva-Maslareova and Heinonen, 2001).

The Maillard reaction or non-enzymatic browning is a cascade of complex, competitive reactions between amino acids, peptides, and proteins on one side and reducing sugars on the other (Arnoldi, 2003). The Maillard reaction was first reported by the French physician Louis-Camille Maillard (Maillard, 1912). In the early stage of Maillard reaction, interactions between sugars and amino groups take place first. This is followed by an intermediate stage in which fissions, cyclisations, dehydrations, condensations, and oligomerizations happen, generating flavors and off-flavors (Arnoldi, 2003).

Ingredients in the food matrix may cause reactions that produce off-flavors. Preservatives can also be a source of off-flavors, an example being sulfites in wine stimulating the synthesis of 2-aminoacetophenone that causes untypical aging off-flavor (Hoenicke et al. 2002). Antioxidants such as gallic acid can stimulate the decomposition of lipid hydroperoxides to volatile oxidation products (Spinnler, 2003). EDTA, an efficient antioxidant, can reduce the size of fat globules in mayonnaise, giving rise to off-flavors (Jacobsen et al. 2001).

Some raw materials can be a source of off-flavors in finished products, due to some microorganisms. The bacterium *Alicyclobacillus acidophilus* isolated from apple juice and orange juice can synthesize gaicol, responsible for off-flavors. Polyphenols and peptides cause bitterness in dairy products like cheese (Lemieux and Simard, 1991).

Food additives may cause off-flavors when they come in contact with enzymes and microbes. The fishy off-flavor in coffee cream is an example of such a reaction (Eyer et al. 1990). Sorbic acid, an antimicrobial, can also cause off-flavors. A kerosene off-flavor found in Feta cheese was traced to the compound1, 3-pentadiene. Bacterial activity produced this compound from decarboxylation of sorbic acid (Horwood et al. 1981).

Vanilla-flavored ice cream is unstable and on storage a cardboard off-flavor appears in the product. This off-flavor was earlier attributed to auto-oxidation of the packing material. However, it is now known that xanthine oxidase, an enzyme present in milk, is the cause. This enzyme, through a series of steps produces the flavor compounds (E)-2-nonenal or heptanal, responsible for the cardboard off-flavor (Gassenmeier, 2002). Denaturing the xanthine oxidase by heat treatment of the ice cream premix prevents the appearance of the cardboard off-flavor.

When an off-flavor appears in a food product, the compounds responsible for the off-flavor are identified through sensory, chemical, and microbiological analyses. On completion of the analyses, the formulator should identify changes in product formulation or manufacturing process and compare the defective product with products having normal flavor. The formulator also needs to have good understanding of the structure and functionality of the compounds suspected to cause off-flavors and how they can interact with the food matrix (Spinnler, 2003).

6.5.2.3.1 *Masking of off-flavors*

6.5.2.3.1.1 Use of flavoring agents Flavoring agents are added to food and beverages to make them more pleasant to consume. When a flavor is added to food, the food assumes the flavor of the added agent. In some cases, the addition of a flavor to a food or beverage supplements, fortifies, or intensifies the existing flavor of the product. Examples of such flavor potentiators are disodium-5′-inosinate, disodium-5′-guanlylate and monosodium glutamate. In yet another instance, the flavor of the product is supplanted, masked or covered up by that of the added flavorant. This is the case where a food or beverage has an undesirable flavor (Omobuwajo, 2007).

While adding flavor it is important that the flavoring meets all legal requirements pertaining to safety. The flavoring agent should not impart any undesirable flavor, odor, color, or taste to the food or beverage. It should also withstand processing conditions such as high temperature, ionizing radiation, low pressure or vacuum, and high pressure (Omobuwajo, 2007).

6.5.2.3.1.2 Use of flavor maskers Off flavors can be masked by flavor modifiers or flavor maskers. Masking agents are flavor ingredients having no smell or taste. However, they modify the flavor of food products. They modify the character of off-flavors, improve overall flavor and make the food more pleasant to consume. However, it is to be noted that there is no single ingredient that can solve all problems related to flavors. The solution lies in the right combination of different masking agents (Gascon, 2007).

Masking agents work through adaptation, cross-adaptation, taste blocking, and taste modification. If adaptation to the sweetness of sucrose lowers the sweetness intensity of another sweetener, the phenomenon is called cross-adaptation (Bartoshuk, 1987). Adaptation to one taste may lower or increase the perception threshold of other taste perceptions. It is reported that while bitter adaptation does not reduce saltiness, sour adaptation reduces bitterness (McBurney, 1974). Adaptation to citric acid and bitter substances did not reduce sweetness, but enhanced its perception (Shallenberger, 1993).

Another gustatory phenomenon helpful in the design of masking agents is taste blocking. The compound gymnemic acid present in the Indian medicinal plant *Gymnema sylvestre* suppresses the perception of sweetness (Kolodny and Kennedy, 1988). The plant is known as *gurmar* in Hindi, meaning "killer of jaggery." Lower concentrations of gymnemic acid suppress only sweetness, with no effect on sourness, saltiness, or bitterness. But at higher concentrations the compound suppresses all tastes (Kurihara, 1971).

Taste modification is another phenomenon involved in taste masking. The protein miraculin, present in the West African miracle fruit (*Synsepalum dulcificum*), by itself does not evoke a sweet response. However, it turns sour tastes into sweetness. A slice of lemon can be eaten without detecting the intense sourness (Faus and Sisniega, 2003).

Ingredients used in the formulation of masking agents are those that possess intensive sweetness and those that exhibit no sweetness. Glycyrrhizin, isolated from the plant *Gycyrrhiza glabra*, neohesperidin dihydrochalcone from citrus fruit, and thaumatin from *Thaumatococcus daniellii* are among such compounds that exhibit high- potency sweetness. Miraculin, maltol, ethyl maltol, alanine, glycine, and lysine are the other ingredients having no sweetness response. Masking agents always function as additive ingredients because they are added on top of the undesirables. It is quite possible that some of the components of a masking agent may react with other components in the food system. It is therefore necessary to evaluate the entire food or beverage system, including processing and packaging. All of these variables may affect the performance of the masking agent (Gascon, 2007).

6.5.2.4 Improving taste with texturants

The properties of a food or beverage perceived by the eyes, skin, and muscles of the mouth, including characteristics such as roughness, smoothness, and graininess, after its ingestion are collectively known as *mouthfeel* or texture. Mouthfeel is related to properties such as density, viscosity, and surface tension. Stabilizers such as carboxymethyl cellulose, gelatin, xanthan gum, alginates, and emulsifiers such as polysorbates and mono- and diglycerides, improve texture. All stabilizers hold water and give body to the finished product (Chaudhari and Fanion, 2008).

Texture of food or beverages is dependent on the number, size, shape, and arrangement of particles. The body and texture influence the consumer acceptance of the product. In addition to the regular ingredients, the particle size of specific fortificants is of great importance in imparting mouthfeel. The negative effects of particle size can be reduced by milling and micropulverizing. Particle size should be fine in the case of products with smooth mouthfeel, while large particle size will be advantageous where crunchiness is desired (Chaudhari and Fanion, 2008).

6.5.2.5 *Improving taste with encapsulation technologies*

Many food ingredients cannot be immediately incorporated into food in their regular form. These include flavors, antimicrobial agents, omega-3 fatty acids, carotenoids, phytosterols, dietary fibers, minerals, and so on. To cite an example, omega-3 fatty acids cannot be simply blended with a beverage base and water to formulate a fortified beverage, as the oil will quickly separate on account of its immiscibility. To overcome this problem omega-3 oil must be first converted into emulsified droplets, which will remain as a stable dispersion within the beverage. This technique protects such food ingredients against chemical, physical, and biological degradation, masks off-flavors, delivers them to a particular site of action, improves storage, handling, and extends shelf-life (McClements, 2012). There are several active compounds that need to be encapsulated. Some important food ingredients that are usually encapsulated for use in food industry are presented in Table 6.1.

6.5.2.5.1 *Flavors* Flavoring agents are used in foods in an encapsulated from. Such flavoring agents include salts, sugars, artificial sweeteners, vinegar, and citrus oil. Encapsulation prevents their volatilization during storage, inhibits chemical degradation, improves ease of handling, and controls the flavor release profile (McClements, 2012).

6.5.2.5.2 *Antioxidants* Antioxidants are used in food technology to slow down the rate of lipid oxidation. The hydrophilic, lipophilic, or amphiphilic nature of the antioxidant determines its location and environment within the food system. Encapsulation of antioxidants improves their ease of handling, enhances compatibility with the food matrix, and prevents chemical degradation. β-carotene can be encapsulated to prevent its exposure to light and oxygen (McClements, 2012)

6.5.2.5.3 *Antimicrobials* Antimicrobials, which are used to inhibit the growth of bacteria and mold, work through different mechanisms such as transition metal chelation and membrane disruption. Encapsulation of antimicrobials increases their compatibility with the food matrix, improves efficacy, controls release, masks off-flavors, and increases ease of storage, transport, and use (McClements, 2012).

6.5.2.5.4 *Bioactive lipids* Bioactive lipids such as acylglycerols, fatty acids, phospholipids, carotenoids, phytosterols, and oil-soluble vitamins

Table 6.1 Some important food ingredients that are usually encapsulated for use in the food industry

Category	Ingredient	Advantages of encapsulation
Flavors	Citrus oils	Allows integration into aqueous medium
		Facilitates storage
		Slows down chemical degradation
		Controls flavor release profile
Antimicrobials	Essential oils	Improves matrix compatibility
		Enables storage and utilization
		Slows down chemical degradation
		Masks off-flavors
		Increases potency
Antioxidants	Carotenoids	Facilitates incorporation into aqueous medium
		Enables storage
		Slows down chemical degradation
		Improves efficacy
Bioactive carbohydrates	Dietary fibers	Improves textural properties
		Enables delivery
		Increases stability

Source: From McClements, D.J., *Encapsulation Technologies and Delivery Systems for Food Ingredients and Nutraceuticals*, Woodhead Publishing Ltd, Cambridge, England, 2012

are encapsulated. Low water solubility, high melting point, and chemical instability make their encapsulation challenging (McClements, 2012).

6.5.2.5.5 Bioactive carbohydrates Dietary fibers are the major class of bioactive carbohydrates that need to be incorporated into food. They are known to reduce cholesterol, modulate blood glucose levels, prevent some types of cancers, and prevent constipation (Redgwell and Fischer, 2005). Dietary fibers form colloidal solutions, affecting the texture of food. They are, therefore, encapsulated for efficient delivery (McClements, 2012).

6.5.2.5.6 Fabrication of delivery systems Delivery systems for active components can be fabricated from different materials such as lipids, surfactants, proteins, carbohydrates, minerals, and water, using many kinds of different processing operations. In the food industry, the ingredients used to construct delivery systems should be food grade and inexpensive. Additionally, the fabrication method must be cost-effective, reproducible, and robust (McClements, 2012).

The methods used to fabricate delivery systems can be classified into different groups such as top-down, bottom-up, or combination methods. In the top-down method a bulk material is broken down into smaller particles that form the delivery system. An example is homogenization of oil and water to form microscopic oil droplets dispersed in water. Such methods can be primarily characterized according to the processing operation used to reduce the size. Delivery systems are prepared by assembling molecules or colloidal particles into particulate structures in bottom-up methods. The assembly process may be spontaneous, as in micelle formation, or directed, as in the electrostatic deposition. Most of the methods developed to create delivery systems are in fact combinations of the topdown and bottom-up approaches. Multilayer emulsions, for example, are formed by blending bulk oil and water phases together in the presence of a charged emulsifier to form an emulsion using a homogenizer (top-down), and then adopting electrostatic deposition to coat the resulting droplets with a biopolymer (bottom-up) (McClements, 2012).

6.5.2.5.7 Applications of encapsulated ingredients The characteristics of phytonutrients intended for food fortification can be improved with encapsulation technology. Acidulants such as malic acid, citric acid, fumaric acid, and tartaric acid are used as flavor modifiers, preservatives, or processing aids (Debevere, 1988; Berry, 2001; Resch et al., 2005). Food acids that are unencapsulated may undergo degradation by heat and pH. They can also interact with other ingredients during formulation and processing, causing undesirable effects such as reduced shelf-life, loss of flavor, color degradation, and separation of ingredients. Microencapsulation overcomes these undesirable effects and improves physical properties and handling characteristics of the phytonutrient (Augustin and Sanguansri, 2012).

Fumaric acid is used to lower the pH of tortilla (a type of soft, thin flatbread made from finely ground wheat, popular in South America), permitting calcium propionate and sorbic acid to work as effective antimicrobials, improving the shelf-life. Encapsulation of fumaric acid prevents its release during the preparation of dough, providing increased dough extensibility and leavening time (LaBell, 1999; Augustin and Sanguansri, 2012).

Phytonutrients require delivery systems to mask their unpleasant odor and taste and safeguard them from degradation during processing and storage. Encapsulated phytonutrients can be added to foods at high concentrations without affecting organoleptic properties. The undesirable sensory properties of ginseng in beverages have been masked using cyclodextrins (Tamamoto et al. 2010). Encapsulation by spray drying in a maltodextrin/apple pectin-based matrix was used successfully to mask the unpleasant odor of functional extracts from *Fadogia ancylantha, Melissa officinalis,* and *Tussilago farfara* (Sansone et al. 2011).

Lutein is a phytonutrient beneficial to the eye. However, it is sensitive to light, oxygen, and moisture. When encapsulated in complex coacervates of gelatin and gellan gum, lutein was less susceptible to degradation in light and humid conditions than unencapsulated lutein (Qv et al; 2011).

Esmaili et al. (2011) studied the use of β-casein micelles as a carrier system for a hydrophobic compound like curcumin. Loading curcumin into β-casein micelles enhanced its stability, bioavailability, and antioxidant activity.

6.5.2.5.8 Encapsulation of phytonutrients During processing of food, storage, distribution, and consumption, food components are prone to degradation and destruction by exposure to the adverse surrounding environments, reducing their functionality. This is especially true in the case of bioactive components. Many food components can react with others, causing alteration or loss of functional properties (Fang and Bhandari, 2012). For example, polyphenols can combine with proteins to form complexes of colloidal nature, causing turbidity of beverages and limiting the shelf-life of the product (Siebert et al; 1996; Siebert, 1999). In the production of juices, beer, and wine, polyphenols may cause the formation of protein precipitates and the appearance of negative sensory characteristics (Galloa et al. 2013). Some bioactive components of food have undesirable taste and flavor even in their natural forms. Therefore, there is a need to protect these ingredients throughout their shelf-life without jeopardizing the sensory properties of the food (Fang and Bhandari, 2012).

Microencapsulation is used for protection and delivery of food components in fortified food. Microencapsulation is a process of packaging or immobilizing an active (core) material in a state of solid, liquid, or gas, within a more stable, protective secondary (wall) material that can be released at controlled rates under specific conditions. Several techniques are available for encapsulation of food ingredients and phytonutrients. Encapsulation technique for a specific application is selected based on parameters such as mean particle size required, physical and chemical properties of both core and coating materials, application of the microencapsulated material, release mechanisms employed, scale-up potential of the process, and cost-effectiveness (Fang and Bhandari, 2012).

It should however, be noted that none of the available techniques can be considered universally applicable processes. Individual food ingredients demonstrate great differences in molecular weight, polarity, solubility, and stability, implying that different encapsulation approaches have to be adopted to meet the specific physicochemical and molecular requirements for a particular phytonutrient (Augustin and Sanguansri, 2008; Fang and Bhandari, 2012). Encapsulants (materials used for enclosing the phytonutrient) to be used in food fortification are selected from a wide range of natural food components such as proteins, sugars, starches, gums, lipids, cellulosic material, or other ingredients that have generally regarded as safe (GRAS) status. Examples are cyclodextrin, chitosan, low-molecular weight emulsifiers such as Tweens, and mineral salts. They are used alone or in combination. The composition of the encapsulant and processing technology significantly influences the functional properties of the final microcapsule (Augustin and Sanguansri, 2008).

6.5.2.5.8.1 Physical processes

6.5.2.5.8.1.1 Spray drying Spray drying is most commonly used in the food industry to encapsulate polyphenols, probiotics, fats, oils, flavors, essential oils, and other oil-soluble phytonutrients. Water-soluble ingredients can also be encapsulated by spray drying. In this process the core material is first dispersed into a solution of the encapsulant such as protein or carbohydrate. The mixture is thereafter atomized into the drying chamber. Water from the mixture evaporates and powder microcapsules are formed. For encapsulating oils and oil-soluble phytonutrients, an emulsion is prepared before spray drying. By adjusting and controlling the processing conditions, microcapsules with desired powder properties such as particle size, moisture content, bulk density, flowability, dispersibility, appearance, and structural strength can be obtained (Reineccius 2001; Augustin and Sanguansri, 2008; Fang and Bhandari, 2012).

6.5.2.5.8.1.2 Spray chilling Spray chilling (spray cooling, spray congealing) is widely used in the pharmaceutical industry. However, in the food industry it is gaining popularity. Spray cooling technology can be divided into two steps. In the first step, the bioactive compound is added to the carrier material, which is a lipophilic material such as palm oil, beeswax, or cocoa butter. The incorporation is achieved by mechanically dispersing the bioactive compound into the encapsulating matrix. The second step involves atomization of the mixed material through a heated atomizing nozzle into a refrigerated chamber. Due to heat transfer between the molten material and the cold air, solidification of the carrier takes place and particles are formed (Killeen, 1993). The droplets stay in the spray cooling chamber only for a few seconds. The fine particles are transported by air into a cyclone and stored in another vessel (Figure 6.2). Spray chilling technology is simple to apply and scale up, without involving the use of organic solvents (Okuro et al. 2013).

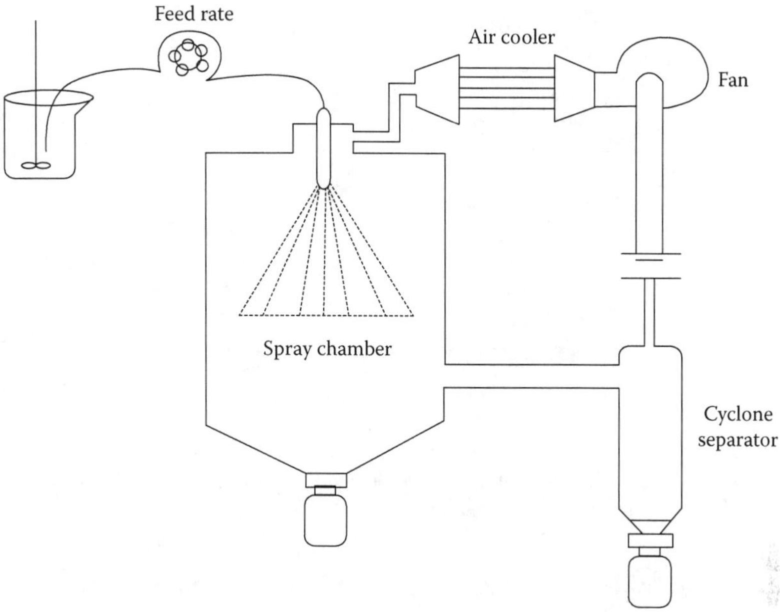

Figure 6.2 Spray chilling equipment. (Reproduced with permission from Okuro, P.K. et al. *Food Technol. Biotechnol.* 51: 171–182, 2013.)

6.5.2.5.8.1.3 Fluidized bed coating Spray drying produces no uniform microcapsules. It produces very fine powder which needs further processing. Moreover, the technique is not suitable for heat-sensitive materials. To overcome these problems, spray drying powders can be agglomerated using fluidized bed technology, which is a three step-process (Madene et al. 2006).

First, the particles to be coated are fluidized in the hot atmosphere of the coating chamber. Thereafter, the coating material is sprayed onto the particles and formation of film is initiated. This is followed by a succession of wetting and drying stages. Small droplets of the sprayed liquid spread on the surface of the particles and merge. The solvent is evaporated by hot air and the coating material adheres to the surface of the particles (Figure 6.3) (Madene et al. 2006). Chua and Chou (2003) are of the opinion that the fluidized bed technology is a low-cost drying technology for developing countries, when compared to other state-of-the-art technologies

6.5.2.5.8.1.4 Centrifugal Extrusion Encapsulation Centrifugal extrusion encapsulation (coaxial extrusion processing) is a liquid coextrusion process. It uses an assembly of cylindrical nozzles consisting of concentric orifices located at the outer circumference of a rotating

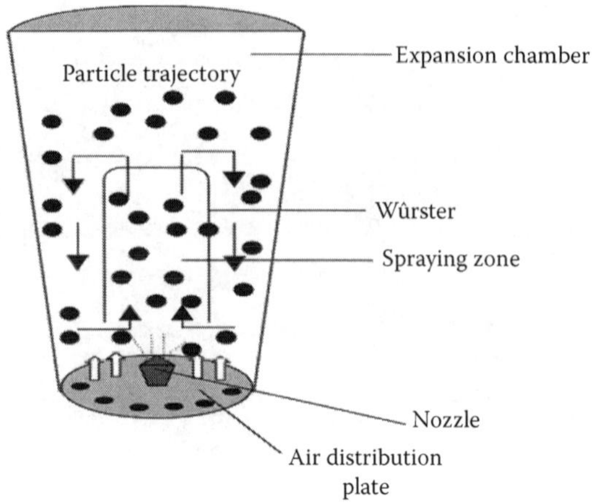

Figure 6.3 Fluidized bed coating. (Reproduced with permission from Madene, A. et al. *Int. J. Food Sci. Tech.* 41: 1–21, 2006.)

cylinder. A liquid bioactive core is pumped through the inner orifice, and the liquid encapsulant material is pumped through the outer orifice both of which are located in the cylindrical head. During this process a co-extruded liquid jet of the bioactive core material is surrounded by the encapsulant. During the rotation of the cylindrical head the extruded liquid jet breaks into droplets and forms microcapsules. Various techniques such as drying, cooling, chelation, gelation, chemical reaction, and cross-linking are adopted for hardening the microcapsules, depending on the nature of the encapsulant material (Augustin and Sanguansri, 2008).

This encapsulation technology is suitable for specialty applications requiring protection of food ingredients. It offers a process for formulating with a variety of shell materials such as gelatin, alginates, carrageenan, starches, fats, and waxes. For obtaining the desired characteristics, shell systems consisting of a blend of two or more polymers may be used (Schlameus, 1995).

6.5.2.5.8.1.5 Spinning-disk coating Spinning-disk coating (centrifugal suspension-separation coating) is a physical coating process involving the suspension of solid core particles in a liquid encapsulating material (Sparks et al. 1995). The encapsulant formulation may be a solution, suspension, or a molten material, applied directly without using any solvents. The core suspension is then passed over a rotating disk to form a thin film around the core particles (Augustin and Sanguansri, 2008).

6.5.2.5.8.1.6 Pressure extrusion Extrusion processes make use of the application of pressure to a mass to make it flow through an orifice under controlled conditions. A droplet generator and a droplet hardening bath are the important parts of an extruder (Rabiskova 2001). Microencapsulation by extrusion involves projecting an emulsion of the core and coating materials through a die at high pressure (Augustin and Sanguansri, 2008).

6.5.2.5.8.1.7 ***Hot melt extrusion*** Hot melt extrusion (HME) is the technology of applying heat and pressure to melt a polymer and force it though an orifice in a continuous process. HME was developed in the 1930's to produce polymer products of uniform shape and density. HME is used in the pharmaceutical industry to mix active pharmaceutical ingredients with polymers to enhance the ingredient's bioavailability (Crowley et al., 2007; Tiwari et al., 2016). More recently this technology has been applied in the food industry.

HME has been applied to the entrapment of flavors for their controlled release and masking the grittiness of minerals and vitamins. HME has unique advantages, such as extruders being multifaceted systems that can provide optimum processing temperature and shear rates by varying screw design, barrel heating, mixing speed, feed rate, moisture content, and plasticizers. Actives and other ingredients can be incorporated at different points of the extrusion process. The encapsulated products can be recovered in desired shapes or sizes such as pellets, rods, and ropes (Lakkis, 2016).

In a typical extrusion encapsulation process, the encapsulating matrix (a mixture of sucrose and maltodextrin) is dry-fed and melted by applying heat and shear in the extruder barrel. During this process the crystalline structure is transformed into amorphous phase. The flavor or active ingredient is added through an orifice in a cooled barrel situated toward the die end of the barrel. The amorphous mixture leaves the die in the form of a rope that is cooled quickly by air or liquid nitrogen to form a solid and glassy material. This material can be ground to compact microparticles with desired particle size (Lakkis, 2016).

6.5.2.5.8.1.8 ***Supercritical fluid technology*** Encapsulation of heat-sensitive core materials can be achieved using supercritical fluids. The supercritical encapsulation techniques are based on the solubilization of active compounds and wall materials in supercritical fluids, more commonly, supercritical CO_2. In the rapid expansion of a supercritical solution (RESS) process, a dispersion of the active compound and dissolved or swollen shell material is prepared in the supercritical fluid. As supercritical CO_2 is nonpolar in nature only shell materials such as fat or wax will solubilize in it. The homogeneous mixture is thereafter rapidly expanded in a container at atmospheric pressure. On account of the sudden change in pressure, the supercritical fluid loses its solvent power and the dissolved material precipitates (Jung and Perrut, 2001; Silva and Meireles, 2014).

The RESS technique is suitable only for compounds having low polarity or moderate solubility in supercritical CO_2. Therefore, a modified method was developed. It included the addition of a cosolvent to increase the solubility of the solute in supercritical CO_2. The method is known as rapid expansion of a supercritical solution with a nonsolvent (RESS-N) process. Another method applied a liquid solvent in the precipitation container to prevent the growth of particles during jet expansion and thus obtain smaller particles. This is the rapid expansion of a supercritical solution in a liquid solvent (RESOLV) process. Still another one specifically used an aqueous solution containing a surfactant instead of a liquid solvent as a stabilizing agent. This method is known as Rapid expansion of a supercritical solution in an aqueous solution (RESSAS) process (Silva and Meireles, 2014).

The supercritical encapsulation process using supercritical CO_2 has limited application in the area of food technology, as substances such as fats, vegetable oils, and vitamins are only moderately soluble in supercritical CO_2 (Weidner, 2009). Some isolated food ingredients, such as rutin and a jabuticaba-skin extract which is rich in anthocyanins, have been encapsulated using the RESS-N approach. In this method, polyethylene glycol was used as the wall material and ethanol was the cosolvent (Santos and Meireles, 2013; Santos et al. 2013).

6.5.2.5.8.2 Chemical processes

6.5.2.5.8.2.1 Coacervation Coacervation is the phase separation in colloidal systems, resulting in a more concentrated phase which is known as the coacervate. Coacervation can be simple or complex. In simple coacervation, separation of phases is achieved by adding a desolvating agent such as alcohol or salt. Phase separation can also be achieved by altering temperature or pH. However, simple coacervation is used seldom to encapsulate active ingredients.

Coacervation has three basic steps. First, phase separation occurs in a suspension or emulsion of active ingredient, leading to a three-phase system consisting of a polymer-rich liquid phase (coacervate), a polymer-poor liquid phase, and a solid or liquid phase containing the active ingredient. Second, the coacervate phase is deposited onto the dispersed particles. Finally, the coating is hardened (Zuidam and Shimoni, 2010).

Complex coacervates can be made from an o/w emulsion of gelatin and gum arabic at a 1:1 w/w ratio and at a 2%–4% w/w of each polymer dissolved in the water phase while adjusting the pH from neutral to about 4 with stirring at a temperature above 35°C. Consequently, three immiscible phases (oil, polymer-rich, and polymer-poor phase) will be formed and the polymer-rich phase droplets will deposit on the emulsion surfaces. Factors such as concentrations of the polymers, pH, turbulence of the system, size of the emulsion, ionic strength, and temperature affect the preparation process. After cooling, the shell can be cross-linked with glutaraldehyde or transglutaminase. The coacervates are then isolated, washed, and dried by spray-drying or fluid bed drying. Gum arabic can be replaced by other negatively charged molecules such as carboxymethylcellulose, pectin, carrageenan, alginate and alginate derivatives, or polyphosphate. Similarly gelatin can be replaced by whey (Zuidam and Shimoni, 2010).

6.5.2.5.8.2.2 ***Solvent evaporation*** Solvent evaporation technique has been applied successfully to develop polymeric microcapsules containing drugs (Suzuki and Price, 1985; Jalil and Nixon, 1990; Wang and Schwendeman, 1999). Several variables such as solubility of the active ingredient, internal morphology, type of solvent, diffusion rate, temperature, polymer composition, and viscosity can influence the properties of the microspheres (Bodmeier and McGinity, 1988a; 1988b; Jalil and Nixon, 1990; Bodmeier et al. 1994; Jaraswekin et al. 2007). The efficiency of solvent evaporation method is dependent on the successful entrapment of the active ingredient within the particles. Therefore, the technique is most successful with ingredients that are either insoluble or poorly soluble in water, which forms the continuous phase (Bodmeier and McGinity, 1987). The choice of solvent evaporation method that can encapsulate efficiently depends on the hydrophilicity or hydrophobicity of the active ingredient (Muhaimin, 2013).

6.5.2.5.8.2.3 ***Single emulsion process*** This process makes use of oil-in-water (O/W) emulsification. The O/W emulsion consists of an organic phase composed of a volatile solvent with dissolved polymer and the active to be encapsulated, emulsified in an aqueous phase containing a dissolved surfactant. For insoluble or sparingly water-soluble ingredients, the O/W method is frequently used. This method is a simple one. It has four major steps (Figure 6.4). First, the hydrophobic ingredient is dissolved in an organic solvent containing the polymer. This organic phase,

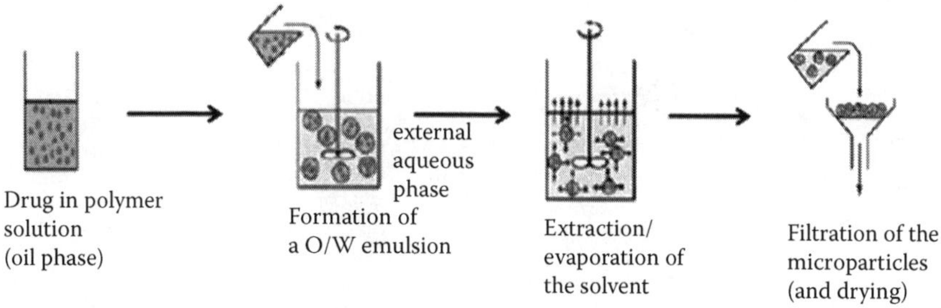

Figure 6.4 A schematic overview of the four principal steps in microsphere preparation by single emulsion method. (Reproduced with permission from Muhaimin, M., Study of microparticle preparation by the solvent evaporation method using Focused Beam Reflectance Measurement [FBRM]. Dissertation for the academic degree of Doktors der Naturwissenschaften, Freie Universität Berlin, 2013.)

called the dispersed phase, is emulsified in an aqueous phase called the continuous phase. The solvent from the dispersed phase is extracted by the continuous phase, accompanied by solvent evaporation. During this process, droplets of the dispersed phase are transformed into solid particles. Finally the microspheres are recovered and dried to remove the residual solvent (Muhaimin, 2013).

6.5.2.5.8.2.4 Double emulsion process The O/W method is not suitable for the encapsulation of actives with high hydrophilicity. An alternative is too employ the water-in-oil-in water (W/O/W) emulsion process (Figure 6.5). An aqueous solution of the active is added to an organic phase composed of the polymer and organic solvent with vigorous stirring to form the first W/O emulsion. This emulsion is then dispersed in another aqueous phase having more surfactant and forms the W/O/W emulsion. A number of hydrophilic actives have been successfully encapsulated by this method (Muhaimin, 2013).

6.5.2.5.8.2.5 Liposomes Liposomes have been used in the pharmaceutical industry for drug delivery. However, they also have many applications in the food industry (Taylor et al. 2005). They are hollow spheres whose size can range from a few nanometers to a few microns. Liposomes are generally made from molecules of phospholipid. The polar head group of phospholipid is water soluble (hydrophilic) and the fatty acid chain is oil-like (hydrophobic). So when phospholipid is added to water, the water soluble part interacts with water and the oily part avoids water (Mirafzali et al. 2014).

The phospholipids align themselves side by side with their oil-like portions orienting themselves toward each other. This is known as a

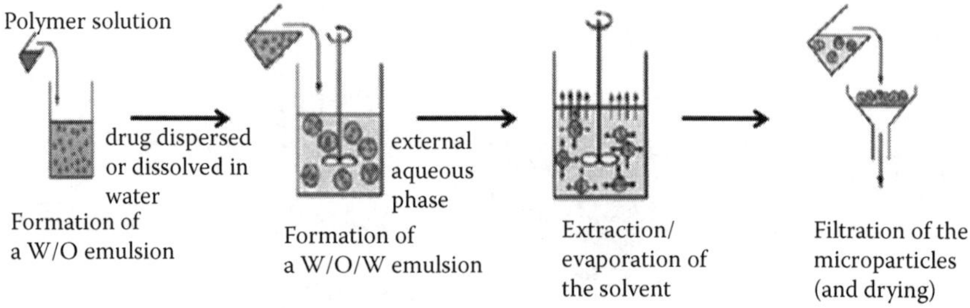

Figure 6.5 Schematic overview of the four principal process steps in microsphere preparation by the double emulsion method. (Reproduced with permission from Muhaimin, M., Study of microparticle preparation by the solvent evaporation method using focused beam reflectance measurement [FBRM]. Dissertation for the academic degree of Doktors der Naturwissenschaften, Freie Universität Berlin, 2013.)

phospholipid bilayer. This bilayer extends itself in water like a sheet, and then curls into a liposome. The inside of liposomes is filled with water and therefore water soluble molecules can be encapsulated inside the liposome. A very important property of liposomes is that molecules that are not water soluble but oil-like can be entrapped in the oil-like part of the phospholipid bilayer. Thus liposomes can act as carriers for water soluble as well as water-insoluble compounds (Morafzali et al. 2014).

Liposomes can be formed from a single type of phospholipid or by mixtures of different phospholipids. By varying the types of phospholipids they can be engineered for many useful properties. The properties of liposomes can be changed by adding non-phospholipid components such as cholesterol, fatty acids, and other lipid soluble compounds (Mirafzali et al. 2014).

One major application of liposomes in the food and nutraceutical industry is their ability to dissolve both water-soluble and lipid-soluble molecules at the same time. An example is tocopherol and ascorbic acid, two powerful antioxidants. Ascorbic acid can be encapsulated inside the core of liposome and tocopherol into the lipid bilayers of the liposomes. One liposome can contain both compounds and can deliver them at the same time (Mirafzali et al. 2014).

Liposomes have been successfully used to deliver oil soluble bioactives. Banville et al. (2000) reported that incorporation of Vitamin D was improved with the use of liposomes. However, after storage for 3-5 months the stability of encapsulated Vitamin D was diminished. Liposomal encapsulation of several phytonutrients such as lutein, β-carotene, lycopene, canthaxanthin (Tan et al. 2013; 2014), curcumin (Jin et al. 2016), resveratrol (Balanč et al. 2015), rutin, and naringenin (Kerdudo et al. 2014) have been reported.

6.5.2.5.8.2.6 Inclusion complexation Cyclodextrins have the ability to form inclusion complexes (Muñoz-Botella et al. 1995; Hedges, 1998; Baudin et al. 2000; Kumar et al. 2001; Koukiekolo et al. 2001; Lu and Chen, 2002). Cyclodextrin is a molecule with hydrophilic outside that can dissolve in water, and a nonpolar cavity that provides a hydrophobic matrix or a micro-heterogeneous environment (Figure. 6.6). Because of this cavity, cyclodextrins can form inclusion complexes with many kinds of hydrophobic guest molecules such as fats, flavors, and colors (Figure 6.7) (Del Valle, 2004). Cyclodextrins are used in food industry for flavor protection and flavor delivery. Most of the flavors are volatile oils or liquids and complexation with cyclodextrins offers an alternative to encapsulation for flavor protection. Cyclodextrins protect the flavor molecules during rigorous food processing methods such as freezing, thawing, and microwaving. Thus they allow flavor quality and quantity to be preserved for a longer period compared to other encapsulants. For more than two decades cyclodextrins have been used in Japan as modified starch for food applications.

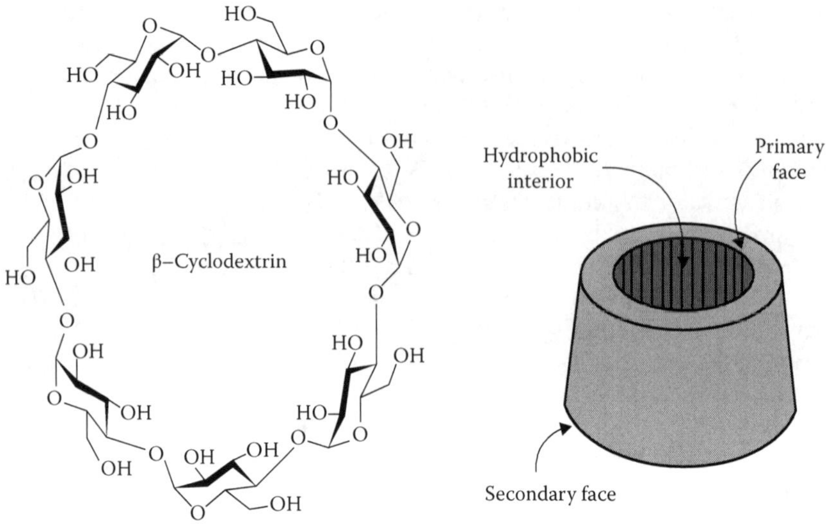

Figure 6.6 Chemical structure of β–cyclodextrin. (Reproduced with permission from Del Valle, E. M. M., *Process Biochem.* 39:1033–1046, 2004.)

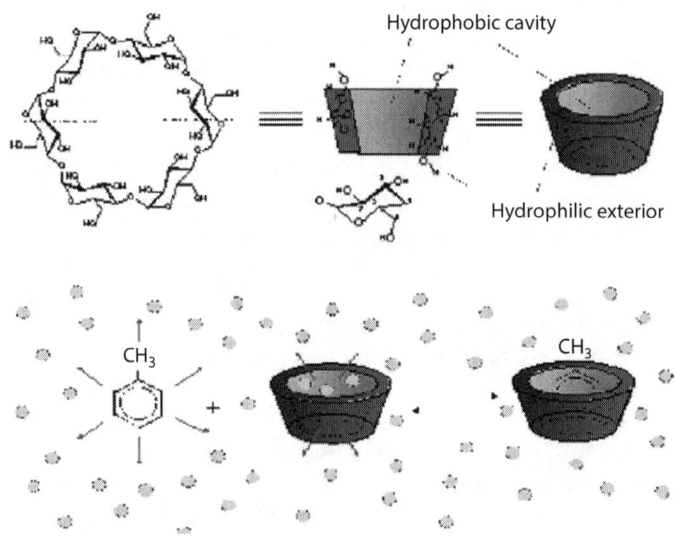

Figure 6.7 Structure of β–cyclodextrin and inclusion complex formation. (Reproduced with permission from Del Valle, E. M. M., *Process Biochem.* 39:1033–1046, 2004.)

6.6 Demonstration of functional effects

In order to give a stamp of authenticity to the functional food product, it is necessary to prove its functional nature using objective parameters. This can be accomplished by assessing the potential of the functional food in modifying target functions, as these target functions are directly related to a state of improved health or reduced proneness to a disease. All markers, whether they are biochemical, physiological, or behavioral in nature, should be *feasible, valid, reproducible, sensitive,* and *specific* (Anonymous, 1999; Nowicka and Naruszewicz, 2004). Ultrasound measures, anthropometric measures and bone mineral density can be the possible markers for skeletal development. Growth and body composition can be judged by anthropometry, body fat mass, total body water, procollagen propeptide excretion, and urinary creatinine excretion. Similarly, cellular and noncellular immune markers can assess immune function (Anonymous, 1999).

The functional nature of many fortified foods has been proven in this way. Jensen et al. (2011) conducted an open-label, clinical pilot study to assess the effect of oral consumption of a fruit and berry blend on pain and range of motion (ROM). The study involved 14 study participants. Study participants consumed 120 mL of MonaVie Active fruit juice daily for 12 weeks. Participants were assessed at baseline and 2, 4, 8, and 12 weeks by structured nurse interviews, questionnaires of pain and activities of daily living (ADL), blood samples, and ROM assessment. Composite ROM and strength evaluation were carried out using J-Tech Tracker Freedom system that employs dual digital inclinometry protocols of the American Medical Association and wireless instruments. Serum antioxidant status was monitored by the cell-based antioxidant protection in erythrocytes (CAP-e) assay. Serum lipid peroxidation and high- C-reactive protein were also measured. The study demonstrated significant pain reduction following consumption of the beverage.

Hongu et al. (2014) investigated the dietary effect of pigmented rice bran with or without plant sterols on lipid profiles during energy restriction–induced weight loss in overweight and obese adults not on cholesterol-lowering medication. Additionally, the study investigated the effect of the intervention on biomarkers of oxidative stress and inflammation. Twenty-four overweight and obese adults were randomized to a 25% calorie-restricted diet containing either pigmented rice bran (RB) or the RB with addition of plant sterols snack bars for 8 weeks. Anthropometrics, blood pressure, blood lipids, glucose, urinary F_2-isoprostanes, C-reactive protein, insulin, and leptin were measured at baseline and after 8 weeks of intervention. The study showed that a nutrient-balanced and energy-restricted diet supplemented with rice bran and plant sterols caused a significant decrease in total and LDL cholesterol in overweight and obese adults.

In order to confirm whether biscuits could be a good matrix to deliver hydroxytyrosol, the compound found predominantly in olive leaves, Mateos et al. (2016) performed a crossover, randomized, double-blind study. On two separate days, 13 subjects consumed 30g of non-enriched biscuits or hydroxytyrosol-enriched biscuits (5.25mg hydroxytyrosol) after overnight-fasting. Blood and urine collected at different intervals were analyzed by accurate-mass quadrupole time-of-flight LC/MS. After consumption of the hydroxytyrosol-enirched biscuits, levels of plasma metabolites rose between 0.5 and 1h and were extensively excreted in urine. Hydroxytyrosol sulfate and 3,4-dihydroxyphenylacetic acid sulfate were the main metabolites, followed by several minor ones. Consumption of the enriched biscuits reduced postprandial oxidised-LDL concentrations, suggesting that hydroxytyrosol is a promising functional ingredient that can be used in the fortification of biscuits, to prevent LDL oxidation.

As the market for functional foods grows, communication of the advantages of such foods becomes important. Health benefits of functional foods can be communicated through health professionals, educators, the media, and the food industry. Of all forms of communication, the various claims made on the label or package or supporting information are the most important. It is essential that such claims be based on unbiased scientific information and are valid, unambiguous, and clear to the consumer (Anonymous, 1999). The term *health claims* is defined differently in different countries. But the widely accepted definition is that of Codex Alimentarius (1991). Codex Alimentarius (1997) has classified and defined four different forms of claims. They are claims related to dietary guidelines, nutrient content claims, comparative claims, and nutrient function claims (Anonymous, 1999). In addition to these four, the European Commission Concerted Action on Functional Food Science in Europe (FUFOSE) supports the development of two further claims—Type A enhanced function claims and Type B reduction of disease risk claims (Anonymous, 1999; Roberfroid, 2005). An example of Type A claims is the statement that caffeine can improve cognitive performance. The statement "Folate can reduce a woman's risk of having a child with neural tube defects" or "Sufficient calcium intake may help to reduce the risk of osteoporosis in later life" are examples of Type B claims (Anonymous, 1999).

A working group of FAO/WHO met in London, Ontario, Canada on April 30 and May 1, 2002 and prepared a joint report on the conditions for health claims for probiotics (microorganisms that are believed to confer health benefit when ingested). The requirements indicated in this document impose on manufacturers the obligation to conduct placebo-controlled clinical studies and to evaluate their results in four phases such as Phase 1 (safety), Phase 2 (efficiency), Phase 3 (effectiveness) and Phase 4 (surveillance). If the manufacturer receives positive results from one research center, the findings should be confirmed by other investigators and the results are to be published in peer-reviewed journals (Anonymous, 2006). Nowicka and Naruszewicz (2004) are of the opinion that similar conditions are to be imposed with respect to all fortified foods.

6.7 Bioavailability of nutraceuticals

Bioactives extracted from herbs are, in many cases, complex mixtures of organic compounds that are difficult to purify. In addition to that many of these ingredients are insoluble in water and their incorporation into aqueous food matrices is a formidable challenge. Both water extracts and organic solvent extracts are used in the formulation of fortified food and beverages. Most of the organic solvent extracts are not soluble in food-grade solvents or in vegetable oils. In some cases they may not dissolve either in water or oil. The nutritional effects of the fortified food and beverage depend very much on the bioavailability of the extracted bioactives used in their formulation (Garti and Yuli-Amar, 2008).

When a fortified food or beverage is consumed by individuals, the degree and duration of the physiological response evoked may vary. The physical form of the product (liquid, soft solid, hard solid, paste, etc.) may also result in partial absorption of the bioactives. There are several definitions for bioavailability. However, Garti and Yuli-Amar (2008) define bioavailability as the fraction of an ingested nutrient available for utilization in normal physiological functions or for storage.

Bioavailability of nutraceuticals is assessed mainly by measuring the component in serum or plasma (Castenmiller and West, 1998; Bramley et al., 2000). The nutraceutical is solubilized in the bile salts present in small intestine and absorbed. It is then bound to chylomicrons and secreted into the intestinal lymph en route to different tissues (van het Hof et al. 1998). Some factors affect the overall bioavailability of the bioactive by interfering with the rates of each absorption step. For example, the molecular configuration (*cis/trans*) of the bioactives is important. The bioavailability of *cis*-isomer is more than that of the *trans*-isomer. This is because the *cis*-isomer has greater solubility in mixed micelles and have lower tendency to aggregate (Castenmiller and West, 1998; Bramley et al., 2000). Particle size reduction is another factor that improves bioavailability. This is evidenced by increased bioavailability of lycopene when tomato is made into a paste (Paiva and Russel, 1999). The matrix of the fortified food also affects bioavailability. For example, the relative bioavailability of lutein is lower from green leafy vegetables than from other vegetables. This may be because lutein is entrapped and complexed to proteins in chloroplasts within the leaf cell (van het Hof et al. 1998). Ingestion of the fortified food along with vegetable oils improves bioavailability (van het Hof et al. 1998; 2000). As bile salts are required for the absorption of the compounds, bioactives administered as dietary supplements should be taken along with food and not on an empty stomach, as ingestion of food stimulates bile secretion (Gallo-Torres, 1970).

6.7.1 The NuBACS

From a review of the major factors influencing the gastrointestinal fate of nutraceuticals, McClements et al. (2015) proposed a new classification scheme—the nutraceutical bioavailability classification scheme—to characterize the major factors that limit their oral bioavailability. The authors were encouraged to develop NuBACS by the success of the biopharmaceutical classification scheme (BCS) widely used in pharmaceutical industry to characterize the major factors that limit the oral bioavailability of drugs, such as low solubility or permeability (Amidon et al. 1995; Dahan et al. 2009). NuBACS categorizes the factors limiting the bioavailability of nutraceuticals into three groups based on their bioaccessibility, absorption and transformation inside the gastrointestinal tract (McClements et al. 2015; Table 6.2). Each of these three major classes has subclasses related to specific physicochemical and physiological changes influencing bioavailability (McClements et al., 2015).

In the NuBACS a bioactive compound with bioavailability above 75% can be classified as $B^*(+)$. Similarly, a bioactive compound with poor bioavailability may be classified as $B^*(-)_L$, $B^*(-)_S$ or $B(-)^*_I$ depending on whether the bioaccessibility is limited by liberation, solubilization or interactions. The absorption of a bioactive compound by the epithelial lining of gastrointestinal tract may be limited by one or more factors, based on its molecular and physiological properties. To cite an example, a bioactive compound may be classified as $A^*(-)_{ML}$, $A^*(-)_{BP}$, $A^*(-)_{TJ}$, $A^*(-)_{AT}$, or $A^*(-)_{ET}$

Table 6.2 The nutraceutical bioavailability classification scheme (NuBACS)

Major classes	Subclasses
Bioaccessibility (B*)	Liberation
	Solubilization
	Interactions
Absorption (A*)	Mucus layer
	Tight junction transport
	Bilayer permeability
	Active transporters
	Efflux transporters
Transformation (T*)	Chemical transformations
	Metabolism

Source: From McClements, D.J., et al., *Annual Review of Food Science and Technology* 6:13.1–13.29, 2015.

when its absorption is limited respectively by mucus layer transport, bilayer permeability, tight junctions, active transporters, or efflux transporters. Similarly, a bioactive compound may be classified as $T^*(-)_C$, $T^*(-)_M$, or $T^*(-)_{CM}$ if its bioaccessibility is limited respectively by chemical degradation, metabolism, or both. Information on the mechanisms limiting the bioavailability of a nutraceutical helps in the effective design of delivery system and food matrices that enhance its bioavailability (McClements et al., 2015).

6.7.2 *Improving oral bioavailability of bioactives*

In spite of their ability to reduce risks of multiple chronic diseases, many bioactives have poor oral bioavailability, which lowers their value as disease-preventing agents (Porter et al., 2007; McClements, 2013; McClements and Xiao, 2014; Yao et al., 2014). The latest and effective way to enhance oral bioavailability of bioactives is to utilize nanotechnology to encapsulate them in engineered nanoparticles (ENs)-based delivery systems (Porter et al., 2008; McClements, 2010; Yao et al., 2014). Depending on the presence or absence of lipids as the major components of the systems, ENs can be grouped as lipid-based or non-lipid-based (Yao et al., 2015; Table 6.3). It is to be noted that unlike the ENs employed in the pharmaceutical industry, ENs for the food industry have to be manufactured with 100% food grade ingredients such as edible lipids, proteins, carbohydrates, and surfactants. This has considerably increased the challenges in developing effective delivery systems (Yao et al., 2015).

6.7.2.1 *ENs improve bioaccessibility*

During its movement through the mouth, stomach, and small intestine, a bioactive compound is exposed to considerable changes in the composition, structure, and flow behavior of its environment. These conditions cause changes in the physical structure and chemistry of the compound, resulting in reduction of its bioaccessibility. ENs are now designed to safeguard bioactive compounds from adverse gastrointestinal conditions. The green tea polyphenol (-)-epigallocatechin gallate (EGCG) is unstable in the pH conditions of small intestinal fluid. Encapsulation of EGCG in nanolipopsomes decreases its degradation by 10-fold (Zou et al., 2014).

6.7.2.2 *ENs enhance absorption of bioactives*

After oral ingestion, most of the bioactive phytocompounds are absorbed in the small intestine (Oehlke et al., 2014). Lipid-based ENs like nanoemlusions are frequently employed to encapsulate lipophilic bioactives like β-carotene and curcumin to increase their absorption (Yao et al., 2015). Digestible carrier oils in ENs are hydrolyzed in the gastrointestinal tract by lipases and produce free fatty acids and monoacylglycerols. These

Table 6.3 Some ENs-based delivery systems

Delivery system	Bioactive compound	Ingredients	Reference
Non-lipid-based ENs			
Biopolymeric nanogels, antisolvent precipitation	Omega-3 fatty acids	Miscible solvents, biopolymers, surfactants	Matalanis et al. (2011)
Biopolymeric nanoparticles	Omega-3 fatty acids	Water, dextrin	Xu et al. (2013)
Biopolymeric nanoparticles	Curcumin	Water, β-cyclodextrin, modified starch, surfactant	Paramera et al (2011)
Organogel-based nanoemulsion	Curcumin	Water, organogel, surfactant	Yu and Huang (2012)
Micelles	Curcumin	Water, surfactant	Schiborr et al. (2014)
Lipid-based ENs			
Nanoemulsion	β-carotene	Water, oil, surfactant	Borel et al. (1998) Herrera and Barbas (2001) Qian et al. (2012) Gong et al. (2012) Yang and McClements (2013)
Liposome	Curcumin, resveratrol	Water, phospholipids, cholesterol	Mignet et al. (2013)
Nanoliposome	(-)-epigallocatechin gallate	Water, phospholipids, cholesterol	Zou et al. (2014)
Microemulsion	Curcumin	Water, surfactants, oil	Xiao et al. (2013)
Micelles	Lycopene	Oil, water, surfactant, lecithin	Chen et al. (2014)

Source: From Yao, M., et al. *Current Opinion in Food Science* 2:214–219, 2015.

compounds interact with bile salts and phospholipids to form mixed micelles in the small intestine (Yao et al., 2014). Mixed micelles from digestion of nanoemulsions carry lipophilic bioactives across the aqueous mucus layer of the small intestine. This has been found to be the case with 5-hydroxylnobiletin, a flavonoid in citrus fruits (Yao et al., 2013).

6.7.2.3 ENs decrease first-pass metabolism of bioactives

When a fortified food or nutraceutical is ingested, the bioactive compound is metabolized by many enzymes present in the gut and liver. This breaking down of the bioactive is known as first-pass metabolism. As a result of this process only a fraction of the ingested bioactive is available in the systemic circulation, thus lowering its bioavailability. ENs are now designed to bypass first-pass metabolism and have increased bioavailability (Yao et al., 2014; 2015).

6.8 Shelf-life of fortified food and beverages

A food product enjoys acceptance by consumers when its quality and nutritional content are maintained from the time of manufacture through distribution and storage until it reaches the consumer. Guidelines for determining product stability and ensuring label claims exist in the case of food and pharmaceutical products. But such guidelines are not available for nutraceutical products. Nevertheless, to maintain consumer acceptance and avoid possible governmental action, nutraceuticals should also be subjected to stability studies so as to ensure shelf-life and label claims. A nutraceutical or fortified food is of value only if it contains the bioactives in the required concentration (Bell, 2007).

There are several definitions of shelf-life (Hough, 2010). However, The IFST guidelines (1993) identify the key factors to be considered when assessing shelf-life. According to it, shelf-life is the time during which the food product will (1) remain safe; (2) retain desired sensory, chemical, physical, and microbiological characteristics; and (3) comply with any label declaration of nutritional data, when stored under the recommended conditions.

Several intrinsic or extrinsic factors influence shelf-life. Intrinsic factors are the properties of the final product and include water activity (available water) (a_w), pH value, total acidity, redox potential (E_h), available oxygen, nutrients, surviving microbiological counts, enzymes, chemical reactants, and preservatives (Valero et al., 2012). Extrinsic factors are those encountered by the final product as it moves through the food chain. They include the time–temperature profile during processing; temperature control during storage and distribution; relative humidity during processing, storage, and distribution; exposure to ultraviolet and infrared light during processing, storage, and distribution; composition of atmosphere within packaging; subsequent heat treatment such as reheating or cooking; and consumer handling (Valero et al., 2012). The interaction of these intrinsic and extrinsic factors inhibits or stimulates many processes that limit shelf-life. These processes can be microbiological, chemical, physical, and temperature-related (Kilcast and Subramaniam, 2000).

6.8.1 Factors affecting shelf-life of a food product

Evaluation of shelf-life of a food product begins with identification of the characteristics of the ingredients, the manufacturing process, and storage conditions that will have an influence on its shelf-life. During the shelf-life evaluation of chilled yogurt and other dairy desserts, Lewis and Dale (1994) observed that shelf-life of chilled dairy desserts is influenced by raw materials, product formulation, processing parameters, implementation of good manufacturing practice, filling and packing, storage, and distribution and handling by consumer. Monitoring and control of these factors ensure satisfactory shelf-life.

For example, ten raw materials such as milk, cream, sugar, bacterial cultures, milk concentrates, milk powders, fruits, stabilizers, flavors, and colors are used in the manufacture of yogurt. These ingredients can introduce microorganisms and chemicals that may influence the quality of the finished product. By working with approved suppliers and agreed specifications, the quality of the product can be maintained. Changes in the source of these ingredients will vary the factors that influence shelf-life (Lewis and Dale, 1994).

The proteins, lactose, fat, and microbiological flora of milk vary between different breeds of cattle, different geographical regions, and seasons. The quality of cream is dependent on the quality of the milk and the method of handling before and after pasteurization. Quality of milk concentrates depends on the quality of the raw milk used and handling techniques. Management of the bacterial cultures is vital to quality of the final product. The source of the other ingredients, the identification of critical control points, and standards of hygiene are also important factors influencing shelf-life (Lewis and Dale, 1994).

Many functional ingredients are used in the formulation of yogurt. To ensure stability of the final product, the formulator should have an understanding of the synergistic and antagonistic reactions that happen when such ingredients are used. Filling operation and packing material are critical to short shelf-life products like yogurt, which has high microbiological sensitivity. Similarly, storage and distribution are also of critical significance. Yogurt may spoil during storage and distribution due to growth of microorganisms and chemical changes such as oxidation, development of rancidity, and moisture migration. Microbiological and chemical changes can be greatly reduced by storage at low temperatures. Several measures need to be taken to achieve desired temperature standards in the distribution chain. Finally, to ensure stability, the end consumer should be educated on the need of temperature control, as all efforts taken by the manufacturer can be futile if the product is handled badly by the consumer (Lewis and Dale, 1994).

6.8.2 Shelf-life measurement

6.8.2.1 Sensory evaluation

Sensory evaluation uses a set of techniques for accurate measurement of human responses to foods while minimizing the potentially biasing effects of brand identity and other influences on consumer perception. Sensory evaluation attempts to isolate the sensory properties of foods and provides important and useful information to product developers, food scientists, and managers about the sensory characteristics of their products. Changes in the eating quality of stored food can be measured with sensory techniques, for which trained panels and naïve consumers are used. The application of sensory evaluation in shelf-life testing is detailed by Kemp et al. (2009) and Lawless and Heymann (2010).

6.8.2.2 Instrumental methods

Instrumental methods are used to measure sensory quality factors. But they are reliable only when the measured parameter has been validated against sensory measurements. Computerized texture analyzers (Phatthalung et al., 2008), electromyographs (Funami et al., 2014), rheometers (Shewfelt et al., 2016), carbon dioxide sensors (Puligundla et al., 2012) electronic noses, and electronic tongues (Persaud, 2016) are valuable only when the measured parameters are correlated with sensory attributes.

6.8.2.3 Physical measurements

Measuring the changes in the texture of products is one of the most commonly used physical tests. These changes are brought about by the interplay of intrinsic and extrinsic factors. For example, moisture may migrate from the environment into the product, through the packaging. Texture is one of the parameters commonly tested to assess the stability of food products. Similarly, properties such as hardness and crispness are also measured (Szczesniak, 1973; Bourne, 1982; Gunasekaran and Ak, 2002). More sophisticated methods such as measurement of food-crushing sounds, sonic resonance testing, and image analysis techniques have also been reported for measuring different aspects of food texture (Kilcast, 2001).

6.8.2.4 Chemical measurements

Many chemical reactions take place during the storage of food. Rancidity is one such change happening in fat-containing foods through lipolytic/hydrolytic reactions, oxidative reactions, and flavor reversion reactions. Foods containing intense sweeteners may undergo chemical hydrolysis, consequently reducing sweetness. Exposure to light can result in color loss. Some chemical tests indicating changes in a particular quality attribute can be applied to different types of products. An example is the measurement of peroxide value and free fatty acid levels as indicators of rancidity of food products. Accurate measurement of these parameters helps in accurate assessment of shelf-life (Kilcast and Subramaniam, 2000).

6.8.2.5 Microbiological measurements

The microbiological stability of a food product can be determined on the basis of the microbial growth leading to spoilage and the growth of microbial pathogens. The extent of the microorganisms that are likely to grow in a food product depends on the water activity, storage temperature, duration of storage, and pH. The "time of spoilage" is determined by storing the food at the appropriate temperature and measuring the microbial load at staged intervals. The time taken to reach a predetermined level of microbial load is considered the end point. Generally, 70% of the time to spoilage is taken as the storage life (Kilcast and Subramaniam, 2000).

6.8.3 Prediction of shelf-life

Food manufacturers introduce new and attractive products with minimum delay. Knowledge of the storage characteristics over the intended shelf-life period is essential to achieve success. Therefore, as in the pharmaceutical industry, accelerated shelf-life studies are carried out. Such studies are designed on the assumption that by changing a storage condition, the chemical or physical process that leads to deterioration is accelerated. However, the validity of any accelerated condition is to be tested against known deterioration characteristics under ambient storage conditions. If it is not possible to identify the ambient storage characteristics of a product due to time pressure, then a comparison is to be made between the test product and an equivalent product with a similar structure and for which a shelf-life has already been established. Mizrahi (2011) describes in detail the study of the accelerated stability of food products.

6.9 Biological effects of fortified food and beverages

6.9.1 Functional confectionery

Functional confectionery has been in existence since ancient times. The formula of a sweet confection for curing an intestinal worm infestation is described in a manuscript excavated from Thebes, Egypt, dating to 3400 B.C. The production of cane sugar provided an impetus to the manufacture of sugar-based confectionery (Pickford and Jardine, 2000). Sugar, sweetened condensed milk, milk powder, butter, butter oil, whey, vegetable fats, gums, emulsifiers, colors, and flavors are the ingredients of confectionery (Edwards, 2000). Chocolates, which are an important class of confectionery, are made of cocoa liquor, sugar, cocoa butter, milk fat, and milk powder (Beckett, 2009). Functional confectionery is formulated by choosing a suitable confectionery vehicle, incorporation of the functional ingredients into the product, manipulation of ingredients considering product taste, shelf-life or quality, masking of undesirable tastes, and assessment of the effect of functional ingredients on the critical parameters of the end product (Pickford and Jardine, 2000).

Functional confectionery provides a unique vehicle for delivering health-promoting compounds. Fisher (2011) developed a novel starch-based confection containing freeze-dried strawberries to provide sustained, targeted release of phytochemicals to the oral mucosa for promoting oral health. Optimized starch-based confection was formulated by mixing modified corn starch, corn syrup, and distilled water over heat (Table 6.4). The mixture was stirred and heated on a hot plate to form a gel, indicated by Brix between 65 to 68 and a final temperature of 90°C. On cooling to 60°C at room temperature, freeze-dried strawberry powder was incorporated into the gel. Confection prepared without strawberry powder was used as control formulation.

A clinical trial was conducted to evaluate the efficacy of the confectionery in the prevention of oral disease in 36 smoking and non-smoking men and women. Estimation of inflammatory markers (IgA, cortisol, 8-hydroxydeoxyguanosine) from a paraffin-stimulated saliva sample, analysis of urinary polyphenols and urine cotinine, and analysis of urinary biomarkers of genetic damage and inflammation (8-hydroxydeoxyguanosine and 8-epi-prostaglandin F2α) were carried out to evaluate the effect of consumption of functional confectionery on salivary inflammatory markers and gene expression profiles in oral mucosa. It was observed that the confectionery demonstrated great potential as a novel vehicle for delivering fruit bioactives to oral tissue. It was well-tolerated and there was good subject

Table 6.4 Confectionery formulation used in the clinical trial

FDS confection*	% Wet basis	Control confection	% Wet basis
Freeze-dried fruit powder	48.5	Corn syrup	49.2
Corn syrup	24.3	Modified starch	24.6
Modified corn starch	10.1	Water	25.2
Water	17.1	Flavor	0.12
Total	100	Total	100

**FDS = Freeze-dried strawberry*

Source: Reproduced with permission from Fisher, L.A., Physicochemical characterization of a novel strawberry confection for delivery of fruit bioactives to human oral mucosa. Master of Science thesis, The Ohio State University, 2011. With permission.)

compliance. The novel starch-based confection could be conveniently consumed without mastication, a feature advantageous to those with difficulty in eating due to loss of teeth, oral sores, and other oral maladies.

6.9.1.1 Chocolate

Cocoa beans have the highest content of flavan-3-ols (Arts et al., 1999; Lee et al., 2003a). Epidemiological studies show an inverse relationship between the consumption of a flavonoid-rich diet and the risk of hypertension. A short term intake of cocoa polyphenols is reported to lower blood pressure and improve endothelium-dependent vasodilatation (Grassi et al., 2005a, 2005b; Taubert et al., 2007; Davison et al., 2008). This beneficial effect of cocoa polyphenols seems to be brought about by an increase in the nitric oxide synthase activity in endothelial cells, leading to an increase in nitric oxide concentration (Karim et al., 2000; Heiss et al., 2003; 2005; Keen et al., 2005; Balzer et al., 2006; Berry et al., 2010).

Daily consumption of 40 g of dark chocolate for 14 days reduced the urinary excretion of the stress hormone cortisol and catecholamines in 30 stressed human volunteers. Stress-related differences in energy metabolism and gut microbial activities were also normalized by the therapy (Martin et al. 2010).

Improvements in cognitive function following a single dose of chocolate or cocoa flavanols were demonstrated in two clinical trials (Scholey et al., 2010; Field et al., 2011). Effects on information processing speed and working memory were observed in these studies within hours of consumption of cocoa flavanols or dark chocolate. The cocoa, cognition, and aging (CoCoA) study shows that daily consumption of cocoa flavanols improves cognitive function in healthy, elderly subjects. Improvements in processing speed and attentional tasks were observed following 8-weeks of consumption of a moderately high daily dose of cocoa flavanols (Mastroiacovo et al., 2015).

Crichton et al. (2016) investigated whether habitual chocolate intake is associated with improved cognitive function, with adjustment for cardiovascular, lifestyle, and dietary factors. Cross-sectional analyses undertaken on 968 community-dwelling participants, aged 23–98 years, showed that habitual chocolate intake was related to cognitive performance measured with several neuropsychological tests. More frequent chocolate consumption improved global composite scores, visual-spatial memory and organization, working memory, scanning and tracking, abstract reasoning, and the Mini-Mental State Examination.

An interventional trial on 20 peripheral arterial disease patients was carried out to find out the acute effect of 40 g of dark chocolate or white chocolate. Flow-mediated dilation, serum levels of isoprostanes, nitrite/nitrate, sNOX2-dp, maximal walking distance (MWD), and maximal walking time (MWT) were measured at baseline and 2 h after chocolate ingestion. MWD, MWT, and sNOX2-dp were significantly increased after the consumption of dark chocolate. However, milk chocolate failed to produce any of these effects (Loffredo et al. 2014).

Chronic supplementation with 40 g dark chocolate resulted in a higher gas exchange threshold and enhanced time-trial performance of nine moderately-trained cyclists. Ingestion of dark chocolate reduced the oxygen cost of moderate intensity exercise. This may be an effective ergogenic aid for short-duration moderate intensity exercise (Patel et al., 2015).

The two major pathological characteristics of Alzheimer's disease are the formation of protein aggregates in the form of extracellular amyloid-β (Aβ) plaques and intracellular tau neurofibrillary tangles. Oligomers of Aβ peptides and tau protein are toxic (Klein, 2002; Cleary et al., 2005; Santacruz et al., 2005; Berger et al., 2007; Shankar et al., 2008). Reducing these oligomer species is a potential mode of intervention. Wang et al. (2014) tested three different cocoa extracts on $A\beta_{40}$ and $A\beta_{42}$ oligomerization using the photoinduced cross-linking of unmodified proteins technique. The extracts could prevent the oligomerization of Aβ.

Cocoa beans have antioxidant activity higher than that shown by green tea and red wine (Lee et al., 2003a; Subhashini et al., 2010). This antioxidant activity can modify the course of cardiovascular diseases, cancer, and many chronic conditions (Park et al., 2014). Recent studies show that cocoa consumption can improve skin health (Park et al., 2014; Scapagnini et al., 2014). Cocoa provides beneficial effects on skin structure and dermal microcirculation (Neukam et al., 2007; Katz et al., 2011). Long-term ingestion of cocoa also pacifies aberrant skin conditions by improving blood flow to cutaneous and sub-cutaneous tissues (Heinrich et al. 2006). Cocoa has the ability to inhibit skin cancer growth and skin inflammation *in vitro* and *in vivo* (Lee et al., 2006a; Kang et al., 2008; Kim et al., 2010). Kim et al., (2016) reported that cocoa extract may offer a protective effect against photoaging by inhibiting the breakdown of dermal matrix, which leads to an overall reduction in wrinkle formation in hairless mouse skin.

Administration of cocoa flavanols through food may be an effective strategy for alleviation of metabolic syndrome and glucose intolerance in particular. The complex array of flavanols interact with a variety of molecules, allowing many opportunities to ameliorate metabolic diseases. Flavanols can antagonize digestive enzymes and glucose transporters, thereby reducing glucose levels, which helps to maintain glucose homeostasis. Unabsorbed flavanols, and those that undergo enterohepatic recycling, proceed to the colon where they can exert prebiotic effects on the gut microbiota. Interactions with the gut microbiota may result in reduced endotoxin absorption. Insulin signaling may also be influenced, by relieving insulin-signaling pathways from oxidative stress and inflammation and/or via a heightened incretin response (Strat et al., 2015).

Cocoa extracts containing polyphenolic compounds show the ability to scavenge ROS and protect human HepG2 liver cells (Martìn et al., 2008), colonic cancer cells (Caco-2 cells) (Carnésecchi et al., 2002), and rat adrenal pheochromocytoma cells (PC12 cells) (Cho et al., 2008) against oxidative stress. But these effects cannot be solely attributed to polyphenols, as cocoa and cocoa products also contain methylxanthines, peptides, biogenic amines, and micronutrients that can modulate the health effects of cocoa products by enhancing or reducing their biological activity (Abbe Maleyki and Amin, 2008; Visioli et al., 2009). Belščak-Cvitanović et al. (2012) studied the relation of polyphenols, methylxanthines, and minor and major elements of several cocoa products with their cytotoxic activity and reactive oxygen species formation on one human laryngeal carcinoma (HEp2) cell line. The cocoa products containing higher non-fat cocoa solids exhibited higher total polypohenol content and methylxanthines content. Results revealed that milk chocolate containing the lowest non-fat cocoa solids had no effect on HEp2 cells survival, while the highest growth inhibition (27%) of cells was induced by cocoa liquor, after 2 hours of treatment. The authors inferred that the observed prooxidant activity of dark chocolate and cocoa liquor may be attributed to higher contents of methylxanthines and transition metals present in these products.

Recent clinical trials suggest that ingestion of cocoa flavanol mitigates acute hemodialysis-induced and chronic endothelial dysfunction in patients with end-stage renal disease (ESRD), improving vascular function in this high-risk population (Rassaf et al., 2016).

6.9.1.2 Functional chewing gum

Chewing gum is a soft substance designed to be chewed without being swallowed. Chewing gums are made from butadiene-based synthetic rubber. Survey of recent literature shows that chewing gum may increase alertness and improve aspects of performance and increase relaxation (Smith, 2009). Onyper et al (2011) found strong evidence of improvement for working memory, episodic memory and perceptual speed of processing following gum-chewing. Nevertheless, the improvements were only evident when the gum was chewed prior to cognitive testing. This finding suggests that the effect of chewing gum is domain-specific. The cognitive improvements after a period of chewing gum last for 15–20 minutes and decline afterwards. Scholey (2004) is of the opinion that enhancement of memory performance while chewing gum is a fairly robust phenomenon. However, Tucha and Koerts (2012) advise that because of the lack of scientific information and because detrimental effects of gum chewing were repeatedly documented, gum chewing should not be considered as an aid or cognitive enhancer.

Chewing gum may relieve stress and depression. Erbay et al. (2013) conducted a clinical study, in 30 patients with mild to moderate depression.

They were given for six weeks either medication combined with chewing gum, or medication only. A Turkish adaptation of Hamilton Rating Scale for Depression (HAM-D) was used to measure depression levels. Patients who were administrated chewing gum responded better to the treatment than patients who took medication alone. The most beneficial effect observed on gastrointestinal symptoms such as loss of appetite and flatulence, indicate that chewing gum may reduce the symptoms originating from depression.

Some interesting functional chewing gums have also made their appearance recently. The stem bark of the magnolia has been used in the treatment of coughs, diarrhea, and allergic rhinitis in the traditional medicine of China, Japan, and Korea. Recent research indicates that magnolol and honokiol in the bark have strong anti-inflammatory and antimicrobial activities. They are active against an array of organisms such as *E. coli, Pseudomonas aeruginosa, Trichophyton mentagrophytes, Porphyromonas gingivalis, Epidermophyton floccosum, A. niger, Cryptococcus neoformans,* and *Candida albicans* (Lee et al., 2009). Considering these activities, Wrigley has been granted novel food approval in the European Union for *Magnolia officinalis* extract to be used in chewing gums and mints with perceived breath-freshening benefits (Anonymous, 2011). Chewing gum is also intended to be a dosage form to deliver the peptide YY (PYY) hormone that is reported to promote a feeling of fullness and thus act as a weight loss agent (Fazen et al., 2011).

The Danish medicinal chewing gum manufacturer, Fertin Pharma A/S, Denmark, has come up with an immunity-enhancing chewing gum containing *Echinacea purpurea* extract. A clinical trial was conducted in 246 subjects with the common cold. It was observed that treating them with chewing gum containing 13.56 mg of *E. purpurea* extract, three times daily for 7 days, caused cold symptoms to disappear more than when treated with a placebo. The gum is sweetened with xylitol, sorbitol, aspartame, and acesulfame-K. Fertin Pharma has also developed a chewing gum for stress relief and weight management. It contains saffron (*Crocus sativus*) extract (Anonymous, 2013a). The company offers chewing gums as "a dosage form that delivers active ingredients in an effective and consumer-friendly way" (Anonymous, 2013b).

In 2013 Wrigley introduced chewing gums sweetened with fruit powders. Sucrose which is usually used in chewing gums is cariogenic and may lead to dental caries, with additional impact on glucose levels of those suffering from diabetes. Polyol-based bulking agents such as maltitol and sorbitol are used as sugar alternatives. But polyols are associated with gastrointestinal disturbances. Therefore fruit powders are alternative for conventional sweetening agents (Nieburg, 2013).

Between 2009 and 2013 the global sugar-free chewing gum segment registered a compound annual growth rate (CAGR) of 3% to reach $10.6

billion. During the same period the functional chewing gum category grew at a CAGR of 4% to reach $2.6 billion in 2013. The functional chewing gum niche is expected to grow 14% by 2018 to $3 billion. The Korean confectionery giant Lotte recently came up with Walking Plus capsiate chewing gum that is fortified with capsicum extract for causing weight loss (Nieburg, 2014).

6.9.2 *Cheese*

Cheese is a dairy product rich in protein and fat. It is produced in numerous flavors, textures, and forms. It is formed by coagulation of the milk protein, casein. During cheese production the milk is acidified and mixed with the enzyme rennet, resulting in coagulation. The solids are separated and molded into final form (Fox et al., 2000). On account of the high content of salt and fats, cheese is not generally recommended in heart-healthy diets. However, Nilsen et al. (2014) questioned 168 male and female participants from one Norwegian town about their dietary habits and other health-related factors. On the basis of their responses and measurements of their blood pressure, the authors observed that the intake of the traditional Norwegian cheese Gamalost was inversely associated with systolic blood pressure and an increase in a frequency unit of Gamalost corresponded to a reduction in systolic blood pressure of 0.72 mmHg.

Lutein is one of the 600 known naturally occurring carotenoids. Many studies have shown that there exists a direct relationship between lutein intake and pigmentation in the eye (Johnson et al., 2000; Berendschot et al., 2000; Johnson et al., 2005). Administration of lutein can prevent the appearance of age-related macular degeneration (Seddon et al., 1994; Snodderly, 1995; Yao et al., 2013). Jones et al. (2005) incorporated various amounts of lutein from corn into cheddar cheese and evaluated its stability during storage. A significant quantity of lutein could be recovered and there was no evidence of lutein disintegration. The authors suggest that cheese is a good matrix for the delivery of lutein.

6.9.3 *Pasta*

Pasta, which originated in Italy, has gained wide popularity as a convenient and nutritionally palatable, low glycaemic food (Petitot et al., 2009). Traditionally pasta is made from durum wheat semolina, mixed with water or eggs and formed into sheets. Pasta is then dried and stored. It is cooked by boiling. Pasta is a generic name that includes among many others, macaroni, spaghetti, and vermicelli (De Vita, 2009).

Though it is popularly believed that pasta is responsible for weight gain, a recent study has reported that pasta is good food for weight management. Based on data obtained from 23,366 subjects, Pounis et al. (2016)

reported that when consumed in moderation as a traditional component of Mediterranean diet, with plenty of vegetables and olive oil, pasta was negatively associated with body mass index, waist circumference, and waist-to-hip ratio and with a lower prevalence of overweight and obesity.

Isoflavones are naturally occurring phytocompounds belonging to the class of phytoestrogens. Epidemiological and laboratory studies are highly suggestive of beneficial effects of isoflavaones on human health (Setchell and Cassidy, 1999). Soy beans (*Glycine max*) are rich in isoflavones (Dixit et al., 2011). Clerici et al. (2007) compared a novel soy isoflavone-enriched pasta with a conventional one for effects on serum lipids and cardiovascular risk markers such as high sensitivity C-reactive protein (hsCRP), urinary isoprostanes, and brachial artery flow-mediated vasodilatation. In this randomized, controlled, parallel study, 62 adults with hypercholesterolemia consumed a diet that included one 80-g serving/d of pasta for four weeks. The pasta reduced total and LDL cholesterol, arterial stiffness, hsCRP, and urinary isoprostanes. The results suggest that an isoflavone-enriched soy germ pasta delivering levels of isoflavones consistent with those consumed in Asian countries exerts beneficial effects on markers of cardiovascular disease.

Clerici et al. (2011) carried out a randomized, controlled, double-blind, crossover study comparing one serving per day of soy germ pasta and conventional pasta for 8 weeks. The parameters chosen were brachial artery flow-mediated vasodilation, blood pressure, plasma lipids, oxidized LDL cholesterol, 8-iso-PGF2α, total antioxidant capacity, glutathione, and homocysteine. Isoflavone-enriched pasta improved all these parameters consistent with a reduction in oxidative stress. The study shows that pasta enriched with biologically active isoflavones improves endothelial function with beneficial effects on cardiovascular risk markers in patients with type 2 diabetes.

Gastroparesis is a chronic gastric disorder characterized by delayed gastric emptying of solid and semi-solid foods in the absence of mechanical obstruction. It affects nearly 50% of chronic type 2 diabetics. Setchell et al. (2013) conducted a randomized, double-blind, placebo-controlled study comparing soy germ pasta with conventional pasta for effects on gastric emptying. Ten patients suffering from delayed gastric emptying consumed one serving per day of each pasta for 8 weeks, with a 4-week washout. Gastric emptying time was measured using the [^{13}C] octanoic acid breath test. The major finding of this study is that consumption of isoflavone-enriched pasta significantly accelerates gastric emptying, Dietary intervention with isoflavone-enriched pasta can be considered in the management of diabetic gastroparesis, as currently there is no effective therapy for this disorder.

The effect of inulin-fortified pasta on gut peptides and gastric emptying rates was studied by Russo et al. (2011) in twenty healthy young volunteers over a period of five weeks. The results support the hypothesis that inulin plays an active role in mechanisms affecting the release of the gut peptides, neurotensin, somatostatin, and corticotrophin-releasing factor that may modulate gastric emptying.

Based on a randomized, double-blind crossover study involving twenty healthy, young male volunteers over a 5-week period Russo et al. (2012) concluded that consumption of 11% inulin-enriched pasta improves intestinal permeability and modifies the circulating levels of zonulin and glucagon-like peptide 2 (GLP-2). The inulin-enriched pasta group had lower zonulin serum levels and significantly higher GLP-2 basal values in comparison with the baseline and control pasta groups. Zonulin is the only physiological mediator known to regulate intestinal permeability reversibly by modulating intercellular tight junctions (Fasano, 2000; Wang et al., 2000). It is overexpressed in autoimmune disorders such as celiac disease and type 1 diabetes, in which tight junction dysfunction is central (Fasano et al., 2000; Drago et al., 2006; Sapone et al., 2006). GLP-2 is an intestinotrophic hormone (Jeppesen, 2003). Therefore, enrichment with a prebiotic like insulin can be applied in the prevention of gastrointestinal diseases and metabolic disorders.

Considering the nutritional value and medicinal properties of the blue-green alga *Arthrospira platensis* (*Spirulina*) Zouari et al. (2011) studied the effects of pasta fortification with Spirulina at 1, 2, and 3 g/100 g of semolina on the color, cooking properties, firmness, free radical scavenging activity, and sensory characteristics. Fortification with microalgae (2 g microalgae/100 g of semolina) bestowed higher free radical scavenging property to the product compared to controls. This may be attributed to the high content of vitamin E, carotenoids, chlorophyll. and phycobiliproteins present in *Spirulina* (Gad et al. 2010).

Sęczyk et al. (2015; 2016a) fortified wheat pasta with 1%–4% of powdered leaves of parsley (*Petroselinum crispum*). The bioaccessible fraction of pasta fortified with 4% parsley leaves had 67% increased content of phenolics. It exhibited 146% higher antioxidant activity and 220% additional reducing power. Concomitantly the fortified pasta had augmented antiproliferative effect on Walker-256 carcinoma cells. Ultra performance liquid chromatography–mass spectrometry (UPLC/MS) analyses showed that the parsley leaf extracts contained derivatives of apigenin, diosmetin, isorhamnetin, and catechin. As these compounds were bioaccessible after *in vitro* digestion, the authors suggest that these flavonoids enhance the potential bioactivity of the fortified pasta (Patel et al. 2007). Enhancement of antioxidant activity has also been reported in pasta fortification with oregano leaf, carrot leaf (Boroski et al., 2011), grape skin (Sant'Anna et al., 2014) and carob flours (Sęczyk et al., 2016b).

Consumption of fortified pasta is reported to bring about beneficial effects. Capraro et al. (2014) fortified pasta with γ-conglutin, a glucose-lowering protein from *Lupinus albus* seeds, an extract of the other main lupin storage proteins and ovalbumin at a ratio corresponding to 125 mg of pure protein per 100 g of pasta. Hyperglycemic rats were fed with the fortified pasta for 3 weeks. On termination of the treatment there was a significant reduction in food intake in rats fed γ-conglutin concentrate-supplemented pasta and a significant reduction in body weight increase in rats fed α, β and δ-conglutin extract-supplemented pasta. the food conversion indices remained unchanged. There was also a reduction in glycaemia upon glucose overload, in animals fed with the γ-conglutin concentrate-supplemented pasta at a dose of 45 mg per kg body weight. The study shows that pasta fortified with seed proteins can be consumed for controlling body weight gain and blood sugar.

Consumption of foods containing flour of sorghum (*Sorghum bicolor*) enhances antioxidant status and beneficially modulates markers of oxidative stress. Some varieties of sorghum have the highest polyphenolic content. *In vitro* studies show that these sorghum polyphenols function as strong antioxidants (Dlamini et al., 2007). A lone *in vivo* study conducted on Wistar rats showed that a diet containing sorghum flour reduced markers of oxidative stress and inflammation (Moraes et al., 2012). Considering the paucity of information in humans, Khan et al. (2015) conducted a clinical study to investigate the effect of sorghum-containing flour on antioxidant status and markers of oxidative stress. In a randomized crossover design, 20 healthy subjects consumed three test meals of control pasta, 30% red sorghum pasta or 30% white sorghum pasta, 1–2 wk apart. The 2 h post-prandial levels of plasma polyphenols, antioxidant capacity, and superoxide dismutase activity following the red sorghum pasta meal were significantly higher while the protein carbonyl level was significantly lower, indicating reduced oxidative stress. The study demonstrated that pasta containing red wholegrain sorghum flour enhanced antioxidant status and improved markers of oxidative stress in healthy subjects.

6.9.4 Beverages

6.9.4.1 Fruit juices

Fruit juices are generally believed to be healthy drinks, as they are rich sources of vitamins, amino acids, minerals, and antioxidants. Though fruit juices are rich in sugars, they also contain many phytochemicals having health-promoting properties. These include anthocyanidins, flavonoids, carotenoids, coumarins, and phytosterols (Li et al., 2016). By virtue of the nutritional profile, juices of fruits such as açai, mangosteen, pomegranate, noni, guarana, cupuacu, goji, blackcurrant, blueberry, bilberry, cranberry, and raspberry are increasingly becoming popular in the nutraceutical world (Gruenwald, 2009). Fruit juices are reported to have analgesic (Jensen et al., 2011), weight reducing (Evans et al., 2014a), anti-inflammatory (Nemzer et al., 2011), and anti-diabetic (Chudnovskiy et al., 2014) activities. They also exert beneficial effects on urinary markers of coronary artery disease (Mullen et al., 2011; Evans et al., 2014b; Kumar, 2016c).

Mertens-Talcott et al. (2006) investigated the absorption and antioxidant activity of pomegranate in healthy human volunteers after the acute consumption of 800 mg of standardized extract. Ellagic acid from the extract was bioavailable, and the plasma metabolites urolithin A, urolithin B, hydroxyl-urolithin A, urolithin A-glucuronide, and dimethyl ellagic acid-glucuronide were identified by HPLC-MS. The antioxidant capacity was increased with a maximum effect of 32% after 0.5 hour, while the generation of reactive oxygen species remained unaffected. Similar results were reported by Gouda et al. (2016) who conducted a clinical trial on 35 healthy adults. Consumption of pomegranate juice for 21 days significantly increased the plasma and urinary antioxidative activities and reduced the urinary excretion of thiobarbituric acid-reacting species.

Many epidemiological and preclinical studies have shown that an inverse relationship exists between regular consumption of fruit juices and risks of various cancers (Terry et al., 2001; Temple and Gladwin, 2003). For example, pomegranate juice showed the greatest antiproliferative activity in human oral, colon, and prostate cancer cells in comparison with individual compounds such as punicalgin, ellagic acid, and total pomegranate tannins (Seeram et al., 2005). Similarly, a combination of pomegranate juice compounds such as luteolin, ellagic acid, and punicic acid reduced the migratory and chemotactic properties of human breast cancer cells (Rocha et al., 2012). Ellagitannin, another major constituent of pomegranate juice, is hydrolyzed into ellagic acid and then to urolithin by colonic bacteria. A mixture of ellagic and urolithin–A inhibited the proliferation and induced apoptosis in human prostate cancer (DU-145 and PC3) cells (Vicinanza et al., 2013). Schaefer et al. (2006) studied the effects of reconstituted mixtures of five major constituents of apple juice rutin, phloridzin, chlorogenic acid, caffeic acid, and epicatechin on oxidative DNA damage in human colon cancer (Caco-2 and HT-29) cells. The reconstituted mixture demonstrated higher triolox equivalent antioxidative capacity (TEAC) and was more effective in preventing menadione-induced oxidative DNA damage. Similarly, the whole orange juice showed more free radical and superoxide anion scavenging activity compared to the individual polyphenol fractions (Barreca et al., 2014).

Barth et al. (2007) studied the antigenotoxic effects of cloudy apple juice and its fractions using a rat colon carcinogenesis model. They administered cloudy apple juice, or its fractions such as polyphenol fraction or cloud fraction or the combination of polyphenol and cloud fractions for 7 weeks starting 1 week prior to challenge with 1,2-dimethylhydrazine (DMH). DMH-induced genotoxicity was significantly attenuated by cloudy apple juice as a whole, but not by the polyphenol or cloud fractions or their combinations. Compared to polyphenol or cloud fractions, the cloudy apple juice significantly inhibited DMH-induced proliferation of colonocytes. Cloudy apple juice, but not its fractions, reduced the number of large aberrant crypt foci formation in DMH-challenged rats. Considering the functional properties of these juices, they can be used in the fortification of beverages.

Berries are a good source of polyphenols such as anthocyanins, micronutrients, and fiber. Epidemiological and clinical studies show that these constituents are associated with improved cardiovascular risk profiles. Significant improvements in LDL oxidation, lipid peroxidation, total plasma antioxidant capacity, dyslipidemia, and glucose metabolism are reported with anthocyanin extracts (Basu et al., 2010). From a randomized, double-blind, crossover study based on twenty-five overweight or obese males, aged 14–18 years, Djurica et al. (2016) concluded that consumption of strawberry powder can provide vascular health benefits to heavier adolescent males.

Maqui (*Aristotelia chilensis* [Mol.] Stuntz) is an edible berry from central and southern Chile. It has natural colorants due to the presence of anthocyanins. On account of its bioactive components, this fruit has recently become notable as one of the healthiest berries (Céspedes et al., 2008; Schreckinger et al., 2010). High phenolic content has linked maqui with high antioxidant capacity (Rubilar et al., 2011), *in vitro* inhibition of adipogenesis and inflammation (Schreckinger et al., 2010), protection against oxidative stress (Miranda-Rottmann et al., 2002), cardioprotection (Céspedes et al., 2008), and antidiabetic effects demonstrated *in vitro* and *in vivo* (Rojo et al., 2011; Rubilar et al., 2011). Similarly, Açaí (*Euterpe oleracea* Mart.) is a berry native to Amazon river area in South America, having antioxidant, anti-inflammatory (Jensen et al., 2008), anti-atherosclerotic (Schauss et al., 2009), and antiproliferative properties (Hogan et al., 2010). It reduces selected markers of metabolic disease (Udani et al., 2011) reduces pain and improves mobility (Jensen et al., 2011). Blackthorn (*Prunus spinosa* L.) is a fruit of deciduous shrubs native to Spain, Portugal, and Turkey (Barros et al., 2010), commonly used in the preparation of jams and digestive alcoholic drinks. Fruits have antioxidant activity (Ganhão et al., 2010). Gironés-Vilaplana et al. (2012) designed new blends of beverages by mixing lemon juice with juices of maqui, acai, and blackthorn. Profiling of the red fruits revealed the presence of several bioactive phenolics including anthocyanins, flavonols, 5-O-caffeoylquinic acid, and ellagic acid derivatives. Lemon juice contains flavones, flavanones, flavonols, and hydroxycinnamic acids. The beverage formulation based on lemon juice and maqui berry was found to be the most interesting one in terms of antioxidant activity. The results suggest that lemon juice enriched with maqui berries can be a potential novel functional beverage.

Citrus bergamia Risso (Bergamot orange) is a natural hybrid fruit derived from bitter orange and lemon. It is produced exclusively in the Reggio Calabria region of southern Italy (Mandalari et al., 2006). While bergamot is cultivated exclusively to produce essential oils, the juice is a waste, having no real use in food industry on account of its bitter taste. This causes a serious environmental and economic problem for the industries. Pernice et al. (2009) re-evaluated bergamot juice through its chemical characterization and to explore the possibility of using it to fortify fruit juices. They prepared laboratory-scale samples of apple and apricot juices following both the traditional industrial recipe and with the addition of bergamot juice. The juices were fortified with bergamot juice at 10% or 20%, with or without ascorbic acid and citric acid, two additives normally used in the fruit juice industry. The ascorbic acid content and antioxidant activity were measured during the different phases of juice production and after storage at 37°C for 15 days. Apricot and apple juices fortified with bergamot juice had a significant content of antioxidant properties and reduced degradation of ascorbic acid content. The results show that the addition of bergamot juice to juices of other fruits protects their ascorbic acid content from thermal degradation and enhances the antioxidant activity. Thus a valuable product could be developed out of a waste material.

6.9.4.2 Prebiotics-fortified beverages

Recent research has shown that gut microbiota and the regulation of host immunity influence the development of different conditions like metabolic syndrome and associated disorders (Flint, 2011; Murphy et al., 2012). Therefore, new therapeutic approaches are being developed through the study of gut microbiota in metabolic disease and the influence of prebiotics. Galacto-oligosaccharides are a class of prebiotics having the ability to selectively stimulate the growth of bifidobacteria and lactobacilli (Bouhnik et al., 2004; Depeint et al., 2008; Vulevic et al., 2008; Silk et al., 2009). Costabile et al. (2015) studied the effects of orange juice formulation on prebiotic functionality using an *in vitro* colonic model system. Results showed that orange juice fortified with galacto-oligosaccharides produced positive modulations of the microbiota composition and metabolic activity. Numbers of fecal bifidobacteria and lactobacilli were significantly higher when the galactooligosaccharide-fortified juice was fermented. Findings from this study showed that functionality of galactooligosaccharides was maintained within the fortified juice, supporting the use of prebiotic enriched juice for improving gastrointestinal health.

Inulin-type fructans, which are nondigestible carbohydrates, are capable of decreasing triglycerides by several mechanisms, such as decreased hepatic lipogenesis, increased muscle lipoprotein lipase activity, and increased production of short-chain fatty acids by bacterial fermentation of carbohydrates (Reis et al., 2014). Therefore, Kietsiriroje et al. (2015) conducted a double-blind, randomized, controlled trial on the effect of phytosterols and inulin-enriched soymilk on LDL-cholesterol in Thai subjects. Daily consumption of soymilk containing 2 g of phytosterols and 10 g of inulin reduced total cholesterol and LDL-cholesterol better than standard soymilk. The treatment had no effect on triglycerides and HDL-cholesterol levels compared to standard soymilk.

Cardiovascular disease has become a major health problem in developed and developing countries. Epidemiological studies show that it is associated with high levels of blood cholesterol (Moarreaf, 2004). Metabolic diseases such as obesity and diabetes are also associated with cardiovascular disease. Supplementation of diet with fruits, vegetables, and herbs is an important way to prevent the formation of free radicals that cause cardiovascular and associated metabolic diseases. *Terminalia arjuna* is an important herb used for the treatment of cardiovascular disease in the Indian traditional system of Ayurveda. The bark of *T. arjuna* has antihyperlipidaemic, hypocholesterolaemic, antioxidant, anti-inflammatory, and anticarcinogenic effects (Kumar and Prabhakar, 1987). Sawale et al. (2016) encapsulated 50% ethanolic extract of *T. arjuna* using maltodextrin (8% w/v) and gum acacia (2% w/w). The encapsulated microcapsules were formulated into vanilla-flavored chocolate milk. The functional beverage was administered to high cholesterol-fed Wistar rats for 60 days and its hypolipidaemic and antioxidative properties studied. A significant decrease in the body weight gain of high cholesterol-fed rats receiving the encapsulated herb extract was noted. The fortified drink also caused statistically significant decrease in weights of epididymal fat and liver, triglycerides, total cholesterol, low-density lipoprotein cholesterol and very-low-density lipoprotein cholesterol. There were also increase in reduced glutathione and decrease in thiobarbituric acid reactive substances (TBARS) levels in both liver and red blood cell lysates. The study shows that 50% ethanolic extract of *T. arjuna* can be successfully encapsulated and formulated into a functional dairy beverage, masking the bitter taste and red color of the extract.

A new beverage was developed by Singer et al. (2016) to suppress hunger and improve feelings of satiety in healthy volunteers. Data collected from 269 participants showed that coffee enriched with inulin, dextrin, and whey is safe and has possible benefits with regard to feelings of hunger and satiety 2 hours after ingestion.

Tea is rich in polyphenols and other phenolics that have been widely reported to have beneficial health effects (Gutiérrez-Grijalva et al., 2016). Nevertheless, dietary polyphenols are not completely absorbed from the gastrointestinal tract. They are metabolized by the gut microflora and their metabolites may accumulate to exert physiological effects. Lee et al. (2006b) investigated the influence of the phenolic constituents of tea extract and their aromatic metabolites upon bacterial growth. Fecal homogenates containing bacteria transformed tea phenolics, such as epicatechin, catechin, 3-O-methyl gallic acid, gallic acid, and caffeic acid into aromatic metabolites depending on bacterial species. Growth of some pathogenic bacteria including *Clostridium perfringens, Clostridium difficile,* and *Bacteroides* spp. was significantly inhibited by tea phenolics and their derivatives. Commensal bacteria like *Clostridium* spp., *Bifidobacterium* sp., and probiotic organisms like *Lactobacillus* sp. were not so much affected. This study shows that tea phenolics produce significant effects on the intestinal environment by modulating the intestinal bacterial population, as prebiotics do.

6.9.5 Biscuits

The bone mass of many women decreases after menopause, raising the threat of fractures (Seeman et al. 1988; Kanis et al. 1991). Therefore, research continues to look for ways to prevent menopause-related bone loss and fracture. Hussein et al. (2006) developed a functional biscuit consisting of whey protein and soy bean. It had the following formula: whey protein 20%, soy protein 15%, germinated wheat 32%, carrots 5%, skimmed milk 6%, brewer's yeast 4%, sugar 6%, corn oil 10%, and flavor 2%. It was tested on fourteen osteoporotic elderly women, who consumed 60 g of the biscuit daily for a month. Serum calcium and serum osteocalcin levels increased after ingestion of the biscuit for one month. Concomitantly, urinary deoxypyridoline excretion decreased. The whey protein-soy bean biscuits tested in this study seem to be effective in promoting bone formation and suppressing bone resorption in osteoporotic elderly women.

Boobier et al. (2007) reformulated a traditional biscuit to a functional food by adding B_{12}, folic acid, vitamin C, and prebiotic fiber. The consumption of these fortified biscuits by human volunteers reduced their blood levels of homocysteine and glucose, suggesting these biscuits may reduce risk factors associated with heart diseases such as myocardial infarction, stroke, and venous thrombosis (Hortin, 2006; Boobier et al., 2007).

Bahgaat (2010) and Hassan et al. (2012) attempted to prepare functional prebiotic biscuits for lowering serum blood lipids. Functional biscuits were formulated by replacing either wheat flour by different plant meals such as mustard meal, flaxseed meal, and barley meal at 5, 10, 15, 20, 25, and 30% levels or shortening by flaxseed oil at 25, 50, 75, and 100% levels. Several of the biscuits contained 1.37 and 1.25 times more protein, dietary fibers, and alpha linolenic acid. Consumption of biscuits fortified with barley, flaxseed meal, and flaxseed oil for 8 weeks significantly reduced serum total cholesterol, triglycerides, low density lipoproteins, and very low density lipoproteins. The biscuits did not cause deleterious effects on liver or kidney functions. Rats fed a high-fat high-cholesterol diet showed severe damage to liver, heart, and kidney, while feeding of biscuits containing flaxseed oil, flaxseed, and barley meals to the hypercholesterolemic rats lowered the degree of lesions of the liver. Consumption of bakery products fortified with flaxseed oil, flaxseed, or barley meal could be developed as a useful therapy for hyperlipidemia in humans.

Lupin (*Lupinus albus*) is a protein-rich grain legume containing low levels of isoflavones. The most important of the five cultivated species of lupin is the sweet white lupin. It is commonly found in Mediterranean countries and especially in Egypt, Portugal, Greece, and Italy (Hassanein et al., 2011). Mousa (2015a) examined the use of sweet white lupin oil and flour with/without germination as a source of active healthy ingredients to prepare functional biscuits for lowering blood lipids and controlling body weight gain. Functional biscuits were formulated by substituting wheat flour and butter in biscuit formulae with sweet white lupin flour and oil in the range of 20%–30% (w/w) and 30%–40% (v/w), respectively. Results showed that the feeding of hyperlipidemic rats on diets supplemented with different functional sweet white lupin biscuits for 6 weeks significantly reduced serum total cholesterol, triglycerides, low density lipoproteins, very low density lipoproteins, ratio of total cholesterol/high density lipoproteins cholesterol, ratio of low density lipoproteins/high density lipoproteins, cholesterol, and atherogenic index. Additionally, the treatment significantly reduced the body weight gain of rats. These findings suggest that the addition of 25% germinated sweet white lupin flour and 35% or 40% of oil extracted from germinated sweet white lupin to biscuits give interesting results, such as regulation of blood cholesterol and control of body weight of individuals.

Most of the biscuits in the market suffer from high caloric value, unhealthy saturated fats, and trans-fatty acids. Therefore, food technologists focus on developing low calorie and high-fiber functional foods with healthy fats. Mousa (2015b) formulated biscuits using palm oil as fat replacer and sucralose as sweetener. The highly nutritious germinated sweet white lupin flour was used as partial replacer of wheat flour. The formulated biscuits had 15.2% lower energy and 46.7% less fat content than controls. The saturated fatty acids content showed a significant decrease of 17% in wheat biscuits and 30.3% in lupin biscuits made with palm oil. Trans-fatty acids were not detected in these biscuits. It was observed that feeding of lupin biscuits containing sucralose for four weeks reduced the serum glucose of hyperglycemic rats by about 55%. Cholesterol, triglycerides, low-density lipoprotein cholesterol, creatinine, aspartate amino transferase and alanine amino transferase decreased by 37.9%, 25.0%, 74.1%, 49.7%, 41.8%, and 54.5%, respectively, while high-density lipoprotein increased by 59.7% when alloxan diabetic rats were fed with the newly formulated biscuits. This study demonstrates that reduced-calorie biscuits with healthy fats and hypoglycemic activity can be produced by using wheat-lupin composite flour blended with palm oil and sucralose.

Mateos et al. (2016) explored the possibility of using biscuits as a matrix to deliver hydroxytyrosol, which protects low-density lipoproteins (LDL) against oxidation. They performed a crossover, randomized, double-blind study to evaluate hydroytyrosol bioavailability in hydroytyrosol-enriched biscuits against non-enriched biscuits, and the effects on oxidative postprandial status. On two separate days, 13 subjects consumed 30g of non-enriched biscuits or hydroytyrosol-enriched biscuits containing 5.25mg hydroytyrosol following overnight-fasting. After hydroytyrosol-enriched biscuit consumption, plasma metabolites peaked between 0.5 and 1h and were excreted in urine. Hydroytyrosol sulfate and 3,4-dihydroxyphenylacetic acid-sulfate were the main metabolites. Concentrations of postprandial oxidised-LDL decreased with hydroytyrosol-enriched biscuit consumption. The study shows that biscuits can be fortified with hydroytyrosol for lowering LDL levels.

6.9.6 Bread

Clifton et al. (2004) studied the effect of phytosterol-enriched bread in mildly hypercholesterolemic men and women. On consumption of this bread, the plasma sitosterol content increased by 23% and campesterol by 52%. There was a significant reduction in the serum LDL cholesterol level.

Abd El-Megeid et al. (2009) investigated the protective effect of 2% and 4% green tea-fortified bread on renal failure of rats induced by excessive dietary arginine. Feeding of green tea-fortified bread might ameliorate the pathological effects on kidney enzymes, uric acid, urea nitrogen, and creatinine.

Söderholm et al. (2012) studied the effect of high-fiber rye bread enriched with nonesterified plant sterols on the major serum lipids and apolipoproteins (apo) in sixty-eight normocholesterolemic subjects. Participants were randomized to receive a rye bread enriched with plant sterols. Compliance was monitored with 3-day food diaries and alkylresorcinol metabolite concentrations. Consumption of the fortified bread for 2 weeks significantly reduced serum total and LDL cholesterol, apoB/apoA1, and total cholesterol:HDL cholesterol ratios by 5.1%, 8.1%, 8.3%, and 7.2%, respectively, when compared with controls. The doubling of the dose in the following 2 weeks resulted in a 6.5%, 10.4%, 5.5%, and 3.7% difference.

Hobbs et al. (2013) conducted a randomized clinical trial to study the effect of acute ingestion of beetroot bread on endothelium-independent vasodilation and diastolic blood pressure. Twenty-three healthy men received 200 g of bread containing 100 g of beetroot and postprandial microvascular vasodilation was measured by laser Doppler iontophoresis. Arterial stiffness was measured by pulse wave analysis and blood pressure was measured by a noninvasive ambulatory blood pressure monitor. The authors observed a significantly greater microvascular vasodilation response and a lower diastolic blood pressure after acute consumption of beetroot-fortified bread.

Mildner-Szkudlarz and Bajerska (2013) fortified bread with dried and powdered grape skin and its freeze-dried extract. The phenolic compounds in the fortified breads were predominantly epicatechin and catechin along with appreciable amounts of dimeric procyanidins. Sensory evaluation of the fortified breads showed that a maximum of 6% powdered grape skin and 1.4% of its extract could be incorporated without affecting taste. Feeding of high-cholesterol/cholic acid diet containing 6% powdered grape skin or 1.4% extract-fortified bread increased fresh stool weight and significantly reduced protein and fat digestion without negatively affecting growth of rats. Both types of fortified breads reduced the negative impact of high-cholesterol/cholic acid diet, lowering total cholesterol, low-density lipoprotein cholesterol, lipid peroxidation, glucose and leptin levels, preventing visceral fat accumulation and increasing high-density lipoprotein cholesterol levels. The experimental results suggest that cardiovascular risk can be reduced by consumption of bread fortified with grape skin powder or its extract.

Muammar et al. (2016) fortified bread with 5% and 10% juice of *Aloe vera*. When fed to diabetic rats, these fortified bread was able to bring blood glucose, lipid profiles, and biomarkers of liver function down to normal levels.

Metabolic syndrome is associated with an increased risk for type 2 diabetes mellitus and cardiovascular disease. Treatment of metabolic syndrome includes the replacement of saturated fats and monosaccharides with unsaturated fat. Miller et al. (2016) conducted a prospective, open-label clinical study in thirty-nine men and women to test the hypothesis that an American Heart Association diet enriched in monounsaturated fatty acids improves lipoprotein lipids, insulin resistance, inflammation, and endothelial function. Participants consumed 3 monounsaturated fatty acid-enriched or polyunsaturated fatty acid-enriched muffins daily with additional supplementation to ensure 25%–50% increases in dietary fat intake from these sources. Substitution of saturated fatty acids with polyunsaturated fatty acids in patients with metabolic syndrome caused greater reductions in triglycerides and improvement in endothelial function than monounsaturated fatty acids, suggesting that polyunsaturated fatty acids may be the unsaturated fat of choice to reduce cardiometabolic risk in patients with metabolic syndrome.

6.9.7 *Yogurt*

The cholesterol-lowering effects of lactic acid fermented soy milk, in which part of the soy milk was replaced by soy yogurt, were studied in rats (Kitawaki et al. 2009). The results indicate that soy yogurt is helpful in preventing hepatic lipid accumulation in rats. Based on a study carried out on rabbits, Cavallini et al. (2009) suggest that soy yogurt could be consumed to reduce the risk of cardiovascular disease, as it improves the lipid profile. Their study also shows that isoflavone supplementation enhances the antiatherogenic effect of soy yogurt. The results of two clinical studies suggest that phytosterol-enriched yogurt has the ability to lower commonly measured lipid parameters (Nittynen et al., 2008; Ruiu et al., 2009).

The ability of a functional yogurt fortified with herbal extracts to improve metabolic syndrome was studied by Chang et al. (2011). The test product NY-YP901 was supplemented with mixture of *Streptococcus thermophilus, Lactobacillus acidophilus, Bifidobacterium infantis Bifidobacterium breve* (CBG-C2), *Enterococcus fecalis* FK-23, and extracts of *Pinus densiflora*, rice germ, *Yucca schidigera*, and *Quillaja saponaria*. In this randomized, double-blind, placebo-controlled, parallel study, a treatment group consisting of 53 individuals consumed NY-YP901 and control group consisting of 48 individuals consumed a placebo yogurt for eight weeks. After eight weeks of treatment, statistically significant beneficial changes were observed in body weight, body mass index, and low-density lipoprotein (LDL)-cholesterol in the experimental group consuming NY-YP901.

The impact of inulin-fortified yogurt on metabolic syndrome was further studied by Kaminskas et al. (2013). After consuming the inulin-fortified yogurt for twenty-eight days, individuals with metabolic syndrome showed significant decrease of high-density lipoprotein cholesterol, low density lipoprotein cholesterol, and malondialdehyde. Consumption of inulin-enriched yogurt showed a tendency to lower total cholesterol, but there was no change in triglyceride concentration. There was also reduction of both systolic and diastolic blood pressure. According to these findings, consumption of yogurt enriched with inulin might have a beneficial effect on patients with metabolic syndrome and improve their health.

There is a growing trend to make use of agricultural wastes like pomace left after extracting fruit juices, as alternative low-cost sources of phenolic compounds. Pomegranate is one good example of such a fruit, 50% of whose weight is peel, which is usually discarded as waste. Nevertheless, it has a high content of polyphenols. Therefore, Sakr and Dawood (2015) tried to fortify yogurt with pomegranate juice or pomegranate peel extract to produce a heart-healthy dairy product. Experimental results show that yogurt fortified either with pomegranate juice or water extract of peel has the ability to lower total lipid, total triglycerides, and total cholesterol. Pomegranate juice-fortified yogurt and peel extract-fortified yogurt were able to counter the histological changes caused by hypercholesterolemic diet. It therefore, seems that yogurt fortified with either the juice or peel of pomegranate can help in controlling hypercholesterolemia.

In addition to lowering blood cholesterol, yogurts made with plant-derived lactic acid bacteria have the ability to increase defecation frequency in patients suffering from constipation (Higashikawa et al., 2010). Yogurts prepared from cow or goat's milk are also effective in offering protection against experimental acute liver injury in mice (Haro et al., 2009).

Studies conducted in mice offer evidence for the anti-inflammatory effect of yogurt in inflammatory bowel disease. This effect is believed to be mediated by an increase in the number of immunoglobulin A (IgA)+ cells, a decrease in the CD8+ population, and an enhancement of apoptosis of infiltrative cells in the large intestine (Gobbato et al., 2008).

Recent reports indicate that the consumption of yogurt could offer protection from type 2 diabetes. O'Connor et al. (2014) sampled the EPIC-Norfolk study, a cohort of more than 25,000 men and women from Norfolk, England. The authors compared the weekly food diaries of 752 people who developed new onset type 2 diabetes, over 11 years of follow-up, with 3,502 randomly selected subjects. An analysis of the data showed that the consumption of four and a half standard pots of yogurt per week could reduce the risk of developing type 2 diabetes by a quarter.

Development of eye and brain function in infants is believed to be influenced by dietary ω-3 fatty acids. The favored transport of ω-3 fatty acids from mothers to their infants during both pregnancy and breast feeding may result in depletion of maternal ω-3 fatty acid stores. Dietary supplementation of ω-3 fatty acids helps to reverse depletion of maternal docosahexanoic acid stores (Smithers et al., 2008). Epidemiological studies and intervention studies have established a positive relationship between increasing levels of dietary ω-3 fatty acids and decreased risk of coronary heart disease. ω-3 fatty acids offer protection from coronary heart disease through their effects on lipid metabolism, heart function, vasodilatation, platelet aggregation, and blood clotting (Kris-Etherton et al., 2003). Therefore, food-based delivery of ω-3 fatty acids is an attempt to increase the dietary intake of this important nutrient.

McCowen et al. (2010) developed a stable emulsion of docosahexaenoic acid by mixing algal oil, a vegetable source of ω-3 oils, with an aqueous phase. This emulsion was blended with yogurt, which was then inoculated with freeze-dried starter culture containing *Streptococcus thermophilus* and *Lactobacillus delbruecki* subsp. *bulgaricus* and set in containers containing 22.7% strawberry base. Twelve healthy volunteers were served daily one serving of the yogurt that contained 600 mg of docosahexaenoic acid. Plasma phospholipid docosahexaenoic acid content increased significantly after three weeks of supplementation.

Synbiotic yogurt can be beneficial in alleviating some of the maladies afflicting young children. This aspect was studied by Ringel-Kulka et al. (2015). One hundred and forty-nine healthy children attending child care centers were enrolled in a prospective, double-blind, placebo-controlled clinical trial. The intervention applied was a yogurt drink containing *Streptococcus thermophilus, Lactobacillus bulgaricus, Bifidobacterium animalis* subspecies *lactis* (BB-12), and 1 g of inulin. A similar non-synbiotic-containing acidified milk drink served as placebo . The test product and placebo were administered once daily for sixteen weeks. At the end of the study children receiving synbiotic yogurt had significantly fewer days of reported fever and marked improvement in social functioning and school functioning. The synbiotic group reported ≥ 3 loose/watery stools, which may be due to the accelerating effect of BB-12 and inulin on intestinal transit.

6.9.8 Spreads

Plant sterols are minor constituents of vegetable oils having a cholesterol-like chemical structure (Pollak and Kritchevsky, 1981). When consumed at levels 5–10 times higher than the normal intake, plant sterols lower blood LDL cholesterol levels. Cholesterol can be considerably reduced when plant sterols are consumed along with a healthy diet (Hallikainen et al., 2000; Law, 2000). Dietary plant sterols lower blood cholesterol levels by reducing the absorption of dietary and biliary cholesterol from the gut. Displacing cholesterol from the micelles, limiting the intestinal solubility of cholesterol, or decreasing the hydrolysis of cholesterol esters in the small intestine can also be the possible mechanisms (Ling and Jones, 1995).

Spreads have been considered as a suitable matrix for delivering phytosterols. Phytosterol-containing spreads having the ability to lower cholesterol were launched in several European countries, the United States, Australia and New Zealand in the late 1990s (de Deckere and Verschuren, 2000). Several clinical trials have proved the ability of these products to lower total-and LDL-cholesterol (Sierksma et al., 1999. Neil et al., 2001, Christiansen et al., 2001, Ntanios et al., 2002, Lee et al., 2003b, Skeaff et al., 2005).

Consumption of food products such as a fortified spread containing moderate amounts of vitamin E and carotenoids can also lead to measurable and significant improvements in antioxidant status and biomarkers of oxidative stress, as was evident from a double-blind, placebo-controlled, parallel, 11-week intervention study on one hundred five healthy adults (Upritchard et al., 2003).

6.10 Conclusion

The concept of foods that promote health is not new; 2500 years ago Hippocrates advised that food is medicine and medicine can be food (Wildman, 2000). The traditional Indian medical system of Ayurveda also believes that dietary indiscretions can bring forth diseases and they can be cured by consumption of medicinal food and adoption of healthy eating habits (Kumar, 2016a). Food therapy is an important part of Chinese medicine and its efficacy has been confirmed by modern studies (Shen et al., 2010). Scientific research carried out in recent times shows that many food substances play a beneficial role in the management of some diseases (Hasler, 2002).

Phytonutrients are extracted from herbs using conventional solvent extraction technology or supercritical carbon dioxide extraction technology. While the former method uses benign organic solvents, the latter method uses supercritical carbon dioxide, which is ecofriendly (Kumar, 2016b). With the rise of green chemistry, the solvent extraction industry is urged to use safer solvents and auxiliaries. Research in green chemistry has encouraged the use of many biodegradable, noncorrosive, noncarcinogenic, and non-ozone depleting solvents (Kerton, 2009). One among them is ethyl lactate (ethyl 2-hydroxy-propanoate) and its use has already been demonstrated in the extraction of sclareol from clary sage (Tombokan, 2008), carotenoids from different plant matrices (Ishida and Chapman, 2009; Strati and Oreopoulou, 2011; Wu et al., 2011), γ-linolenic acid from spirulina (Golmakani et al. 2012), caffeine from green coffee beans and green tea leaves (Bermejo et al. 2012), thymol from thyme (Angelov et al., 2013), and the fractionation of squalene and tocopherol from edible oils (Hernández et al., 2011; Vicente et al., 2011).

The search for inexpensive raw material is also on the rise. Many plant hulls or husks such as those of peanut, mung bean, buckwheat, rice, and almond are generally discarded as agro-industrial by-products or waste. But they are in fact, rich in antioxidant polyphenolic compounds (Ramarathnam et al., 1989; Yen and Duh, 1993; Duh et al., 1997; Watanabe et al., 1997; Takeoka and Dao, 2003). The latest addition to the list of such raw materials is pistachio hulls, which are accumulated in high volumes during industrial post-harvest processing of pistachio nuts. Researchers from the Plants for Human Health Institute of North Carolina State University report that pistachio hulls have a phytochemical composition with a mixture of anacdardic acid homologues that are known for their anti-inflammatory and antioxidant activities. Many value-added products with potential applications in food supplement and drug industries can be developed from them (Grace et al., 2016).

Nearly two kilograms of spent coffee grounds are left from every kilogram of instant coffee manufactured and this amounts to six million tons every year all over the world. Martinez-Saez et al. (2016) recently reported that this by-product can be used in many food and health products. According to them spent coffee grounds from industrial instant coffee contains appreciable amounts of antioxidant insoluble dietary fiber, proteins, essential amino acids and low glycemic sugars, qualifying them for use in bakery products. The authors formulated six different sugar-free biscuits with varying quantities of grounds obtained from a Spanish instant coffee manufacturer. Stevia was used as sweetener and oligofructose as enhancer of glucose tolerance. The taste of the coffee grounds was effectively masked by these two ingredients. The study shows that up to 4% of spent coffee grounds can be added to the dough without affecting the quality of the biscuits. Taking a cue from these studies, coconut shells and husks of coconut and arecanut also need to be studied for pharmaceutical and nutraceutical applications.

With the burgeoning of the nutraceutical industry, many exotic plants are assuming greater significance. An example is the baobab tree (*Adansonia digitata*), which is widely distributed in Africa. It is believed to live up to more than 1,000 years and can hold nearly 100,000 liters of water. Several classes of compounds have been identified from fruit pulp, seed oil, leaves, and roots of this tree. They include terpenoids, flavonoids, sterols, vitamins, amino acids, carbohydrates, and lipids. Almost all parts of this tree are used in traditional African medicine (Kamatou et al, 2011). Coca-Cola launched in June, 2016 a soft drink that has baobab tree among its ingredients. Named *Aquarius Vive*, the low-calorie beverage was developed for the Spanish market and has zinc, vitamin B3, and baobab extract. The manufacturer "wanted to have an exotic ingredient which could give new news in the product proposition" (Arthur, 2016).

The popularity of food fortification has brought in many novel products. dietGum formulated with Fertin Pharma's patented bi-layered compressed chewing gum technology is designed to aid weight management. The major ingredients are green coffee bean extract (Svetol®) and green tea extract. Svetol® contains >45% chlorogenic acids and induces lipolysis from human adipocytes (Flanagan et al., 2014).

Green tea has lately made its appearance in breakfast cereal. In October 2013, the South African company Herbex Health introduced their product Slimmers Cereal containing extracts of green tea and *Garcinia cambogia* (Anonymous, 2014a). *G. cambogia* helps the body burn fat and prevents the formation of new fat (Heymsfield et al., 1998). The use of these two ingredients in a breakfast cereal is an innovation that is set to benefit from current global interest in achieving weight loss with natural ingredients (Figure 6.8).

Easy Teasy, an England-based company launched recently a series of tea-infused chocolate products (Yu, 2015; Figure 6.9). Zhaolong Foods, China has obtained patent from Anhui Agricultural University to manufacture China's first chewing gum with organic tea polyphenols. The tea polyphenol is anticarcinogenic and can help the human body absorb more vitamin C (Yu, 2016).

The Tetley brothers started their business in 1837, selling tea from the back of a pack horse in Yorkshire. After 175 years they are the world's second largest manufacturer and distributor of tea. Collaborating with a group of futurologists, Tetley recently issued a *Future of Tea* report that predicts how the industry will be in 2026. The desire for more functional foods and supplements will grow and by 2026, Tetley expects the health benefits of

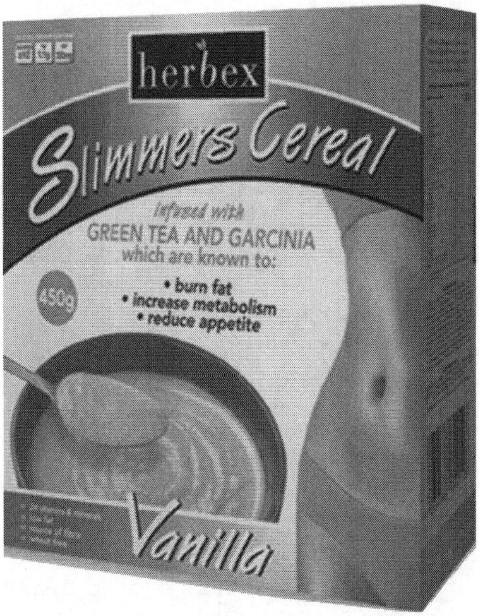

Figure 6.8 Slimmers Cereal, breakfast cereal fortified with green tea and *Garcinia cambogia*. (Reproduced with permission from Herbex, Cape Town, South Africa)

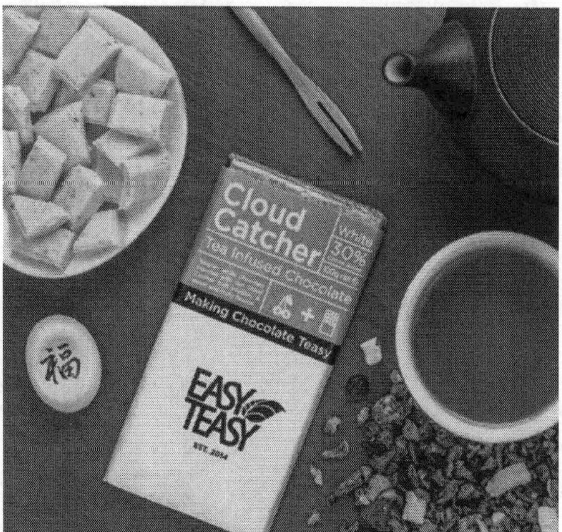

Figure 6.9 Cloud Catcher, tea infused chocolate. (Reproduced with permission from Easy Teasy, Newcastle-upon-Tyne, England)

products to be personalised to each individual. By 2026 Remedy Teas will emerge fortified with medicines, ranging from painkillers to antibiotics. Hangover Tea with added antacids and caffeine, Youthbrew Tea with collagen, Hair Restore Tea with minoxidil, and Virali-Tea with erectile dysfunction medicine are some of the products that are expected to emerge. New tea formats will also appear and for the time-poor, health-seeking, and convenience-hungry populace there will be products such as Tea Shots, Tea Sprays, Tablets, and Strips. Tea will also be presented as Tea Jellies, Sorbets, and Syrups in an array of exotic tastes and flavors (Anonymous, 2016b).

The concept of fortification has been used successfully to correct nutrient inadequacies and deficiencies associated with them. Interest in fortification has now shifted from prevention of deficiencies to improving health. We need to know more about how food intake influences biomarker concentrations. This knowledge is critical so that more appropriate vehicles for food fortification can be identified and better advice given to the food industry. In addition, there is a need for better reporting systems to identify potential adverse effects of excessive nutrient exposures. As the consumption of fortified food, beverages, and dietary supplements is on the rise, more research is needed to investigate the potential health consequences of chronically high intake of nutrients. Similarly, very little is known about the long-term stability of nanoparticles used as fortificants. Their quantification in food and interaction with the gut and the greater immune system also remain largely unknown (Dwyer et al., 2015). Fortification of food and beverages is bound to become a strong means to prevent and manage diseases when advances are made in these areas.

References

Abbe Maleyki, M. J., and Amin, I. 2008. Polyphenols in cocoa and cocoa products: Is there a link between antioxidant properties and health? *Molecules* 13:2190–2219.

Abd El-Megeid, A. A., AbdAllah, I. Z. A., Elsadek, M. F., and Abd El-Moneim, Y. F. 2009. The protective effect of the fortified bread with green tea against chronic renal failure induced by excessive dietary arginine in male albino rats. *World Journal of Dairy & Food Sciences* 4:107–117.

Adlercreutz, H., Mousavi, Y., and Clark J. et al. 1992. Dietary phytoestrogens and cancer: *In vitro* and *in vivo* studies. *Journal of Steroid Biochemistry and Molecular Biology* 41:331–337.

Amidon, G. L., Lennernas, H., Shah, V. P., and Crison, J. R. 1995. A theoretical basis for a biopharmaceutic drug classification: The correlation of *in vitro* drug product dissolution and *in vivo* bioavailability. *Pharmaceutical Research* 12:413–420.

Angelov, I., Bermejo, D. V., Stateva, R. P. Reglero, G., Ibañez, E., and Fornari, T. 2013. Extraction of thymol from different varieties of thyme plants using green solvents. In *III Iberoamerican Conference on Supercritical Fluids*, Cartagena de Indias, Colombia, pp. 1–7.

Anonymous. 1978. *Primary Health Care: Report on the International Conference on Primary Health Care Alma-Ata*, September, 1978, USSR, pp. 6–12 WHO, Geneva, 1–78.

Anonymous. 1999. Scientific concepts of functional foods in Europe consensus document. *British Journal of Nutrition* 81:S1–S27.

Anonymous. 2006. *Probiotics in food—Health and Nutritional Properties and Guidelines for Evaluation*, WHO/FAO, Rome, pp. 1–56.

Anonymous. 2011. Wrigley gains novel food approval for magnolia bark extract in EU.http://www.confectionerynews.com/Regulation-Safety/Wrigley-gains-novel-foodapproval-for-magnolia-bark-extract-in-EU (accessed November 26, 2011).

Anonymous. 2013a. http://www.confectionerynews.com/R-D/Chewing-gum-developed-tobattle-common-cold (accessed May 18, 2013).

Anonymous. 2013b. http://www.fertin.com/Products/Nutraceutical/Pages/default.aspx (accessed December 25, 2013).

Anonymous. 2014a. http://herbexhealth.com/shop/slimmers-cereal/ (accessed February 19, 2014).

Anonymous. 2016a. Sweet Dreams are Made of Cheese. http://www.dailymail.co.uk/health/article-362101/Sweet-dreamscheese.html (accessed January 22, 2016).

Anonymous. 2016b. The Future of Tea Report. https://www.tetley.co.uk/docs/librariesprovider6/default-document-library/future-of-tea-report (accessed on 29 August, 2016).

Arnoldi, A. 2003. The Maillard reaction as a source of off-flavours. In: Baigrie, B. (Ed.). *Taints and Off-flavours in Food*. Boca Raton, FL: CRC Press; pp. 162–175.

Arthur, R. 2016. Coca-Cola turns to baobab in new low calorie soft drink brand. NutraIngredients.com 19 July. http://www.nutraingredients.com/Manufacturers/Coca-Cola-turns-to-baobab-in-new-low-calorie-soft-drink-brand/ (accessed 22 July, 2016).

Arts, I. C., Hollman, P. C., and Kromhout, D. 1999. Chocolate as a source of tea flavonoids. *Lancet* 354:488.

Augustin, M. A., and Sanguansri, L. 2008. Encapsulation of bioactives. In: Aguilera, J.M., and Lillford, P.J. (Eds.). *Food Materials Science: Principles and Practice*. New York, NY: Springer Science + Business Media; pp. 577–601.

Augustin, M. A., and Sanguansri, L. 2012. Challenges in developing delivery systems for food additives, nutraceuticals and dietary supplements. In: Garti, N., and McClements, D.J. (Eds.). *Encapsulation Technologies and Delivery Systems for Food Ingredients and Nutraceuticals*. Cambridge, UK: Woodhead Publishing Ltd; pp. 19–48.

Bai, L. 2007. Analysis of some nutritive and medicinal components in Shiitake (*Lentinus edodes* (Berk.) Singer). *Journal of Zhoukou Normal University* 24:101–102.

Bahgaat, W. K. 2010. Utilization of some functional foods for lowering blood lipids. PhD thesis submitted to Department of Food Science, Faculty of Agriculture, Ain Shams University, Cairo, Egypt.

Balanč, B. D., Ota, A., Djordjević, V. B. et al. 2015. Resveratrol-loaded liposomes: Interaction of resveratrol with phospholipids. *European Journal of Lipid Science and Technology* 117:1615–1626.

Balzer, J., Heiss, C., and Schroeter, H. 2006. Flavanols and cardiovascular health—Efforts on the circulating NO pool in humans. *Journal of Cardiovascular Pharmacology* 47 (Suppl. 2):S122–S127.

Banville, C., Vuillemard, J. C., and Lacroix, C. 2000. Comparison of different methods for fortifying cheddar cheese with vitamin D. *International Dairy Journal* 10:375–382.

Barreca, D., Bellocco, E., Leuzzi, U., and Gattuso, G. 2014. First evidence of C- and O-glycosyl flavone in blood orange (*Citrus sinensis* (L.) Osbeck) juice and their influence on antioxidant properties. *Food Chemistry* 149:244–252.

Barros, L., Carvalho, A. M., Morais, J. S., and Ferreira, I. C. F. R. 2010. Strawberry-tree, blackthorn and rose fruits: Detailed characterisation in nutrients and phytochemicals with antioxidant properties. *Food Chemistry* 120:247–254.

Barth, S. W., Faehndrich, C., Bub, A. et al. 2007. Cloudy apple juice is more effective than apple polyphenols and an apple juice derived cloud fraction in a rat model of colon carcinogenesis. *Journal of Agricultural and Food Chemistry* 55:1181–1187.

Bartoshuk, L. M. 1987. Is sweetness unitary? An evaluation of the evidence for multiple sweets. In: Dobbing, J. (Ed.). *Sweetness*. London: Springer-Verlag; pp. 33–47.

Basu, A., Rhone, M., and Lyons, T. J. 2010. Berries: Emerging impact on cardiovascular health. *Nutrition Reviews* 68:168–177.

Baudin, C., Pean, C., Perly, B., and Goselin, P. 2000. Inclusion of organic pollutants in cyclodextrin and derivatives. *International Journal of Environmental Analytical Chemistry*. 77:233–242.

Beckett, S. 2009. Chocolate manufacture. In: Talbot, G. (Ed.). *Science and Technology of Enrobed and Filled Chocolate, Confectionery and Bakery Products*. Cambridge, UK: Woodhead Publishing Limited; pp. 11–28.

Bell, L. N. 2007. Nutraceutical stability concerns and shelf-life testing. In: Wildman, R. E. C. (Ed.). *Handbook of Nutraceuticals and Functional Foods*. Boca Raton, FL: CRC Press; pp. 467–483.

Belščak-Cvitanović, A., Durgo, K., Cindrić, I. J., Vojvodić, A., Komes, D., and Franekić, J. 2012. Bioactive compounds content, cytotoxic and antioxidant/prooxidant activity of different cocoa products on human laryngeal carcinoma cell line. *Proceedings of 6th Central European Congress on Food*, 23–26 May, Novi Sad, Serbia, pp. 108–113.

Berendschot, T. T. J. M., Goldbohm, R. A., Klöpping, W. A. A. et al. 2000. Influence of lutein supplementation on macular pigment, assessed with two objective techniques. *Investigative Ophthalmology & Visual Science* 41:3322–3326.

Berger, Z., Roder, H., Hanna, A. et al. 2007. Accumulation of pathological tau species and memory loss in a conditional model of tauopathy. *The Journal of Neuroscience* 27:3650–3662.

Bermejo, D. V., Luna, P., Manic, M. S., Najdanovic-Visak, V., Regleroa, G., and Fornari, T. 2012. Extraction of caffeine from natural matter using a bio-renewable agrochemical solvent. *Food and Bioproducts Processing* 91:303–309.

Berry, N. M., Davison, K., Coates, A. M., Buckley, J. D., and Howe, P. R. C. 2010. Impact of cocoa flavanol consumption on blood pressure responsiveness to exercise. *British Journal of Nutrition* 103:1480–1484.

Berry, S. K. 2001. Role of acidulants in food industry. *Journal of Food Science and Technology-Mysore* 38:93–104.

Bodmeier, R., and McGinity, J. W. 1987. The preparation and evaluation of drug-containing poly(dl-lactide) microspheres formed by the solvent evaporation method. *PharmaceuticalResearch* 4:465–471.

Bodmeier, R., and McGinity, J. W. 1988a. Solvent selection in the preparation of poly (D, Llactide) microspheres prepared by the solvent evaporation method. *International Journal of Pharmaceutics* 43:179–186.

Bodmeier, R., and McGinity, J. W. 1988b. Polylactic acid microspheres containing quinidine base and quinidine sulfate prepared by the solvent evaporation method. III. Morphology of the microspheres during dissolution studies. *Journal of Microencapsulation* 5:325–330.

Bodmeier, R., Wang, H., and Hermann, J. 1994. Microencapsulation of chlorpheniramine maleate, a drug with intermediate solubility properties, by a non-aqueous solvent evaporation technique. *STP Pharma Sciences* 4:275–281.

Boobier, W. J., Baker, J. S. Hullen, D., Graham, M. R., and Davies, B. 2007. Functional biscuits and coronary heart disease risk factors. *British Food Journal* 109:260–267.

Borel, P., Tyssandier, V., Mekki, N. et al. 1998. Chylomicron betacarotene and retinyl palmitate responses are dramatically diminished when men ingest betacarotene with mediumchain rather than long-chain triglycerides. *Journal of Nutrition* 128:1361–1367.

Boroski, M., de Aguiar, A. C., Boeing, J. S. et al. 2011. Enhancement of pasta antioxidant activity with oregano and carrot leaf. *Food Chemistry* 125:696–700.

Borzalleca, J. F. 1994. Foods of the future: What will we be eating in the next century. In: Kirby, D. F., and Dudrick, S.J. (Eds.). *Practical Handbook of Nutrition in Clinical Practice.* Boca Raton, FL: CRC Press; pp. 279–288.

Bouhnik, Y., Raskine, L., Simoneau, G. et al. 2004. The capacity of nondigestible carbohydrates to stimulate fecal bifidobacteria in healthy humans: A double-blind, randomized, placebo-controlled, parallel-group, dose-response relation study. *American Journal of Clinical Nutrition* 80:1658–1664.

Bramley, P. M., Elmadfa, I., Kafatos, A. et al. 2000. Vitamin E. *Journal of the Science of Food and Agriculture* 80:913–938.

Buttriss, J. 2012. Plant foods and health. In: Salter, A., Wiseman, H., and Tucker, G. (Eds.). *Phytonutrients.* West Sussex, UK: Wiley-Blackwell; pp. 1–51.

Capraro, J., Magni, C., Scarafoni, A. et al. 2014. Pasta supplemented with isolated lupin protein fractions reduces body weight gain and food intake of rats and decreases plasma glucose concentration upon glucose overload trial. *Food & Function* 5:375–380.

Castenmiller, J. J. M., and West C. E. 1998. Bioavailability and bioconversion of carotenoids. *Annual Review of Nutrition* 118:19–38.

Cavallini, D. C., Abdalla, D. S., Vendramini, R. C. et al. 2009. Effects of isoflavone-supplemented soy yogurt on lipid parameters and atherosclerosis development in hypercholesterolemic rabbits—A randomized double-blind study. *Lipids in Health and Disease* 8:40. doi:10.1186/1476-511X-8-40.

Céspedes, C. L., El-Hafidi, M., Pavon, N., Alarcon, J. 2008. Antioxidant and cardioprotective activities of phenolic extracts from fruits of Chilean blackberry *Aristotelia chilensis* (Elaeocarpaceae), Maqui. *Food Chemistry* 107:820–829.

Chang, B. J., Park, S. U., Jang, Y. S. et al. 2011. Effect of functional yogurt NY-YP901 in improving the trait of metabolic syndrome. *European Journal of Clinical Nutrition* 65:1250–1255.

Chaudhari, R., and Fanion, M. 2008. Technical aspects of micronutrient addition to foods. In: Ottaway, P. B. (Ed.) *Food Fortification and Supplementation.* Boca Raton, FL: CRC Press; pp. 108–125.

Chen, Y. J., Inbaraj, B. S., Pu, Y. S., and Chen, B. H. 2014. Development of lycopene micelle and lycopene chylomicron and a comparison of bioavailability. *Nanotechnology* 25:155102.

Chihara, G. 1993. Medical aspects of lentinan isolated from *Lentinus edodes* (Berk.) *Sing.* In: Chang, S.-T. et al. (Eds.). *Mushroom Biology and Mushroom Products.* Hong Kong, China: The Chinese University Press; pp. 261–265.

Cho, E. S., Lee, K. W., and Lee, H. J. 2008. Cocoa procyanidins protect PC12 cells from hydrogen-peroxideinduced apoptosis by inhibiting activation of p38 MAPK and JNK. *Mutation Research* 640:123–130.

Christiansen, L. I., Lähteenmäki, P. L., Mannelin, M. R., Seppänen-Laakso, T. E., Hiltunen, R. V., and Yliruusi, J. K. 2001. Cholesterol-lowering effect of spreads enriched with microcrystalline plant sterols in hypercholesterolemic subjects. *European Journal of Nutrition* 40:66–73.

Chua, K. J., and Chou, S. K. 2003. Low-cost drying methods for developing countries. *Trends in Food Science & Technology* 14:519–528.

Chudnovskiy, R., Thompson, A., Tharp, K., Hellerstein, M., Napoli, J. L., and Stahl, A. 2014. Consumption of clarified grapefruit juice ameliorates high-fat diet induced insulin resistance and weight gain in mice. *PLOS ONE* 9(10):e108408.

Cleary, J. P., Walsh, D. M., Hofmeister, J. J. et al. 2005. Natural oligomers of the amyloid-β protein specifically disrupt cognitive function. *Nature Neuroscience* 8:79–84.

Clerici, C., Nardi, E., Battezzati, P. M. et al. 2011. Novel soy germ pasta improves endothelial function, blood pressure, and oxidative stress in patients with type 2 diabetes. *Diabetes Care* 34:1946–1948.

Clerici, C., Setchell, K. D. R., Battezzati, P. M. et al. 2007. Pasta naturally enriched with isoflavone aglycons from soy germ reduces serum lipids and improves markers of cardiovascular risk. *Journal of Nutrition* 137:2270–2278.

Clifton, P. M., Noakes, M., Sullivan, D. et al. 2004. Cholesterol-lowering effects of plant sterol esters differ in milk, yoghurt, bread and cereal. *European Journal of Clinical Nutrition* 58:503–509.

Codex Alimentarius. 1991. *Codex General Guidelines on Claims.* 2nd ed. (CAC/GL 1–1979, rev. 1–1991). Geneva: WHO.

Codex Alimentarius. 1997. *Guideline for Use of Nutrition Claims* (CAC/GL 23–1997, Volume 1A, rev.). Geneva: WHO.

Costabile, A., Walton, G. E., Tzortzis, G., Vulevic, J. Charalampopoulos, D., and Gibson, G. R. 2015. Effects of orange juice formulation on prebiotic functionality using an *in vitro* colonic model system. *PLOS ONE* 10 (3):e0121955. doi:10.1371/journal.pone.0121955. eCollection 2015.

Crawford, D. 1973. Garlic-growing and agricultural specialization in Graeco-Roman Egypt. *Chronique d'Egypte* 48:350–363.

Crichton, G. E., Elias, M. F., Alkerwi, A. 2016. Chocolate intake is associated with better cognitive function: The Maine-Syracuse Longitudinal Study. *Appetite* 100:126–132.

Crowley M. M., Zhang F., Repka M. A. et al. 2007. Pharmaceutical applications of hot melt extrusion: Part I. *Drug Development and Industrial Pharmacy* 33:909–926.

Dahan, A., Miller, J. M., and Amidon, G. L. 2009. Prediction of solubility and permeability class membership: Provisional BCS classification of the world's top oral drugs. *AAPS Journal* 11:740–746.

Davison, K., Coates, A. M., Buckley, J. D., and Howe, P. R. C. 2008. Effect of cocoa flavanols and exercise on cardiometabolic risk factors in overweight and obese subjects. *International Journal of Obesity* 32:1289–1296.

Debevere, J. M. 1988. Effect of buffered acidulant systems on the survival of some food poisoning bacteria in medium acid media. *Food Microbiology* 5:135–139.

de Deckere, E. A. M., and Verschuren, P. M. 2000. Functional fats and spreads. In: Gibson, G. R., and Williams, C.M. (Eds.). *Functional foods: Concept to product*, Cambridge, UK: Woodhead Publishing Limited; pp.233–257.

DeFelice, S. L. 1992. The nutraceutical initiative: A recommendation for U.S. economic and regulatory reforms. *Genetic Engineering News* 12:13–15.

Del Valle, E. M. M. 2004. Cyclodextrins and their uses: A review. *Process Biochemistry* 39:1033–1046.

Depeint, F., Tzortzis, G., Vulevic, J., I'Anson, K., and Gibson, G. R. 2008. Prebiotic evaluation of a novel galactooligosaccharide mixture produced by the enzymatic activity of *Bifidobacterium bifidum* NCIMB 41171, in healthy humans: A randomized, double-blind, crossover, placebo-controlled intervention study. *American Journal of Clinical Nutrition* 87:785–791.

De Vita, O. Z. 2009. Voyage in the pasta universe. In *Encyclopedia of Pasta*. Berkeley and Los Angeles: University of California Press; pp. 1–12.

Dixit, A. K., Antony, J. I. X., Sharma, N. K., Tiwari, R. K. 2011. Soybean constituents and their functional benefits. In: Tiwari, V. K. (Ed.). *Opportunity, Challenge and Scope of Natural Products in Medicinal Chemistry*, Trivandrum: Research Signpost; pp. 367–383.

Djurica, D., Holt, R. R., Ren, J., Shindel, A. W., Hackman, R. M., and Keen, C. L. 2016. Effects of a dietary strawberry powder on parameters of vascular health in adolescent males. *British Journal of Nutrition* 116:639–647. doi:10.1017/S0007114516002348.

Dlamini, N. R., Taylor, J., Rooney, L. W. 2007. The effect of sorghum type and processing on the antioxidant properties of African sorghum-based foods. *Food Chemistry* 105:1412–1419.

Drago, S., El Asmar, R., Di Pierro, M. et al. 2006. Gliadin, zonulin and gut permeability: Effects on celiac and non-celiac intestinal mucosa and intestinal cell lines. *Scandinavian Journal of Gastroenterology* 41:408–419.

Duan, Z., Xu, H., and Chen, Y. 1997. The effects of prevention and repair *of Lentinus edodes* on genetic damage induced by radiation in mice. *Chinese Journal of Radiological Health* 6:196–198.

Duh, P., Yen, W. J., Du, P. C., and Yen, G. C. 1997. Antioxidant activity of mung bean hulls. *Journal of the American Oil Chemists' Society* 74:1059–1063.

Dwyer, J. T., Wiemer, K. L., and Dary, O. et al. 2015. Fortification and health: Challenges and opportunities. *Advances in Nutrition* 6:124–131.

Edwards, W. P. 2000. *The Science of Sugar Confectionery*. Cambridge, UK: The Royal Society of Chemistry; pp. 1–166.

Erbay, F. M., Aydın, N., and Satı-Kırkan, T. 2013. Chewing gum may be an effective complementary therapy in patients with mild to moderate depression. *Appetite* 65:31–34.

Esmaili, M., Ghaffaria, S. M., Moosavi-Movahedi, Z. et al. 2011. Beta casein-micelle as a nano vehicle for solubility enhancement of curcumin; food industry application. *LWT - Food Science and Technology* 44:2166–2172.

Evans, M., Wilson, D., and Guthrie, N. 2014b. A randomized, double-blind, placebo-controlled, pilot study to evaluate the effect of whole grape extract on antioxidant status and lipid profile. *Journal of Functional Foods* 7:680–691.

Evans, S. F., Meister, M., Mahmood, M. et al. 2014a. Mango supplementation improves blood glucose in obese individuals. *Nutrition and Metabolic Insights* 7:77–84.

Eyer, H., Gauch, R., and Bosset, J. O. 1990. The fishy off-flavour of coffee cream. *Schweiz Milchwissenschaft und Forschung* 19:43–45.

Fang, Z., and Bhandari, B. 2012. Spray drying, freeze drying and related processes for food ingredient and nutraceutical encapsulation. In Garti, N., and McClements, D. J. (Eds.) *Encapsulation Technologies and Delivery Systems for Food Ingredients and Nutraceuticals*, Cambridge, UK: Woodhead Publishing Ltd; pp. 71–109.

Fasano, A. 2000. Regulation of intercellular tight junctions by zonula occludens toxin and its eukaryotic analogue zonulin. *Annals of the New York Academy of Sciences* 915:214–222.

Fasano, A., Not, T., Wang, W. et al. 2000. Zonulin, a newly discovered modulator of intestinal permeability, and its expression in coeliac disease. *Lancet* 355:1518–1519.

Faus, I., and Sisniega, H. 2003. Sweet-tasting proteins. In: Fahnestock, S. R and Steinbüchel, A. (Eds.). *Biopolymers*, vol. 8. Weinheim, Germany: Wiley-VCH; pp. 203–220.

Fazen, C. H., Valentin, D., Fairchild, T. J., and Doyle, R. P. 2011. Oral delivery of the appetite suppressing peptide hPYY(3–36) through the Vitamin B12 uptake pathway. *Journal of Medicinal Chemistry* 54:8707–8711.

Field, D. T., Williams, C. M., and Butler, L. T. 2011. Consumption of cocoaflavanols results in an acute improvement in visual and cognitive functions. *Physiology & Behavior* 103:255–260.

Fisher, L. A. 2011. Physicochemical characterization of a novel strawberry confection for delivery of fruit bioactives to human oral mucosa. Phd thesis, presented in partial fulfillment of the requirements for the degree Master of Science in the Graduate School of The Ohio State University, pp 1–103.

Flanagan, J., Bily, A., Rolland, Y., and Roller, M. 2014. Lipolytic activity of Svetol®, a decaffeinated green coffee bean extract. *Phytotherapy Research* 28:946–948.

Flint, H. J. 2011. Obesity and the gut microbiota. *Journal of Clinical Gastroenterology* 45:S128–S132.

Foucault, M. 1984. *Histoire de la sexualité. L'usage des Plaisirs*, vol. 2, Paris: Gallimard; pp. 21.

Fox, P. F., Guinee, T. P., Cogan, T. M., and McSweeney, P. L. H. 2000. Cheese: Historical aspects. In *Fundamentals of Cheese Science*. Maryland: Aspen Publishers; 1–9.

Fulushima, M., Ohashi, T., Fuliwara, Y. Sonoyama, K., and Nakano, M. 2001. Cholesterol-lowering effects of Maitake fibre, Shiitake fibre and Enokitake fibre in rats. *Experimental Biology and Medicine* 226:758–765.

Funami, T., Ishihara, S., and Kaoru Kohyama, K. 2014. Use of electromyography in measuring food texture. In: Dar, Y. L., and Light, J. M. (Eds.). *Food Texture Design and Optimization*. West Sussex, UK: John Wiley & Sons; pp.283–307.

Gad, A. S., Khadrawy, Y. A., El-Nekeety, A. A., Mohamed, S. R., Hassan, N. S., and Abdel-Wahhab, M. A. 2010. Antioxidant activity and hepatoprotective effects of whey protein and Spirulina in rats. *Nutrition* 27:582–589.

Gallo-Torres, H. E. 1970. Obligatory role of bile for the intestinal absorption of vitamin E. *Lipids* 5:379–384.

Galloa, M., Vinci, G., Graziani, G., De Simone, C., and Ferranti, P. 2013. The interaction of cocoa polyphenols with milk proteins studied by proteomic techniques. *Food Research Journal* 54:406–415.

Ganhão, R., Estévez, M., Kylli, P., Heinonen, M., and Morcuende, D. 2010. Characterization of selected wild mediterranean fruits and comparative efficacy as inhibitors of oxidative reactions in emulsified raw pork burger patties. *Journal of Agricultural and Food Chemistry* 58:8854–8861.

Garti, N., and Yuli-Amar, I. 2008. Micro- and nano-emulsions for delivery of functional food ingredients. In: Garti, N. (Ed.). *Delivery and Controlled Release of Bioactives in Foods and Nutraceuticals*. Cambridge, England: Woodhead Publishing Limited; pp.149–183.

Gascon, M. 2007. Masking agents for use in foods. In: Taylor, E., and Hort, J. (Eds.). *Modifying Flavour in Food*. Boca Raton, FL: CRC Press; pp. 232–242.

Gassenmeier, K. 2002. A new pathway leading to cardboard off-notes in ice cream and how to protect flavour integrity. *10th Weurman Flavour Research Symposium* June 25–28, Beaune, France.

Gironés-Vilaplana, A., Valentão, P., Andrade, P. B., Ferreres, F., García-Viguera, C., and Moreno, D. A. 2012. Quality and antioxidant capacity of novel beverages based on lemon and exotic berries. *Proceedings of 6th Central European Congress on Food*, May 23–26, Novi Sad, Serbia, pp. 7–12.

Gobbato, N., Rachid, M., and Perdigon, G. 2008. Anti-inflammatory effect of yoghurt in an experimental inflammatory bowel disease in mouse. *Journal of Dairy Science* 75:497–504.

Golmakani, M. T., Mendiola, J. A. Rezaeic, K., and Ibáñez, E. 2012. Expanded ethanol with CO_2 and pressurized ethyl lactate to obtain fractions enriched in γ-linolenic acid from *Arthrospira platensis* (Spirulina). *Journal of Supercritical Fluids* 62:109–115.

Gómez-Pinilla, F. 2008. Brain foods: The effects of nutrients on brain function. *Nature Reviews Neuroscience* 9:568–578.

Gong, Y. H., Wu, Y. K., Zheng, C. L., Fan, L. Y., Xiong, F., and Zhu, J. B. 2012. An excellent delivery system for improving the oral bioavailability of natural vitamin E in rats. *AAPS PharmSciTech* 13:961–966.

Gouda, M., Moustafa, A., Hussein, L., and Hamza, M. 2016. Three week dietary intervention using apricots, pomegranate juice or/and fermented sour sobya and impact on biomarkers of antioxidative activity, oxidative stress and erythrocytic glutathione transferase activity among adults. *Nutrition Journal* 15:52. doi:10.1186/s12937-016-0173-x.

Grace, M. H., Esposito, D., Timmers, M. A. et al. 2016. Chemical composition, antioxidant and anti-inflammatory properties of pistachio hull extracts. *Food Chemistry* 210:85–95.

Grant, M. 2000. *Introduction, Galen on Food and Diet*. London: Routledge; pp. 1–13.

Grassi, D., Lippi, C., Necozione, S. Desideri, G., and Ferri, C. 2005a. Short-term administration of dark chocolate is followed by a significant increase in insulin sensitivity and a decrease in blood pressure in healthy persons. *American Journal of Clinical Nutrition* 81:611–614.

Grassi, D., Necozione, S., Lippi, C. et al. 2005b. Cocoa reduces blood pressure and insulin resistance and improves endothelium-dependent vasodilation in hypertensives. *Hypertension* 46:398–405.

Gruenwald, J. 2009. Fortification of beverages with products other than vitamins and minerals. In: Paquin, P. (Ed.). *Functional and Speciality Beverage Technology*, Cambridge, UK: Woodhead Publishing Limited; pp. 92–106.

Gunasekaran, S., and Ak, M. M. 2002. Fundamental rheological methods. In: Gunasekaran, S., and Ak, M. M. (Eds.). *Cheese Rheology and Texture*. Boca Raton, FL: CRC Press; 31–112.

Gutiérrez-Grijalva, E. P., Ambriz-Pére, D. L., Leyva-López, N., Castillo-López, R. I., and Heredia, J. B. 2016. Review: Dietary phenolic compounds, health benefits and bioaccessibility. *Archivos Latinoamericanos De Nutrición* 66:87–100.

Hallikainen, M. A., Sarkkinen, E. S. Gylling, H., Erkkila, A. T., and Uusitupa, M. I. J. 2000. Comparison of the effects of plant sterol eater and plant stanol ester-enriched margarines in lowering serum cholesterol concentrations in hypercholesterolaemic subjects on a low-fat diet. *European Journal of Clinical Nutrition* 54:715–725.

Hamilton, R. J. 2003. Oxidative rancidity as a source of off-flavours. In: Baigrie, B. (Ed.). *Taints and Off-flavours in Food*. Boca Raton, FL: CRC Press; pp. 140–161.

Haro, C., Lazarte, S., Zelaya, H. Alvarez, S., and Aguero, G. 2009. Yogurt—Effect on leukocytes and blood coagulation in an acute liver injury model. *Journal of Medicinal Food* 12:796–802.

Hasler, C. M. 2002. Functional foods: Benefits, concerns and challenges—A position paper from the American Council on Science and Health. *Journal of Nutrition* 132:3772–3781.

Hassan, A. A., Rasmy, N. M., Foda, M. I., and Bahgaat, W. K. 2012. Production of functional biscuits for lowering blood lipids. *World Journal of Dairy & Food Sciences* 7:1–20.

Hassanein, M. M. M., El-Shami, S. M., and El-Mallah, M. H. 2011. Investigation of lipids profiles of nigella, lupin and artichoke seed oils to be used as healthy oils. *Journal of Oleo Science* 60:99–107.

Hedges, R. A. 1998. Industrial applications of cyclodextrins. *Chemical Reviews* 98:2035–2044.

Heinrich, U., Neukam, K., Tronnier, H. Sies, H., and Stahl, W. 2006. Long-term ingestion of high flavanol cocoa provides photoprotection against UV-induced erythema and improves skin condition in women. *Journal of Nutrition* 136:1565–1569.

Heiss, C., Dejam, A., Kleinbongard, P. Schewe, T. Sies, H., and Kelm, M. 2003. Vascular effects of cocoa rich in flavan-3-ols. *Journal of the American Medical Association* 290:1030–1031.

Heiss, C., Kleinbongard, P., Dejam, A. et al. 2005. Acute consumption of flavanol-rich cocoa and the reversal of endothelial dysfunction in smokers. *Journal of the American College of Cardiology* 46:1276–1283.

Henry, C. J. 2010. Functional foods. *European Journal of Clinical Nutrition* 64:657–659.

Hernández, E. J., Luna, P., Stateva, R. P., Najdanovic-Visak, V., Reglero, G., and Fornari, T. 2011. Liquid–liquid phase transition of mixtures comprising squalene, olive oil, and ethyl lactate—Application to recover squalene from oil deodorizer distillates. *Journal of Chemical & Engineering Data* 56:2148–2152.

Herrera, E., and Barbas, C. 2001. Vitamin E: Action, metabolism and perspectives. *Journal of Physiology and Biochemistry* 57:43–56.

Heymsfield, S. B., Allison, D. B., Vasselli, J. R., Pietrobelli, A., Greenfield, D., and Nunez, C. 1998. *Garcinia cambogia* (hydroxycitric acid) as a potential anti-obesity agent—A randomized controlled trial. *Journal of American Medical Association* 280:1596–1600.

Higashikawa, F., Noda, M., Awaya, T. Nomura, K. Oku, H., and Sugiyama, M. 2010. Improvement of constipation and liver function by plant-derived lactic acid bacteria—A double blind, randomized trial. *Nutrition* 26:367–374.

Hobbs, D. A., Goulding, M. G., Nguyen, A. et al. 2013. Acute ingestion of beetroot bread increases endothelium-independent vasodilation and lowers diastolic blood pressure in healthy men—A randomized controlled trial. *The Journal of Nutrition* 43:1399–1405.

Hoenicke, K., Boerchet, O., Grüning, K., Simat, T. J. 2002. Untypical aging off-flavor in wine: Synthesis of potential degradation compounds of indole-3-acetic acid and kinurenine and their evaluation as precursors of 2-aminoacetophenone. *Journal of Agricultural and Food Chemistry* 50:4303–4309.

Hogan, S., Chung, H., Zhang, L. et al. 2010. Antiproliferative and antioxidant properties of anthocyanin-rich extract from açai. *Food Chemistry* 118:208–214.

Hongu, N., Kitts, D. D., Zawistowski, J. et al. 2014. Pigmented rice bran and plant sterol combination reduces serum lipids in overweight and obese Adults. *Journal of American College of Nutrition* 33:231–238.

Hortin, G. L. 2006. Homocysteine- Clinical significance and laboratory measurement. *Laboratory Medicine* 37:551–553.

Horwood, J. F., Lloyd, G. T., Ramshaw, E. H., and Stark, W. 1981. An off-flavour associated with the use of sorbic acid during Feta cheese maturation. *Australian Journal of Dairy Technology* 36:38–40.

Hussein, H. M., Hussein, M. M., and El-Damohery, S. T. 2006. The effect of natural formulated functional biscuits on elderly bone health. *Journal of Medical Sciences* 6:937–943.

IFST. 1993. *Shelf-life of Foods: Guidelines for its Determination and Prediction*. London: Institute of Food Science & Technology.

Ishida, B. K., and Chapman, M. H. 2009. Carotenoid extraction from plants using a novel, environmentally friendly solvent. *Journal of Agricultural and Food Chemistry* 57:1051–1059.

Jacobsen, C., Hartvigsen, K., Homsen, M. K. et al. 2001. Lipid oxidation in fish oil enriched mayonnaise: Calcium disodium ethylenediaminetetraacetate, but not gallic acid strongly inhibited oxidative deterioration. *Journal of Agricultural and Food Chemistry* 49:1009–1019.

Jalil, R., and Nixon, J. R. 1990. Microencapsulation using poly(dl-lactic acid) I: Effect of preparative variables on the microcapsule characteristics and release kinetics. *Journal of Microencapsulation* 7:229–244.

Jaraswekin, S., Prakongpan, S., and Bodmeier, R. 2007. Effect of poly(lactide-co-glycolide) molecular weight on the release of dexamethasone sodium phosphate from microparticles. *Journal of Microencapsulation* 24:117–128.

Jensen, G. S., Ager, D. M., Redman, K. A., Mitzner, M. A., Benson, K. F., and Schauss, A. G. 2011. Pain reduction and improvement in range of motion after daily consumption of an açai (*Euterpe oleracea* Mart.) pulp-fortified polyphenolic-rich fruit and berry juice blend. *Journal of Medicinal Food* 14:702–711.

Jensen, G. S., Wu, X., Patterson, K. M. et al. 2008. *In vitro* and *in vivo* antioxidant and anti-inflammatory capacities of an antioxidant-rich fruit and berry juice blend. Results of a pilot and randomized, double -blinded, placebo-controlled, crossover study. *Journal of Agricultural and Food Chemistry* 56:8326–8333.

Jeppesen, P. B. 2003. Clinical significance of GLP-2 in short-bowel syndrome. *Journal of Nutrition* 133:3721–3724.

Jiang, B., Mu, W., Obiro, W., and Shi, J. 2011. Traditional Chinese functional foods. In: Shi, J., Ho, C. T., and. Shahidi, F. (Eds.). *Functional Foods of the East*. Boca Raton, FL: CRC Press; pp 13–50.

Jin, H. H., Lu, Q., and Jiang, J. G. 2016. Curcumin liposomes prepared with milk fat globule membrane phospholipids and soybean lecithin. *Journal of Dairy Science* 99:1780–1790.

Johnson, E. J., Hammond, B. R., Yeum, K. J. et al. 2000. Relation among serum and tissue concentrations of lutein and zeaxanthin and macular pigment density. *American Journal of Clinical Nutrition* 71:1555–1562.

Johnson, E. J., Neuringer, M., Russell, R. M. Schalch, W., and Snodderly, D. M. 2005. Nutritional manipulation of primate retinas, III: Effects of lutein or zeaxanthin supplementation on adipose tissue and retina of xanthophyll-free monkeys. *Investigative Ophthalmology & Visual Science* 46:692–702.

Jones, S. T., Aryana, K. J., and Losso, J. N. 2005. Storage stability of lutein during ripening of cheddar cheese. *Journal of Dairy Science* 88:1661–1670.

Jouanna, J. 1983. *Hippocrate, Tome X, 2e partie, Maladies II. Collection des*. Paris, France: Universités de France.

Jung, J., and Perrut, M. 2001. Particle design using supercritical fluids: Literature and patent survey. *Journal of Supercritical Fluids* 20:179–219.

Kamatou, G. P. P., Vermaak, I., and Viljoen, A. M. 2011. An updated review of *Adansonia digitata*: A commercially important African tree. *South African Journal of Botany* 77:908–919.

Kaminskas, A., Abaravičius, J. A., Liutkevičius, A. et al. 2013. Quality of yoghurt enriched by inulin and its influence on human metabolic syndrome. *Veterinarija ir Zootechnika* 64:23–28

Kang, N. J., Lee, K., Lee, D. E. et al. 2008. Cocoa procyanidins suppress transformation by inhibiting mitogen-activated protein kinase kinase. *Journal of Biological Chemistry* 283:20664–20673.

Kanis, J. A., Geusens, P., Christiansen, C. 1991. Guidelines for clinical trials in osteoporosis. A position paper of the European Foundation for Osteoporosis and Bone Disease. *Osteoporosis International* 1:182–188.

Karim, M., McCormick, K., and Kappagoda, C. T. 2000. Effects of cocoa extracts in endothelium-dependent relaxation. *Journal of Nutrition* 130:2105S–2108S.

Katz, D. L., Doughty, K., and Ali, A. 2011. Cocoa and chocolate in human health and disease. *Antioxidants & Redox Signaling* 15:2779–2811.

Keen, C. L., Holt, R. R., Oteiza, P. I., Fraga, C. G., and Schmitz, H. H. 2005. Cocoa antioxidants and cardiovascular health. *American Journal of Clinical Nutrition* 81:298S–303S.

Kemp, S. E., Hollowood, T., and Hort, J. 2009. *Sensory Evaluation- A Practical Handbook*. West Sussex: Wiley-Blackwell; pp. 1–208.

Kerdudo, A., Dingas, A., Fernandez, X., and Faure, C. 2014. Encapsulation of rutin and naringenin in multilamellar vesicles for optimum antioxidant activity. *Food Chemistry* 159:12–19.

Kerton, F. M. 2009. *Introduction*, In *Alternative Solvents for Green Chemistry*, Cambridge: RSC Publishing; pp. 1–22.

Khan, I., Yousif, A. M., Johnson, S. K., Gamlath, S. 2015. Acute effect of sorghum flour-containing pasta on plasma total polyphenols, antioxidant capacity and oxidative stress markers in healthy subjects: A randomised controlled trial. *Clinical Nutrition* 34:415–421.

Kietsiriroje, N., Kwankaew, J., Kitpakornsanti, S., and Leelawattana, R. 2015. Effect of phytosterols and inulin-enriched soymilk on LDL-cholesterol in Thai subjects: A double-blinded randomized controlled trial. *Lipids in Health and Disease* 14:146. doi:10.1186/s12944-015-0149-4.

Kilcast, D. 2001. Modern methods of texture measurement. In: Kress-Rogers, E., and Brimelow, C. J. B. (Eds.). *Instrumentation and Sensors for the Food Industry*. Cambridge, UK: Woodhead Publishing Limited; pp. 518–550.

Kilcast, D., and Subramaniam, P. 2000. Introduction. In: Kilcast, D., and Subramaniam, P. (Eds.). *The Stability and Shelf-Life of Food*. Boca Raton, FL: CRC Press; pp. 1–22.

Killeen, M. J. 1993. The process of spray drying and spray congealing. *Pharmaceutical Engineering* 13:56–64.

Kim, J. E., Son, J. E., Jung, S. K. et al. 2010. Cocoa polyphenols suppress TNF-alpha-induced vascular endothelial growth factor expression by inhibiting phosphoinositide 3- kinase (PI3K) and mitogen-activated protein kinase kinase-1 (MEK1) activities in mouse epidermal cells. *British Journal of Nutrition* 104:957–964.

Kim, J. E., Song, D., Kim, J. et al. 2016. Oral supplementation with cocoa extract reduces UVB-induced wrinkles in hairless mouse skin. *Journal of Investigative Dermatology* 136:1012–1021.

Kitawaki, R., Nishimura, Y., Takagi, N. Iwasaki, M. Tsuzuki, K., and Fukuda, M. 2009. Effects of lactobacillus fermented soymilk and soy yogurt on hepatic lipid accumulation in rats fed a cholesterol-free diet. *Bioscience, Biotechnology and Biochemistry* 73:1484–1488.

Klein, W. L. 2002. Aβ toxicity in Alzheimer's disease—Globular oligomers (ADDLs) as new vaccine and drug targets. *Neurochemistry International* 41:345–352.

Kolodny, D. E., and Kennedy, L. M. 1988. A model system for receptor cell studies with the taste modifier, hodulcin. *Chemical Senses* 13:545–557.

Koukiekolo, R., Desseaux, V., Moreau, Y., Marchis, M. G., and Santimone, M. 2001. Mechanism of porcine pancreatic alpha-amylase inhibition of amylose and maltopentaose hydrolysis by alpha-, beta- and gammacyclodextrins. *European Journal of Biochemistry* 268:841–848.

Kris-Etherton, P. M., Harris, W. S., and Appel, L. J. 2003. Omega-3 fatty acids and cardiovascular disease: New recommendations from the American Heart Association. *Arteriosclerosis, Thrombosis, and Vascular Biology* 23:151–152.

Kubomara, K. 1998. Japan redefines functional foods. *Prepared Foods* 167:129–132.

Kumar, D. S. 2016a. Medical herbalism through the ages. In: *Herbal Bioactives and Food Fortification: Extraction and Formulation*. Boca Raton, FL: CRC Press; pp. 1–28.

Kumar, D. S. 2016b. Extraction of the bioactives. In: *Herbal Bioactives and Food Fortification; Extraction and Formulation*. Boca Raton, FL: CRC Press; pp. 63–127.

Kumar, D. S. 2016c. Food and beverages fortified with phytonutrients. In: *Herbal Bioactives and Food Fortification: Extraction and Formulation*. Boca Raton, FL: CRC Press; pp. 173–238.

Kumar, D. S., and Prabhakar, Y. S. 1987. On the ethnomedical significance of the Arjun tree, *Terminalia arjuna* (Roxb.) Wight & Arnot. *Journal of Ethnopharmacology* 20:173–190.

Kumar, R., Dahiya, J. S., Singh, D., and Nigam, P. 2001. Biotransformation of cholesterol using *Lactobacillus bulgaricus* in glucose controlled bioreactor. *Bioresource Technology* 28:209–211.

Kurihara, K. 1971. Taste modifiers. In: Beidler L.M. (Ed.). Handbook of Sensory Physiology, IV, Chemical Senses. Berlin: Springer-Verlag; pp. 363–378.

LaBell, F. 1999. Encapsulated acid improves flour tortilla quality. *Prepared Foods* 168:91.

Lakkis, J. M. 2016. Introduction. In: Lakkis J. M. (Ed.). *Encapsulation and Controlled Release Technologies in Food Systems.* West Sussex, UK: John Wiley and Sons Ltd; pp. 1–15.

Law, M. 2000. Plant sterol and stanol margarines and health. *British Medical Journal* 320:861–864.

Lawless, H. T., and Heymann, H. 2010. Quality control and shelf-life (stability) testing. In: *Sensory Evaluation of Food: Principles and Practices,* 2nd ed. New York, NY: Springer Sciences + Business Media; pp. 407–432.

Lee, H. C., Jenner, A. M., Low, C. S., and Lee, Y. K. 2006b. Effect of tea phenolics and their aromatic fecal bacterial metabolites on intestinal microbiota. *Research in Microbiology* 157:876–884.

Lee, J., Jung, E., Hur, S., and Park, D. 2009. Antibacterial and anti-inflammatory effects of a magnolia extract. *Cosmetics & Toiletries* 124:53–60.

Lee, K. W., Kim, Y. J., Lee, H. J., and Lee, C. Y. 2003a. Cocoa has more phenolic phytochemicals and a higher antioxidant capacity than teas and red wine. *Journal of Agricultural and Food Chemistry* 51:7292–7295.

Lee, K. W., Kundu, J. K., Kim, S. O., Chun, K. S., Lee, H. J., and Surh, Y. J. 2006a. Cocoa polyphenols inhibit phorbol ester-induced superoxide anion formation in cultured HL-60 cells and expression of cyclooxygenase-2 and activation of NF-kappa B and MAPKs in mouse skin *in vivo. Journal of Nutrition* 136:1150–1155.

Lee, Y. M., Haastert, B. Scherbaum, W., and Hauner, H. 2003b. A phytosterol-enriched spread improves the lipid profile of subjects with type 2 diabetes mellitus--a randomized controlled trial under free-living conditions. *European Journal of Nutrition* 42:111–117.

Lemieux, I., and Simard, R. E. 1991. Bitter flavour in dairy products. I. A review of the factors likely to influence its development, mainly in cheese manufacture. *Le Lait* 71:599–636.

Lewis, M., and Dale, R. H. 1994. Chilled yogurt and other dairy desserts. In: Man, C. M. D., and Jones, A. A. (Eds.). *Shelf-life Evaluation of Foods.* Dordrecht, the Netherlands: Springer-Science + Business Media; pp. 127–155.

Li, S., Shahidi, F., Ho, C. T. 2016. Chemistry of functional beveragesr. In: Shahidi, F., and Alsalvar, C. (Eds.). *Handbook of Functional Beverages and Human Health.* Boca Raton, FL: CRC Press; pp. 35–46.

Lin, Z., and Huang, Y. 1987. Protective action of *Lentinus edodes* polysaccharide on experimental liver injury. *Journal of Peking University (Health Sciences)* 19:93–95.

Ling, W. H., and Jones, P. J. H. 1995. Dietary phytosterols: A review of metabolism, benefits and side effects. *Life Sciences* 57:195–206.

Liu, D., Qian, J. Y., and Bu, M. 2002. Current research in anti-tumor activities of lentinan. *Edible Fungi of China* 22:6–7.

Loffredo, L., Perri, L., Catasca, E. et al. 2014. Dark chocolate acutely improves walking autonomy in patients with peripheral artery disease. *Journal of the American Heart Association* 3: e001072. doi:10.1161/JAHA.114.001072.

Lord, T. 2003. Packaging materials as a source of taints. In Baigrie, B. (Ed.). *Taints and Off-flavours in Food*. Boca Raton, FL: CRC Press; 64–111.

Lu, X., and Chen, Y. 2002. Chiral separation of amino acids derivatized with fluoresceine-5-isothiocyanate by capillary electrophoresis and laser-induced fluorescence detection using mixed selectors of beta-cyclodextrin and sodium taurocholate. *Journal of Chromatography A* 955:133–140.

Madene, A., Jacquot, M., Scher, J., and Desobry, S. 2006. Flavour encapsulation and controlled release—A review. *International Journal of Food Science and Technology* 41:1–21.

Maillard, A. C. 1912. Action des acides amines sur les sucres. Formation des melanoidines par voie methodologique. *Comptes Rendus de l'Académie des Sciences* 154:66–68.

Mandalari, G., Bennett, R. N., Bisignano, G. et al. 2006. Characterization of flavonoids and pectins from bergamot (*Citrus bergamia* Risso) peel, a major byproduct of essential oil extraction. *Journal of Agriculture and Food Chemistry* 54:197–203.

Martin, F. J., Rezzi, S., Trepat, E. P. et al. 2010. Metabolic effects of dark chocolate consumption on energy, gut microbiota and stress-related metabolism in free-living subjects. *Journal of Proteome Research* 8:5568–5579.

Martín, M. A., Ramos, S., Mateos, R. et al. 2008. Protection of human HepG2 cells against oxidative stress by cocoa phenolic extract. *Journal of Agricultural and Food Chemistry* 56:7765–7772.

Martinez-Saez, N., García, A. T., Pérez, I. D. et al. 2016. Use of spent coffee grounds as food ingredient in bakery products. *Food Chemistry* 216:114–122.

Masatomo, H., Naoto, S., Tomotake, N. Kazuo, F., and Kazuko, T. 1999. Three kinds of antibacterial substances from *Lentinus edodes* (Berk.) Sing. (Shiitake, an edible mushroom). *International Journal of Antimicrobial Agents* 11:151–157.

Mastroiacovo, D., Kwik-Uribe, C., Grassi, D. et al. 2015. Cocoa flavanol consumption improves cognitive function, blood pressure control, and metabolic profile in elderly subjects: The Cocoa, Cognition, and Aging (CoCoA) Study- a randomized controlled trial. *American Journal of Clinical Nutrition* 101:538–548.

Matalanis, A., Jones, O. G., McClements, D. J. 2011. Structured biopolymer-based delivery systems for encapsulation, protection, and release of lipophilic compounds. *Food Hydrocolloids* 25:1865–1880.

Mateos, R., Martínez-López, S., Baeza Arévalo, G., Amigo-Benavent, M., Sarriá, B., and Bravo-Clemente, L. 2016. Hydroxytyrosol in functional hydroxytyrosol-enriched biscuits is highly bioavailable and decreases oxidised low density lipoprotein levels in humans. *Food Chemistry* 205:248–256.

Mcburney, D. H. 1974. Are these primary taste for man? *Chemical Senses and Flavor* 1:17–28.

McClements, D. J. 2010. Emulsion design to improve the delivery of functional lipophilic components. *Annual Review of Food Science and Technology* 1:241–269.

McClements, D. J. 2012. Requirements for food ingredient and nutraceutical delivery systems. In: Garti, N., and McClements, D. J. (Eds.). *Encapsulation Technologies and Delivery Systems for Food Ingredients and Nutraceuticals*. Cambridge, UK: Woodhead Publishing Ltd; pp. 3–18.

McClements, D. J. 2013. Utilizing food effects to overcome challenges in delivery of lipophilic bioactives: Structural design of medical and functional foods. *Expert Opinion on Drug Delivery* 10:1621–1632.

McClements, D. J., and Xiao, H. 2014. Excipient foods: Designing food matrices that improve the oral bioavailability of pharmaceuticals and nutraceuticals. *Food & Function* 5:1320–1333.

McClements, D. J., Li, F., and Xiao, H. 2015. The nutraceutical bioavailability classification scheme: Classifying nutraceuticals according to factors limiting their oral bioavailability. *Annual Review of Food Science and Technology* 6:13.1–13.29.

McCowen, K. C., Ling, P. R., Decker, E. et al. 2010. A simple method of supplementation of omega-3 polyunsaturated fatty acids: Use of fortified yogurt in healthy volunteers. *Nutrition in Clinical Practice* 25:641–645.

Mertens-Talcott, S. U., Jilma-Stohlawetz, P., Rios, J., Hingorani, L., and Derendorf, H. 2006. Absorption, metabolism, and antioxidant effects of pomegranate (*Punica granatum* L.) polyphenols after ingestion of a standardized extract in healthy human volunteers. *Journal of Agricultural and Food Chemistry* 54:8956–8961.

Mignet, N., Seguin, J., and Chabot, G. G. 2013. Bioavailability of polyphenol liposomes: A challenge ahead. *Pharmaceutics* 5:457–471.

Mildner-Szkudlarz, S., and Bajerska, J. 2013. Protective effect of grape by-product-fortified breads against cholesterol/cholic acid diet-induced hypercholesterolaemia in rats. *Journal of the Science of Food and Agriculture* 93:3271–3278.

Miller, M., Sorkin, J. D., Mastella, L. et al. 2016. Poly is more effective than monounsaturated fat for dietary management in the metabolic syndrome: The muffin study. *Journal of clinical Lipidology*. doi:10.1016/j.jacl.2016.04.011.

Mirafzali, Z., Thompson, C. S., and Tallua, K. 2014. Application of liposomes in the food industry. In: Gaonkar, A., Vasisht, N., Khare, A., and Sobel, R. (Eds.). *Microencapsulation in the Food Industry: A Practical Implementation Guide*. San Diego, CA: Elsevier; pp. 139–150.

Miranda-Rottmann, S., Aspillaga, A. A., Pérez, D. D., Vasquez, L., Martinez, A. L. F., and Leighton, F. 2002. Juice and phenolic fractions of the berry *Aristotelia chilensis* inhibit LDL oxidation in vitro and protect human endothelial cells against oxidative stress. *Journal of Agricultural and Food Chemistry* 50:7542–7547.

Mizrahi, S. 2011. Accelerated shelf-life testing of foods. In: Kilcast, D., and Subramaniam, P. (Eds.). *Food and Beverage Stability and Shelf-life*. Cambridge, UK: Woodhead Publishing Limited; pp. 482–506.

Moarreaf, A. R. 2004. Risk factor modification of coronary artery disease. *Shiraz E-Medical Journal* 5:1–7.

Moraes, E. A., Natal, D. I. G., Queiroz, V. A. V. et al. 2012. Sorghum genotype may reduce low-grade inflammatory response and oxidative stress and maintains jejunum morphology of rats fed a hyperlipidic diet. *Food Research International* 49:553–559.

Mousa, R. M. A. 2015a. Influence of functional sweet white lupin biscuits on lipid profile and food efficiency of induced hyperlipidemic rats. *Journal of Food Research* 4:14–25.

Mousa, R. M. A. 2015b. Formulation of reduced calorie and trans-free fat biscuits using palm oil and sucralose: Study of their hypoglycemic activity on albino rats. *American Journal of Food and Nutrition* 3:131–140.

Muammar, M. A., Elsadek, M. F., and Shafie, M. E. 2016. Potential effect of fortified pan bread with *Aloe vera* juice on alloxan-induced diabetic rats. *African Journal of Traditional, Complementary and Alternative Medicines* 13.doi:10.4314/ajtcam.v13i1.3457.

Muhaimin, M. 2013. Study of microparticle preparation by the solvent evaporation method using Focused Beam Reflectance Measurement (FBRM). Dissertation for the academic degree of Doktors der Naturwissenschaften (Dr. rer. nat.) filed in the Department of Biology, Chemistry and Pharmacy at Freie Universität Berlin, pp. 1–218.

Mullen, W., Gonzalez, J., Siwy, J. et al. 2011. A pilot study on the effect of short-term consumption of a polyphenol rich drink on biomarkers of coronary artery disease defined by urinary proteomics. *Journal of Agricultural and Food Chemistry* 59:12850–12857.

Muñoz-Botella, S., del Castillo, B., and Martyn, M. A. 1995. Cyclodetrin properties and applications of inclusion complex formation. *ARS Pharmaceutica* 36:187–198.

Murphy, E. F., Cotter, P. D., Hogan, A. et al. 2012. Divergent metabolic outcomes arising from targeted manipulation of the gut microbiota in diet-induced obesity. *Gut* 62:220–226.

Neil, H. A., Meijer, G. W., and Roe, L. S. 2001. Randomized controlled trial of use by hypercholesterolaemic patients of a vegetable oil sterol-enriched fat spread. *Atherosclerosis* 156:329–337.

Nemzer, B. V., Rodriguez, L. C. Hammond, L. DiSilvestro, R., Hunter, J. M., and Pietrzkowski, Z. 2011. Acute reduction of serum 8-iso-PGF2-alpha and advanced oxidation protein products *in vivo* by a polyphenol-rich beverage—A pilot clinical study with phytochemical and *in vitro* antioxidant characterization. *Nutrition Journal* 10:67. doi:10.1186/1475-2891-10-67.

Neukam, K., Stahl, W., Tronnier, H. Sies, H., and Heinrich, U. 2007. Consumption of flavanol-rich cocoa acutely increases microcirculation in human skin. *European Journal of Nutrition* 46:53–56.

Ni, L, Rao P., and Wang, Z. 1997. Isolation and characterization of bioactive peptides in sufu. *Journal of Zhejiang University (Agriculture and Life Science)* 21:93–97.

Nieburg, O. 2013. Wrigley develops gums sweetened-with-dried-fruit-powders (accessed 27 July, 2016). *Confectionery News.com*. http://www.confectionerynews.com/Ingredients/Wrigley-develops-gum-sweetened-with-dried-fruit-powders

Nieburg, O. 2014. Is functional chewing gum the answer to the category's woes? *Confectionery News.com*. http://www.confectionerynews.com/Markets/Functional-chewing-gum-market-opportunities (accessed 31 May, 2016).

Nielsen, T., and Powell, R. A. 2015. Dreams of the *Rarebit Fiend*: Food and diet as instigators of bizarre and disturbing dreams. *Frontiers in Psychology*. doi:10.3389/fpsyg.2015.00047.

Nilsen, R., Pripp, A. H., Høstmark, A. T., Haug, A., and Skeie, S. 2014. Short communication—Is consumption of a cheese rich in angiotensin-converting enzyme-inhibiting peptides, such as the Norwegian cheese Gamalost, associated with reduced blood pressure? *Journal of Dairy Science* 97:2662–2668.

Nowicka, G., and Naruszewicz, M. 2004. Assessing health claims for functional Foods. In: Arnoldi, A. (Ed.). *Functional Foods, Cardiovascular Disease and Diabetes.* Cambridge, UK: Woodhead Publishing Ltd; pp. 10–17.

Nittynen, L. H., Jauhiainen, T. A., Poussa, T. A., and Korpela, R. 2008. Effects of yoghurt enriched with free plant sterols on the levels of serum lipids and plant sterols in moderately hypercholesterolaemic subjects on a high-fat diet. *International Journal of Food Sciences & Nutrition* 59:357–367.

Ntanios, F. Y., Homma, Y., Ushiro, S. 2002. A spread enriched with plant sterolesters lowers blood cholesterol and lipoproteins without affecting Vitamins A and E in normal and hypercholesterolemic Japanese men and women. *Journal of Nutrition* 132:3650–3655.

O'Connor, L. M., Lentjes, M. A. H., Luben, R. N., Khaw, K. T., Wareham, N. J., and Forouhi, N. G. 2014. Dietary dairy product intake and incident type 2 diabetes—A prospective study using dietary data from a 7-day food diary. *Diabetologia* 57:909–917.

Oehlke, K., Adamiuk, M., Behsnilian, D. et al. 2014. Potential bioavailability enhancement of bioactive compounds using food-grade engineered nanomaterials: A review of the existing evidence. *Food & Function* 5:1341–1359.

Okuro, P. K., de Matos, Jr. F. E., and Favaro-Trindade, C. S. 2013. Technological challenges for spray chilling encapsulation of functional food ingredients. *Food Technology Biotechnology* 51:171–182.

Omobuwajo, T. O. 2007. Food flavorings: Principles of application. In: Hui, Y. H., Chandan, R. C., and Clark, S. et al. (Eds.). *Handbook of Food Products Manufacturing.* New Jersey: John Wiley and Sons, Inc; pp. 119–130.

Onyper, S. V., Carr, T. L., Farrar, J. S., and Floyd, B. R. 2011. Cognitive advantages of chewing gum. Now you see them, now you don't. *Appetite* 57:321–328.

Paiva, S. A. R., and Russel, R. M. 1999. β-Carotene and other carotenoids as antioxidants, *Journal of the American College of Nutrition* 18:426–433.

Paramera, E. I., Konteles, S. J., and Karathanos, V. T. 2011. Stability and release properties of curcumin encapsulated in *Saccharomyces cerevisiae*, beta-cyclodextrin and modified starch. *Food Chemistry* 125:913–922.

Park, H. S., Jin, S. P., Lee, Y. et al. 2014. Toll-like receptor 2 mediates a cutaneous reaction induced by repetitive ultraviolet B irradiation in C57/BL6 mice *in vivo*. *Experimental Dermatology* 23:591–595.

Patel, D., Shukla, S., and Gupta, S. 2007. Apigenin and cancer chemoprevention: Progress, potential and promise (Review). *International Journal of Oncology* 30:233–245.

Patel, R. K., Broune, J., and Spendiff, O. 2015. Dark chocolate supplementation reduces the oxygen cost of moderate intensity cycling. *Journal of the International Society of Sports Nutrition* 12:47. doi:10.1186/s12970-015-0106-7.

Pernice, R., Borriello, G., Ferracane, R., Borrelli, R. C. Cennamo, F., and Ritieni, A. 2009. Bergamot: A source of natural antioxidants for functionalized fruit juices. *Food Chemistry* 112:545–550.

Persaud, K. 2016. Electronic noses and electronic tongues in the food industry. In: Méndez, M. L. R. (Ed.). *Electronic Noses and Tongues in Food Sciences.* San Diego, CA: Academic Press; pp. 3–14.

Petitot, M., Abecassis J., and Micard, V. 2009. Structuring of pasta components during processing: Impact on starch and protein digestibility and allergenicity. *Trends in Food Science and Technology* 20:521–532.

Phatthalung, K. N., Penroj P., and Samuhasaneetoo, S. 2008. Shelf-life extension of Thai noodles. *Asian Journal of Food and Agro-Industry*1:167173.

Pickford, E. F., and Jardine, N. J. 2000. Functional confectionery. In: Gibson, G. R., and Williams, C. M. (Eds.). *Functional Foods: Concept to Product*. Boca Raton, FL: CRC Press; pp. 258–286.

Pietta, P. 2000. Phytomedicines: Creating safer choices. In: Watson, R. R. (Ed.). *Vegetables, Fruits and Herbs in Health Promotion*. Boca Raton, FL: CRC Press; pp. 73–84.

Pollak, O. J., and Kritchevsky, D. 1981. Sitosterol. In: *Monographs on Atherosclerosis*. Basel, Switzerland: Karger; pp.60–163.

Porter, C. J., Trevaskis, N. L., and Charman, W. N. 2007. Lipids and lipid-based formulations: Optimizing the oral delivery of lipophilic drugs. *Nature Reviews Drug Discovery* 6:231–248.

Porter, C. J. H., Pouton, C. W., Cuine, J. F., and Charman, W. N. 2008. Enhancing intestinal drug solubilisation using lipid-based delivery systems. *Advanced Drug Delivery Reviews* 60:673–691.

Potter, P. 2012. *Hippocrates*, vol. X. Cambridge, MA: Harvard University Press

Pounis, G., Di Castelnuovo, A., Costanzo, S. et al. 2016. Association of pasta consumption with body mass index and waist-to-hip ratio: Results from Moli-sani and INHES studies. *Nutrition & Diabetes* 6:e218. doi:10.1038/nutd.2016.20.

Puligundla, P., Jung, J., and Ko, S. 2012. Carbon dioxide sensors for intelligent food packaging applications. *Food Control* 25:328–333.

Qian, C., Decker, E. A., Xiao, H., and McClements, D. J. 2012. Nanoemulsion delivery systems: Influence of carrier oil on beta-carotene bioaccessibility. *Food Chemistry* 135:1440–1447.

Qv, X. Y., Zeng, Z. P., and Jiang, J. G. 2011. Preparation of lutein microencapsulation by complex coacervation method and its physicochemical properties and stability. *Food Hydrocolloids* 25:1596–1603.

Rabiskova, M. 2001. Extrusion technology. In Vilstrup, P. (Ed.). *Microencapsulation of Food Ingredient*, Surrey, UK: Leatherhead Publishing; pp. 224–248.

Ramarathnam, N., Osawa, T., Namiki, M., and Kawakishi, S. 1989. Chemical studies on novel rice hull antioxidants. 2. Identification of isovitexin, a C-glycosyl flavonoid. *Journal of Agricultural and Food Chemistry* 37:316–319.

Rassaf, T., Rammos, C., and Hendgen-Cotta, U. B. et al. 2016. Vasculoprotective effects of dietary cocoa flavanols in patients on hemodialysis: A double-blind, randomized, placebo-controlled trial. *Clinical Journal of the American Society of Nephrology* 11:108–118.

Redgwell, R. J., and Fischer, M. 2005. Dietary fiber as a versatile food component: An industrial perspective. *Molecular Nutrition & Food Research* 49:521–535.

Reineccius, G. A. 2001. The spray drying of food ingredients. In: Vilstrup, P. (Ed.). *Microencapsulation of Food Ingredients*. Surrey, UK: Leatherhead Publishing; pp. 151–179.

Reis, S. A., Conceicao L. L., Rosa D. D., Dias, M. M., and Peluzio Mdo, C. 2014. Mechanisms used by inulin-type fructans to improve the lipid profile. *Nutricion Hospitalaria* 31:528–534.

Ren, H., Liu, H., Endo, H. Takagi, Y., and Hayashi, T. 2006. Anti-mutagenic and anti-oxidative activities found in Chinese traditional soybean fermented products furu. *Food Chemistry* 95:71–76.

Resch, J. J., Daubert, C. R., and Foegeding, E. A. 2005. The effects of acidulant type on the rheological properties of beta-lactoglobulin gels and powders derived from these gels. *Food Hydrocolloids* 19:851–860.

Ringel-Kulka, T., Kotch, J. B., Jensen, E. T., Savage, E., and Weber, D. J. 2015. Randomized, double-blind, placebo-controlled study of synbiotic yogurt effect on the health of children. *Journal of Pediatrics* 166:1475–1481.

Roberfroid, M. 2005. Inulin: A Fructan, In: *Inulin-Type Fructans: Functional Food Ingredients*. Boca Raton, FL: CRC Press; pp. 39–60.

Roberfroid, M. B. 2008. Defining functional foods. In: Gibson, G. R., and Williams, C. M. (Eds.). *Functional Foods- Concept to Product*. Boca Raton, FL: CRC Press; pp. 9–27.

Rocha, A., Wang, L., Penichet, M., and Martins-Green, M. 2012. Pomegranate juice and specific components inhibit cell and molecular processes critical for metastasis of breast cancer. *Breast Cancer Research and Treatment* 136:647–658.

Rojo, L. E., Ribnicky, D., Logendra, S. et al. 2011. *In vitro* and *in vivo* anti-diabetic effects of anthocyanins from Maqui Berry (*Aristotelia chilensis*). *Food Chemistry* 131:387–396.

Rubilar, M., Jara, C., Poo, Y. et al. 2011. Extracts of maqui (*Aristotelia chilensis*) and murta (*Ugni molinae* Turcz.): Sources of antioxidant compounds and α-glucosidase/α-amylase inhibitors. *Journal of Agricultural and Food Chemistry* 59:1630–1637.

Ruiu, G., Pinach, S., Veglia, F. et al. 2009. Phytosterol-enriched yogurt increases LDL affinity and reduces CD36 expression in polygenic hypercholesterolemia. *Lipids* 44:153–160.

Russo, F., Clemente, C., Linsalata, M. et al. 2011. Effects of a diet with inulin-enriched pasta on gut peptides and gastric emptying rates in healthy young volunteers. *European Journal of Nutrition* 50:271–277.

Russo, F., Linsalata, M., Clemente, C. et al. 2012. Inulin-enriched pasta improves intestinal permeability and modifies the circulating levels of zonulin and glucagon-like peptide 2 in healthy young volunteers. *Nutrition Research* 32:940–946.

Sakr, S. S., and Abou Dawood, S. A. 2015. Hypocholesterolemic effect of pomegranate's peel (water extract) supplemented yoghurt in hypercholesterolemic rats. *Indian Journal of Dairy Science* 68:14–19.

Sansone, F., Mencherini, T., Picerno, P., D'Amore, M., Aquino, R. P., and Lauro, M. R. 2011. Maltodextrin/pectin microparticles by spray drying as carrier for nutraceutical extracts. *Journal of Food Engineering* 105:468–476.

Santacruz, K., Lewis, J., Spires, T. et al. 2005. Tau suppression in a neurodegenerative mouse model improves memory function. *Science* 309:476–481.

Sant'Anna, V., Christiano, F. D. P., Marczak, L. D. F., Tessaro, I. C., Thys, R. C. S. 2014. The effect of the incorporation of grape marc powder in fettuccini pasta properties. *LW T- Food Science & Technology International* 58:497–501.

Santos, D. T., Albarelli, J. Q., Beppu, M. M., Meireles, M. A. A. 2013. Stabilization of anthocyanin extract from jabuticaba skins by encapsulation using supercritical CO_2 as solvent. *Food Research International* 50:617–624.

Santos, D. T., and Meireles, M. A. A. 2013. Micronization and encapsulation of functional pigments using supercritical carbon dioxide. *Journal of Food Process Engineering* 36:36–49.

Sapone, A., de Magistris, L., Pietzak, M. et al. 2006. Zonulin upregulation is associated with increased gut permeability in subjects with type 1 diabetes and their relatives. *Diabetes* 55:1443–1449.

Sassi, M. M. 2001. *The Science of Man in Ancient* Greece (Translated from the Italian by P. Tucker. With a foreword by Sir G. Lloyd), 142. Chicago and London: University of Chicago Press.

Sawale, P. D., Pothuraju, R., Hussain, S. A. Kumar, A. Kapila, S., and Patil, G. R. 2016. Hypolipidaemic and anti-oxidative potential of encapsulated herb (*Terminalia arjuna*) added vanilla chocolate milk in high cholesterol fed rats. *Journal of the Science of Food and Agriculture* 96:1380–1385.

Scapagnini, G., Davinelli, S., Di Renzo, L. et al. 2014. Cocoa bioactive compounds: Significance and potential for the maintenance of skin health. *Nutrients* 6:3202–3213.

Schaefer, S., Baum, M., Eisenbrand, G., and Janzowski, C. 2006. Modulation of oxidative cell damage by reconstituted mixtures of phenolic apple juice extracts in human colon cell lines. *Molecular Nutrition & Food Research* 50:413–417.

Schauss, A. G., Jensen, G. S., and Wu, X. 2009. Increased antioxidant capacity and inhibition of lipid peroxidation in healthy adults consuming an açai (*Euterpe oleracea*) fruit-based juice. *Acta Horticulturae* 841:97–100.

Schiborr, C., Kocher, A., Behnam, D. Jandasek, J. Toelstede, S., and Frank, J. 2014. The oral bioavailability of curcumin from micronized powder and liquid micelles is significantly increased in healthy humans and differs between sexes. *Molecular Nutrition & Food Research* 58:516–527.

Schlameus, W. 1995. Centrifugal extrusion encapsulation. In: Risch, S. J and G. A. Reineccius. *Encapsulation and Controlled Release of Food Ingredients*. Washington DC: American Chemical Society; pp. 96–103.

Scholey, A. 2004. Chewing gum and cognitive performance: A case of a functional food with function but no food? *Appetite* 43:215–216.

Scholey, A. B., French, S. J., Morris, P. J., Kennedy, D. O., Milne, A. L., and Haskell, C. F. 2010. Consumption of cocoa flavanols results in acute improvements in mood and cognitive performance during sustained mental effort. *Journal of Psychopharmacology* 24:1505–1514.

Schreckinger, M. E., Wang, J. Yousef, G., Lila, M. A., and De Mejia, E. G. 2010. Antioxidant capacity and *in vitro* inhibition of adipogenesis and inflammation by phenolic extracts of *Vaccinium floribundum* and *Aristotelia chilensis*. *Journal of Agricultural and Food Chemistry* 58:8966–8976.

Sęczyk, L, Swieca, M, and Gawlik-Dziki, U. 2015. Changes of antioxidant potential of pasta fortified with parsley (*Petroselinum crispum* Mill.) leaves in the light of protein - phenolics interactions. *Acta Scientiarum Polonorum Technologia Alimentaria* 14:29–36.

Sęczyk, L., Świeca, M., Gawlik-Dziki, U., Luty, M., and Czyż, J. 2016a. Effect of fortification with parsley (*Petroselinum crispum* Mill.) leaves on the nutraceutical and nutritional quality of wheat pasta. *Food Chemistry* 190:419–428.

Sęczyk, Ł., Świeca, M., and Gawlik-Dziki, U. 2016b. Effect of carob (*Ceratonia siliqua* L.) flour on the antioxidant potential, nutritional quality, and sensory characteristics of fortified durum wheat pasta. *Food Chemistry* 194:637–642.

Seddon, J. M., Ajani, U. A., Sperduto, R. D. et al. 1994. Dietary carotenoids, vitamins A, C, and E, and advanced age-related macular degeneration. Eye disease case control study group. *Journal of the American Medical Association* 272:1413–1420.

Seeman, E., Cooper, M. E., Hopper, J. L. Parkinson, E. McKay, J., and Jerums, G. 1988. Effect of early menopause on bone mass in normal women and patients with osteoporosis. *American Journal of Medicine* 85:213–216.

Seeram, N. P., Adams, L. S., Henning, S. M. et al. 2005. *In vitro* antiproliferative, apoptotic and antioxidant activities of punicalagin, ellagic acid and a total pomegranate tannin extract are enhanced in combination with other polyphenols as found in pomegranate juice. *The Journal of Nutritional Biochemistry* 16:360–367.

Setchell, K. D. R., and Cassidy, A. 1999. Dietary isoflavones: Biological effects and relevance to human health. *Journal of Nutition* 129:758S–767S.

Setchell, K. D. R., Nardi, E., Battezzati, P. M. et al. 2013. Novel soy germ pasta enriched in isoflavones ameliorates gastroparesis in Type 2 diabetes. *Diabetes Care* 36:3495–3497.

Shallenberger, R. S. 1993. *Taste Chemistry*. New York, NY: Chapman & Hall; pp. 1–613.

Shankar, G. M., Li, S., Mehta, T. H. et al. 2008. Amyloid-β protein dimers isolated directly from Alzheimer's brains impair synaptic plasticity and memory. *Nature Medicine* 14:837–842.

Shen, C., Pang, S. M., Kwong, E. W., and Cheng, Z. 2010. The effect of Chinese food therapy on community dwelling Chinese hypertensive patients with Yin-deficiency. *Journal of Clinical Nursing* 19:1008–1020.

Shewfelt, R. L., Orta-Ramirez, A., and Clarke, A. D. 2016. Food engineering. In: *Introducing Food Science*, 2nd ed. Boca Raton, FL: CRC Press; pp. 321–344.

Siebert, K. J. 1999. Effects of protein–polyphenol interactions on beverage haze, stabilization and analysis. *Journal of Agricultural and Food Chemistry* 47:353–362.

Siebert, K. J., Carrasco, A., and Lynn, P. Y. 1996. Formation of protein–polyphenol haze in beverages. *Journal of Agricultural and Food Chemistry* 44:1997–2005.

Sierksma, A., Weststrate, J. A., and Meijer, G. W. 1999. Spreads enriched with plant sterols, either esterified 4,4-dimethylsterols or free 4-desmethylsterols, and plasma total- and LDL-cholesterol concentrations. *British Journal of Nutriton* 82:273–282.

Silk, D. B. A., Davis, A., Vulevic, J., Tzortzis, G., and Gibson, G. R. 2009. Clinical trial: The effect of a.trans-galactooligosaccharide prebiotic on fecal microbiota and symptoms in irritable bowel syndrome. *Alimentary Pharmacology & Therapeutics* 29:508–518.

Silva, E. K., and Meireles, M. A. A. 2014. Encapsulation of food compounds using supercritical technologies: Applications of supercritical carbon dioxide as an antisolvent. *Food and Public Health* 4:247–258.

Singer, J., Grinev, M., Silva, V. Cohen, J., and Singer, P. 2016. Safety and efficacy of coffee enriched with inulin and dextrin on satiety and hunger in normal volunteers. *Nutrition* 32:754–760.

Skeaff, C. M., Thoma, C. Mann, J. Chisholm, A. Williams, S., and Richmond, K. 2005. Isocaloric substitution of plant sterol-enriched fat spread for carbohydrate-rich foods in a low-fat, fibre-rich diet decreases plasma low-density lipoprotein cholesterol and increases high-density lipoprotein concentrations. *Nutrition, Metabolism and Cardiovascular Diseases* 15:337–344.

Smith, A. P. 2009. Chewing gum, stress and health. *Stress and Health* 25:445–451.

Smithers, L. G., Gibson, R. A. McPhee, A., and Makrides, M. 2008. Effect of long-chain polyunsaturated fatty acid supplementation of preterm infants on disease risk and neurodevelopment: A systematic review of randomized controlled trials. *American Journal of Clinical Nutrition* 87:912–920.

Snodderly, D. M. 1995. Evidence for protection against age-related macular degeneration by carotenoids and antioxidant vitamins. *American Journal of Clinical Nutrition* 62:1448S–1461S.

Söderholm, P. P., Alfthan, G., Koskela, A. H., Adlercreutz, H., and Tikkanen, M. J. 2012. The effect of high-fiber rye bread enriched with nonesterified plant sterols on major serum lipids and apolipoproteins in normocholesterolemic individuals. *Nutrition, Metabolism & Cardiovascular Diseases* 22:575–582.

Sparks, R. E., Jacobs, I. C., and Mason, N. S. 1995. Centrifugal suspension-separation for coating food ingredients. In: Risch, S. J., and Reineccius, G. A. (Eds.). *Encapsulation and Controlled Release of Food Ingredients.* Washington, DC: American Chemical Society; pp. 87–95.

Spinnler, E. 2003. Off-flavours due to interactions between food components. In: Baigrie, B. (Ed.). *Taints and Off-flavours in Food.* Boca Raton, FL: CRC Press; pp. 176–188.

Srinivasan, K. 2011. Traditional Indian functional foods, In: Shi, J., Ho, C. T., and Shahidi, F. (Eds.). *Functional Foods of the East.* Boca Raton, FL: CRC Press; pp. 51–84.

Strat, K. M., Rowley, IV, T. J., and Smithson, A. T., 2015. Mechanisms by which cocoa flavanols improve metabolic syndrome and related disorders. *The Journal of Nutritional Biochemistry* 35:1–21.

Strati, I. F., and Oreopoulou, V. 2011. Effect of extraction parameters on the carotenoid recovery from tomato waste. *International Journal of Food Science & Technology* 46:23–29.

Subhashini, R., Rao, U. S. M., Sumathi, P., and Gunalam, G. 2010. A comparative phytochemical analysis of cocoa and green tea. *Indian Journal of Science and Technology* 3:188–192.

Suzuki, K., and Price, J. C. 1985. Microencapsulation and dissolution properties of a neuroleptic in a biodegradable polymer, poly(dl-lactide). *Journal of Pharmaceutical Sciences* 74:21–24.

Swinbanks, D., and O'Brien, J. 1993. Japan explores the boundary between food and medicine. *Nature* 364:180.

Szczesniak, A. S. 1973. Instrumental methods of texture measurements. In: Kramer, A., and Szczesniak, A. (Eds.). *Texture Measurements of Foods.* Dordrecht, the Netherlands: D.Reidel Publishing Company; pp. 71–108.

Takeoka, G. R., and Dao, L. T. 2003. Antioxidant constituents of almond [*Prunus dulcis* (Mill.) D.A. Webb] hulls. *Journal of Agricultural and Food Chemistry* 51:496–501.

Tamamoto, L. C., Schmidt, S. J., and Lee, S. Y. 2010. Sensory properties of ginseng solutions modified by masking agents. *Journal of Food Science* 25:S341–S347.

Tan, C., Xia, S., Xue, J. Xie, J. Feng, B., and Zhang, X. 2013. Liposomes as vehicles for lutein: Preparation, stability, liposomal membrane dynamics, and structure. *Journal of Agricultural and Food Chemistry* 61:8175–8184.

Tan C., Xue J., Abbas S., Feng, B., Zhang X., and Xia, S. 2014. Liposome as a delivery system for carotenoids: Comparative antioxidant activity of carotenoids as measured by ferric reducing antioxidant power, DPPH assay and lipid peroxidation. *Journal of Agricultural and Food Chemistry* 62:6726–6735.

Taubert, D., Roesen, R., Lehmann, C. Jung, N., and Schömig, E. 2007. Effects of low habitual cocoa intake on blood pressure and bioactive nitric oxide. *Journal of the American Medical Association* 298:49–60.

Taylor, T. M., Davidson, P. M., Bruce, B. D., and Weiss, J. 2005. Liposomal nanocapsules in food science and agriculture. *Critical Reviews in Food Science and Nutrition* 45:587–605.

Temkin, O. 1953. Greek medicine as science and craft. *Isis* 44:213–225.

Temple, N. J., and Gladwin, K. K. 2003. Fruit, vegetables, and the prevention of cancer: Research challenges. *Nutrition* 19:467–470.

Terry, P., Terry, J. B., and Wolk, A. 2001. Fruit and vegetable consumption in the prevention of cancer: An update. *Journal of Internal Medicine* 250:280–290.

Tiwari, R. V., Patil, H., and Repka, M. A. 2016. Contribution of hot-melt extrusion technology to advance drug delivery in the 21st century. *Expert Opinion on Drug Delivery* 13:451–464.

Tombokan, X. C. 2008. Ternary phase equilibria of the sclareol-ethyl lactate-CO_2 system and its application in the extraction and isolation of sclareol from Clary Sage. PhD thesis, North Carolina State University.

Totelin, L. 2015. When foods become remedies in ancient Greece: The curious case of garlic and other substances. *Journal of Ethnopharmacology* 167:30–37.

Tucha, L., and Koerts, J. 2012. Gum chewing and cognition: An overview. *Neuroscience & Medicine* 3:243–250.

Udani, J. K., Singh, B. B., Singh, V. J., and Barrett, M. L. 2011. Effects of Açai (*Euterpe oleracea* Mart.) berry preparation on metabolic parameters in a healthy overweight population: A pilot study. *Nutrition Journal* 10 (1). doi:10.1186/1475-2891-10-45.

Upritchard, J. E., Schuurman, C. R., Wiersma, A. et al. 2003. Spread supplemented with moderate doses of vitamin E and carotenoids reduces lipid peroxidation in healthy, nonsmoking adults. *American Journal of Clinical Nutrition* 78:985–992.

Valero, A., Carrasco, E., and Garcia-Gimenco, R. M. 2012. Principles and methodologies for the determination of shelf-life in foods. In: Eissa, A. H. A. (Ed.). *Trends in Vital Food and Control Engineering*, Croatia: InTech; pp. 3–42.

van het Hof, K. H., Gärtner, C., West, C. E., and Tijburg, L. B. 1998. Potential of vegetable processing to increase the delivery of carotenoids to man. *International Journal for Vitamin and Nutrition Research* 68:366–370.

van het Hof, K. H., West, C. E., Weststrate, J. A., and Hautvast, J. G. A. J. 2000. Dietary factors that affect the bioavailability of carotenoids. *Journal of Nutrition* 130:503–506.

Verma, R. L., and Keswani, N. J. 1974. Unani medicine in medieval India- its teachers and texts. In: Keswani, N. H. (Ed.) *The Science of Medicine and Physiological Concepts in Ancient and Medieval India*. New Delhi, India: All India Institute of Medical Sciences; pp.125–142.

Vicente, G., Paiva, A., Fornari, T., and Najdanovic-Visak, V. 2011. Liquid–liquid equilibria for separation of tocopherol from olive oil using ethyl lactate. *Chemical Engineering Journal* 172:879–884.

Vicinanza, R., Zhang, Y., Henning, S. M., and Heber, D. 2013. Pomegranate juice metabolites, ellagic acid and urolithin a, synergistically inhibit androgen-independent prostate cancer cell growth via distinct effects on cell cycle control and apoptosis. *Evidence-Based Complementary and Alternative Medicine* 2013. Article ID 247504, doi:10.1155/2013/247504.

Visioli, F., Bernaert, H., Corti, R. Ferri, C. Heptinstall, S., and Molinari, E. 2009. Chocolate, lifestyle, and health. *Critical Reviews in Food Science and Nutrition* 49:299–312.

Vulevic, J., Drakoularakou, A., Yaqoob, P. Tzortzis, G., and Gibson, G. R. 2008. Modulation of the fecal microflora profile and immune function by a novel trans-galactooligosaccharide mixture (B-GOS) in healthy elderly volunteers. *American Journal of Clinical Nutrition* 88:1438–1446.

Wang, J., Lu, Z., Chi, J. et al. 1997. Multicenter clinical trial of the serum lipid-lowering effects of a *Monascus purpureus* (red yeast) rice preparation from traditional Chinese medicine. *Current Therapeutic Research* 58:964–978.

Wang, J., and Schwendeman, S. P. 1999. Mechanisms of solvent evaporation encapsulation processes: Prediction of solvent evaporation rate. *Journal of Pharmaceutical Sciences* 88:1090–1099.

Wang, J., Varghese, M., Ono, K. et al. 2014. Cocoa extracts reduce oligomerization of amyloid—Implications for cognitive improvement in Alzheimer's disease. *Journal of Alzheimer's Disease* 41:643–650.

Wang, L., Li, L., Fan, J., and Qi, T. 2004. Antioxidative activity evaluation study on fermented tofu extracts by scavenging DPPH. *Food Science (China)* 25:169–172.

Wang, L., Saito, M., Tatsumi, E., and Li, L. 2003. Antioxidative and angiotensin I-converting enzyme inhibitory activities of sufu (fermented tofu) extracts. *Japan Agricultural Research Quarterly* 37:129–132.

Wang, W., Uzzau, S., Goldblum, S. E., and Fasano, A. 2000. Human zonulin, a potential modulator of intestinal tight junctions. *Journal of Cell Science* 113:4435–4440.

Watanabe, M., Ohshita, Y., and Tsushida, T. 1997. Antioxidant Compounds from Buckwheat (*Fagopyrum esculentum* Möench) Hulls. *Journal of Agricultural and Food Chemistry* 45:1039–1044.

Wei, H., Wei, L., Frenkel, K. Bowen, R., and Barnes, S. 1993. Inhibition of tumor promoter-induced hydrogen peroxide formation *in vitro* and *in vivo* by genistein. *Nutrition and Cancer* 20:1–12.

Weidner, E. 2009. High pressure micronization for food applications. *Journal of Supercritical Fluids* 47:556–565.

Whitfield, F. B. 2003. Microbiologically derived off-flavours. In: Baigrie, B. (Ed.). *Taints and Off-flavours in Food*. Boca Raton, FL: CRC Press, 112–139.

Wildman, R. E. C. 2000. Nutraceuticals: A brief review of historical and teleological aspects. In: Wildman, R. E. C. (Ed.). *Handbook of Nutraceuticals and Functional Foods* Boca Raton, FL: CRC Press; pp. 1–12.

Wright, L. T., Nancarrow, C., and Kwok, P. M. H. 2001. Food taste preferences and cultural influences on consumption. *British Food Journal* 103:348–357.

Wu, J. 2002. Medical and health function of edible fungi and its improvement of food structure. *Edible Fungi of China* 22:9–11.

Wu, W., Lu, M., and Yu, L. 2011. A new environmentally friendly method for astaxanthin extraction from *Xanthophyllomyces dendrorhous*. *European Food Research and Technology* 232:463–467.

Wu, X., and Chen, S. 2002. Development of the cultivation of Xianggu in China. *Journal of Zhejiang Forest Science and Technology* 22:14–18, 2002.

Xiao, Y., Chen, X., Yang, L. et al. 2013. Preparation and oral bioavailability study of curcuminoid-loaded microemulsion. *Journal of Agricultural and Food Chemistry* 61:3654–3660.

Xu, J., Zhao, W. X., Ning, Y. W. et al. 2013. Improved stability and controlled release of omega 3/omega 6 polyunsaturated fatty acids by spring dextrin encapsulation. *Carbohydrate Polymers* 92:1633–1640.

Yang, Y., and McClements, D. J. 2013. Vitamin E bioaccessibility: Influence of carrier oil type on digestion and release of emulsified α- tocopherol acetate. *Food Chemistry* 141:473–481.

Yanishlieva-Maslarova, N. V., and Heinonen, I. M. 2001. Sources of natural antioxidants: Vegetables, fruits, herbs, spices and teas. In: Pokorny, J., Yanishlieva, N., and Gordon, M. (Eds.). *Antioxidants in Food: Practical Applications*. Boca Raton, FL: CRC Press; pp. 210–263.

Yao, M. F., Chen, J. J., Zheng, J. K., Song, M. Y., McClements, D. J., and Xiao, H. 2013. Enhanced lymphatic transport of bioactive lipids: Cell culture study of polymethoxyflavone incorporation into chylomicrons. *Food & Function* 4:1662–1667.

Yao, M., McClements, D. J., and Xiao H. 2015. Improving oral bioavailability of nutraceuticals by engineered nanoparticle-based delivery systems. *Current Opinion in Food Science* 2:214–219.

Yao, M. F., Xiao, H., and McClements, D. J. 2014. Delivery of lipophilic bioactives: Assembly, disassembly, and reassembly of lipid nanoparticles. *Annual Review of Food Science and Technology* 5:53–81.

Yao, Y., Qiu, Q. H., Wu, X. W., Cai, Z. Y., Xu, S., and Liang, X. Q. 2013. Lutein supplementation improves visual performance in Chinese drivers—1-year randomized, double-blind, placebo-controlled study. *Nutrition* 29:958–964.

Yen, G. C., and Duh, P. D. 1993. Antioxidative properties of methanolic extracts from peanut hulls. *Journal of the American Oil Chemists' Society* 70:383–386.

Yu, D. 2015. Loose-leaf tea infused chocolate launched by UK startup Easy Teasy. http://www.confectionerynews.com/Manufacturers/Loose-leaf-tea-infused-chocolate-launched-by-UK-startup-Easy-Teasy (accessed 27 July, 2016).

Yu, D. 2016. Zhaolong Foods to produce China's first gum with organic tea ingredient. http://www.nutraingredients.com/Ingredients/Minerals/Zhaolong-Foods-to-produce-gum-with-organic-tea polyphenols/ (accessed 27 July, 2016).

Yu, H. L., and Huang, Q. R. 2012. Improving the oral bioavailability of curcumin using novel organogel-based nanoemulsions. *Journal of Agricultural and Food Chemistry* 60:5373–5379.

Zhang, F., Zhang, S., Sun, F. Liu, Z., and Chen, X. 2006. Anti-virus effect of lentinan. *Journal of Changchun University of Traditional Chinese Medicine* 22:11–12.

Zhang, R., Li, L., Li, J. Fu, H., and Rao, P. 1998. A study of hypocholesterolemic effect of tofuru. *Journal of Fuzhou University (Natural sciences edition)* 26:132–135.

Zou, L. Q., Peng, S. F., Liu, W. et al. 2014. Improved *in vitro* digestion stability of (-)-epigallocatechin gallate through nanoliposome encapsulation. *Food Research International* 64:492–499.

Zouari, N., Abid, M., Fakhfakh, N. et al. 2011. Blue-green algae (*Arthrospira platensis*) as an ingredient in pasta: Free radical scavenging activity, sensory and cooking characteristics evaluation. *International Journal of Food Sciences and Nutrition* 62:811–813.

Zuidam, N. J., and Shimoni, E. 2010. Overview of microencapsulates for use in food products or processes and methods to make them. In: Zuidam, N. J., and Nedović, V. A. (Eds.). *Encapsulation Technologies for Active Food Ingredients and Food Processing*. New York, NY: Springer; pp. 3–29.

chapter seven

Fortification of dietary fibers in foods

Ami Patel, Ankit Goyal, Nihir Shah, and Manvesh Sihag

Contents

7.1 Introduction

Dietary fibers (DFs) or prebiotics could be defined as indigestible carbohydrates, mainly polysaccharides (e.g., celluloses, hemicelluloses, gums, and pectins), oligosaccharides (inulin), lignin and associated plant substances (e.g., waxes, suberin), which support the growth of beneficial lactic acid bacteria (LAB) in the colon and exert antagonism or enmity to pathogenic microorganisms limiting their abundance. The term *prebiotics* was coined by Gibson and Roberfroid in 1995 and Figure 7.1 represents the general classification scheme of DFs. The importance of dietary fibers in foods is heading toward the enlargement of a prospective market for fiber-rich products in recent years (Dhingra et al., 2012). The DFs market continues to grow due to great response in most countries and the intensifying market prospects. The analysts predict the global DF market to grow at a compound annual growth rate (CAGR) 16.54% in terms of revenue and 15.64% in terms of volume from 2014–2019 and is proposed to reach $4.31 billion by 2020 (Business wire, 2016).

The general recommendation for adequate intake of dietary fibers varies from individual to individual depending on their age, gender, and

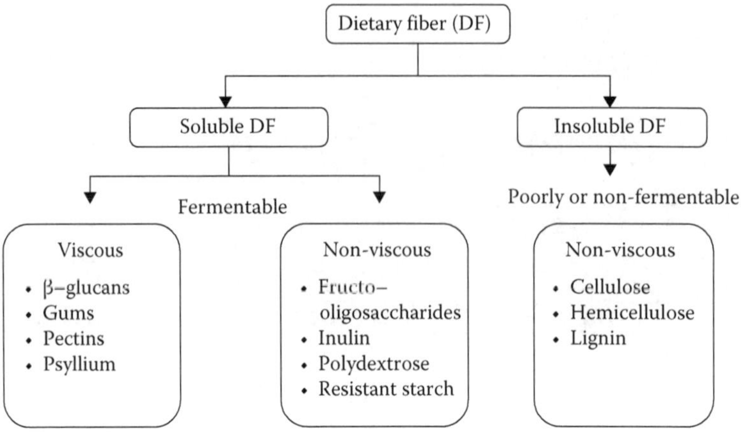

Figure 7.1 Dietary fiber classification based on chemical properties.

energy intake. The recommended daily intake of dietary fiber for adult women and adult men is 28g and 36g if their daily energy intake is 2000 Kcal and 2600 Kcal, respectively (Witwer, 2008). Many health benefits are being provided through DF intake. Their intake lessens the prevalence of obesity (Moyano et al., 2016), diabetes (InterAct consortium, 2015), coronary heart disease (Huang and Zhang, 2015), stroke (Threapleton et al., 2015), hypertension (Urushidani and Kuriyama, 2015) and certain gastrointestinal disorders such as gastric and oesophageal cancer (Sun et al., 2015), gastro-oesophageal reflux disease (Ness-Jensen et al., 2016), disease of gall bladder (Timmanpyati et al., 2015), peptic ulcer and diverticular diseases (Aldoori et al., 1997), haemorrhoids (Lohsiriwat, 2012), and constipation (Abdullah et al., 2015).

Currently, there is a trend of finding the new sources of dietary fibers for food industry and the low fiber foods are being accompanied with ones rich in fiber. The main functionality of fibers isolated from plants are oil adsorption, water binding capacity, solubility, viscosity, gel forming ability, and mineral and organic molecule binding capacity, which affects the product quality and sensory attributes. Dehydrated fruit and vegetable fibers provide high water and oil binding capacity, colonic fermentability, and low phytic acid contents and energy. By-products of the fruits and vegetables industry are also a potential source as novel ingredients for enhancing the fiber content of diet (O'Shea et al., 2012). Supplementation of DF in dairy products (Tseng and Zhao, 2013), canned meat, frozen foods (Almeida et al., 2013), chocolates (Norhayati et al., 2013; Konar et al., 2015), and beverages (Thongsombat et al., 2007; Buriti et al., 2014) has also been investigated recently, but the major focus still remains on cookies, crackers, and other cereal-based products (Foschia et al., 2013). Therefore, this chapter emphasizes recent developments and findings on fortification of

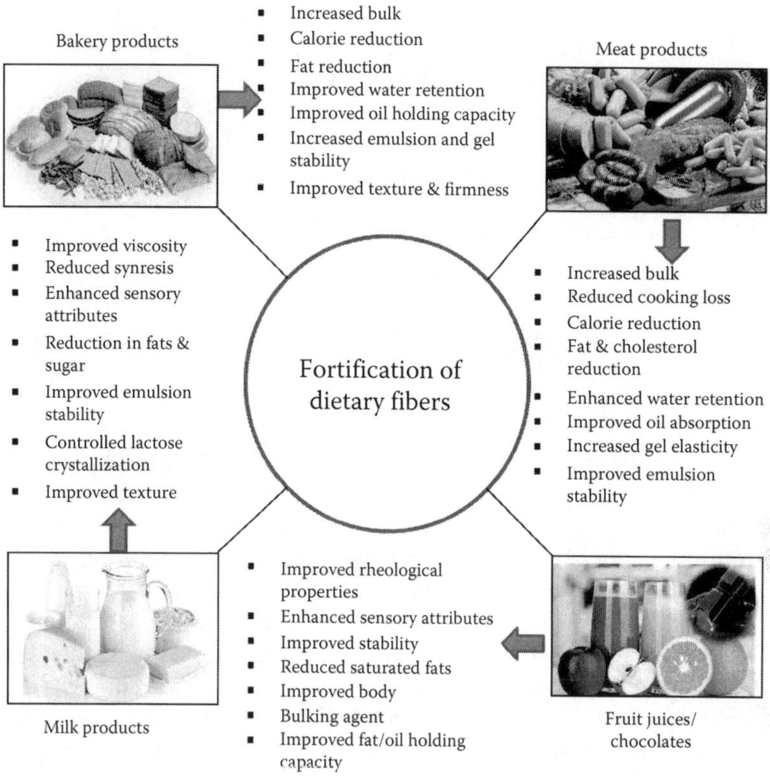

Figure 7.2 Effect of dietary fiber fortification on techno-functional properties of various food products.

bakery items, dairy products, meat and meat products, juices, beverages, and chocolates with dietary fiber. The general functions and significance of DF in different food types are depicted in Figure 7.2.

7.2 Fortification of dietary fibers

7.2.1 In bakery products

Bakery products are among the most popular food products consumed by all age-groups on a regular basis. High content of calories, fats, and cholesterol; and lower shelf-life of some baked goods (such as cake, bread) has diverted the attention of researchers and scientists toward the functional bakery products. A rapid change in rheological properties, physical structure (such as firmness, hardness, springiness, etc.), and oxidative stability (peroxide value) during processing and storage of baked goods has always been a challenge for food processors. As a functional ingredient, DFs not only increase the bulk and reduce the calories, fat content, and cholesterol but also provide a solution for negative changes that occurs during storage. A wide range of literature has suggested that incorporation of soluble DFs improved the structural and functional properties such as water retaining capacity, oil holding capacity, emulsion and gel stability of bakery products (Elleuch et al., 2011). Several workers have reported improved texture profile, mouthfeel, firmness, and physical stability on supplementation of DFs in bread (Waters et al., 2012), pasta (Martinez et al., 2014), noodles (Menon et al., 2015), cake (Jun et al., 2014), muffins (Sudha et al., 2015), and chips (Kayacier et al., 2014). Various food and by-products such as apple pomace, fruits' peel and kernel powder, dried fruits' flour, de-oiled legume flour, oat and barley flour, wheat, oat and rice bran, and so on, could be utilized as a potential source of DFs which have been successfully incorporated in different bakery products as discussed in Table 7.1.

Soluble DFs demonstrate several advantages over the insoluble fibers, for example, greater viscosity, better gel forming ability, emulsifying capacity without any off-flavor and bad texture. Some non-starch polysaccharides have also been reported to possess antioxidative properties. Zha et al., (2009) observed antioxidant activity of polysaccharides fractions from rice bran against superoxide radical, hydroxyl free radical and lipid peroxidation. Similarly, López-Vargas et al., (2013) and Martínez et al., (2012) determined the antioxidant properties of DF powder obtained from yellow passion fruit (*Passiflora edulis* var. *flavicarpa*) co-products and mango, guava, pineapple, and passion fruit, respectively, concluding that these DFs have significant antioxidant activity, could be utilized as a functional ingredients for the preservation of freshness of bakery and meat products, as well as in pharmaceutical industry due to its health promoting benefits.

Bread is the most common bakery product fortified with DFs. Fruit fiber concentrates, oat, barley, and maize fibers, rice bran, and so on have been incorporated in dough to replace a significant amount of fat and flour and to improve water holding capacity, loaf volume, water swelling capacity, gas retention, oil binding ability, firmness of the crust and crumb, and shelf-life. Bchir et al., (2014) studied the effect of date fibers on dough performance and bread quality and reported a significant ($P<0.05$) increase in water holding capacity (from 55.5±0.1 to 60.5±0.5%) and dough stability (from 4.0±0.0 to 29.0±1.5 min). Durum wheat bread enriched with bran (5%–30%) was also assessed for nutritional, textural, and sensory properties and found to be of lower quality in terms of sensory scores with an increase in bran content. However, when the dough was incorporated with guar seed flour and modified food-starch (2%), the product (with 30% bran) was completely acceptable (Previtali et al., 2015). Incorporation of prebiotic inulin-type fructans (up to 12%) in dough has been reported to provide

Table 7.1 Recent reports of various bakery products enriched with dietary fibers

Source of DF	Amount supplemented	Fortified food product	Major observations	Reference
Coffee silverskin	5 g/100 g wheat flour	Wheat bread	Improved water-retention capacity, oil-retention capacity, shelf-life, and sensory quality.	Pourfarzad et al., (2013)
Soy flour and rice bran	10%, 15%, 20%, 25% level each	Biscuit	15% soy flour +15% rice bran incorporated biscuit obtained the highest sensory scores; had no significant difference ($p < 0.05$) with control.	Mishra and Chandra, (2012)
Oat meal and Inulin	30% oatmeal and 10% inulin	Wheat flour tortilla	Oatmeal-inuline supplemented tortilla had 45% lesser fat and 71% more DF than control tortilla with same organoleptic and textural characteristics.	Heredia-Olea et al., (2015)
DF and bran from wheat, oat, and rice	10%, 20% and 30%	Cupcakes	Comparable cupcakes could be prepared with 20% DF and 10% cereal bran; DF resulted softer crumb texture and cereal bran improved crumb firmness.	Lebesi and Tzia, (2011)
Apple and apricot powders	10%, 20%, 30% and 40%	Cookies	Hardness significantly increased with higher level of apple powder; however, apricot powder added to cookies showed comparable sensory scores with control and lower hardness than that of apple powder added to cookies.	Özbas et al., (2014)
Brewer's spent grain (BSG)	5%, 10%, 15% and 20%	Bread	Bread added with 10% BSG showed comparable sensory characteristics with improved water absorption and springiness.	Waters et al., (2012)

(*Continued*)

Table 7.1 (Continued) Recent reports of various bakery products enriched with dietary fibers

Source of DF	Amount supplemented	Fortified food product	Major observations	Reference
Mango peel and kernel powder	20%, 30%, and 50%	Cookies	Mango peel and kernel powder (up to 30%) could be used to enhance the nutritional properties of cookies without affecting textural and sensory properties significantly.	Bandyopadhyay et al., (2014)
Apple pomace powder	15% and 20%	Cookies	Fortified cookies were ~44%–59% softer, ~30% more chewy, and ~14% moister than those of the control.	Jung et al., (2015)
Nejayote from white maize	3%, 6%, and 9%	Pan bread	Addition up to 9% Nejayote did not significantly affect the bread quality and baking performance and resulted in ~54% increased fiber content.	Acosta-Estrada et al., (2014)
Pomegranate peel	1.5%, 3.0%, 4.5,% 6.0%, and 7.5%	Cookies	Approximately 80% increase was observed in fiber content with acceptable sensory scores.	Ismail et al., (2014)
Cladodes (stems) from prickly pear	2.5%, 5.0%, and 7.5%	Cookies	Cookies supplemented with 5% cladodes remained organoleptically acceptable at 5-point hedonic scale.	Msaddak et al., (2015)
Watermelon rind waste	10, 20%, and 30%	Cookies	Fortified cookies resulted higher water absorption and oil-holding capacity due to increased fiber content; showed similar sensory scores as control.	Naknaen et al., (2016)

(Continued)

Table 7.1 (Continued) Recent reports of various bakery products enriched with dietary fibers

Source of DF	Amount supplemented	Fortified food product	Major observations	Reference
Wine grape pomace	5%, 10%, 15%, and 20%	Breads, muffins, and brownies	No significant difference in overall acceptability of 5% and 10% fortified bread and muffins; and 15% and 20% fortified brownies as compared to control.	Walker et al., (2014)
Banana flour	10%, 20%, and 30%	Bread	Banana flour (up to 30%) could be fortified in wheat flour with no significant difference in taste, aroma, appearance, and texture of control bread.	Baba et al., (2015)
Amaranth flour	15%, 30%, 40%, and 50%	Pasta	30% amaranth flour was the maximum fortification level obtained with acceptable quality; 40% and 50% fortifications caused some detrimental effects on technology and sensory quality.	Martinez et al., (2014)
Legumes (chickpea, pigeon pea, moong bean, and cow pea) flour	25%	Cookies	Improved water absorption capacity, oil absorption capacity, and swelling property with no significant ($P<0.05$) difference in sensory quality compared with control.	Thongram et al., (2016)
Pigeon pea flour or pigeon pea by-product flour	5%, 10%, 15%, 20%, and 25%	Biscuits	Good quality biscuits with higher protein and DF could be prepared by addition of maximum 15% pigeon pea flour without affecting sensory quality of product.	Tiwari et al., (2011)
Apple peels	3% and 6%	Cake	6% addition reduced the volume with harder texture; however, 3% fortification did not affect the quality significantly.	Jun et al., (2014)

(Continued)

Table 7.1 (Continued) Recent reports of various bakery products enriched with dietary fibers

Source of DF	Amount supplemented	Fortified food product	Major observations	Reference
Apple pomace	3%, 6%, and 9%	Rice based cracker	Crispness decreased with increase in pomace level; sensory value for flavor increased with increase in pomace level up to 6%; overall acceptability was in the range and preferred by consumers.	Mir et al., (2015)
Bengal gram flour and germinated pearl millet flour	6% each	Biscuit	2.87 times higher DF was observed in flour fortified biscuit with no significant difference among the samples and control.	Aggarwal et al., (2016)
Carob (*Ceratonia siliqua* L.) flour	1%–5%	Pasta	No significant difference ($P<0.05$) was observed among the sensory scores of fortified pasta and control.	Sęczyk et al., (2016)
Oat powder	0%, 4%, 8%, 12%, 16%, and 20%	Wheat-semolina pasta	Water uptake and swelling index increased, while optimal cooking time decreased significantly with increase in oat powder content; however, higher levels of fortification caused disruption in physical structure and gluten matrix.	Piwińska et al., (2015)
Corn bran	20%, 40%, and 60%	Rice noodles	Lower expansion ratio, soft noodle texture, and decreased extensibility of the corn bran-incorporated noodles.	Baek et al., (2014)

(*Continued*)

Table 7.1 (Continued) Recent reports of various bakery products enriched with dietary fibers

Source of DF	Amount supplemented	Fortified food product	Major observations	Reference
Apple, pear, and date pomaces concentrates	2%	Bread	Improved water absorption, stability, and tenacity; reduced extensibility and softness of enriched dough; more aerated internal crumb structure; no significant ($P<0.05$) difference in bread crumb and crust texture profiles of sample and control.	Bchir et al., (2014)
Barley flour	10%, 20%, and 30%	Instant noodles	L* (lightness) as well as hardness decreased with an increase in barley flour. Sustagrain and Salute/Radiant (variety) barley flour up to 10% and 20% could be fortified, respectively, when sensory scores were considered.	Hou and Jimenez, (2013)
Banana stem flour	10%	Bread	Lower volume, darker crumb, and lighter crust color than the control bread; product was acceptable in terms of sensory scores.	Ho et al., (2013)
Apple fiber	0%–15%	Wheat chips	Overall acceptability of fortified chips decreased with the increase of frying temperature, but received highest sensory score at low temperature (170°C).	Kayacier et al., (2014)
NUTRIOSE (resistant starch)	10%, 15%, and 20%	Noodles (from sweet potato flour and starch)	Reduced cooking loss; lowest glycemic index and the highest sensory scores were obtained for noodles with 15% NUTRIOSE + 1% gaur gum.	Menon et al., (2015)

better structure and gas retention during proofing and baking, thus improving the specific volume, softer crumb, improved crust, and crumb browning with enhanced sensory properties (Capriles and Areas, 2013).

Along with the bread, several other bakery products play a substantial role in the human diet, for example, cookies, pasta, vermicelli, noodles, biscuits, and cake. Cookies are the traditional and nonperishable snacks. High amounts of saturated fat and calories are the only major disadvantages of consuming cookies. Several researchers have worked and succeeded in replacing a large amount of flour and fat by incorporating DFs in cookies. Fortification of DFs such as bamboo powder (Mustafa et al., 2016), peanut skins (de Camargo et al., 2014), mango peel (Bandyopadhyay et al., 2014), and amaranth flour (Chauhan et al., 2015) could enhanced the crispiness, texture, firmness, sensory attributes, and shelf-life. Chauhan et al., (2015) observed the reduced hardness in cookies fortified with amaranth flour (raw and germinated) as compared to control cookies. Peanut skin is also a rich source of insoluble DFs, which was incorporated at 1.3, 1.8, and 2.5% level in cookies (de Camargo et al., 2014). Authors reported that along with the insoluble fibers (up to 52%), total phenolic content (up to 30%) and thus, antioxidant activities also increased to a significant level.

Biscuits, which can be considered an alternative to cookies, have also been fortified with rice bran, bengal gram flour, germinated pearl millet flour, and pigeon pea flour (Tiwari et al., 2011; Aggarwal et al., 2016). Nagi et al., (2012) supplemented full fat and defatted cereal brans (wheat, oat, and corn) in biscuits and reported that a 20% fortification level was best on the basis of spread ratio and sensory properties. Similarly, Mishra, and Chandra (2012) developed functional biscuits by adding rice bran from levels of 10%–25% and noticed an improved nutritional profile with no significant effect on organoleptic properties.

7.2.2 *In dairy products*

Milk is considered to be a nearly balanced food that supplies various nutrients to meet the recommended daily allowances for the growth and maintenance of the body. Usually, dairy products do not possess DFs. Dairy products and DFs both have established positive roles in improving the health status of individuals irrespective of their opposite intake pattern. Fortification of DFs in fermented or non-fermented dairy products can significantly affect the rheological properties including viscosity and syneresis, overall body-texture (smoothness, creaminess), color, and appearance as well as sensorial properties of the finished product. Researchers speculated that if DF, such as inulin, is present during the milk fermentation and coagulation process, inulin may become a part of the protein structural network by complexion with protein aggregates (Kip et al., 2006). The type of prebiotic, based on the length of their chains, can influence the activity of starter cultures and pH value of the fermented milk products (Aryana and McGrew, 2007).

Incorporation of DF in dairy products had shown to reduce the fat and sugar content from the product without influencing the mouth feel and thus reducing the total caloric value of food. Thus, such dairy products are suitable options as functional dietetic foods. Recently, fortification of dairy products with DF exceeded more to improve functionality and formulate novel functional foods. Diverse DFs obtained from fruits like apple, peach, grapes, and orange; cereals and grains such as rice, maize, wheat, and oat; and fructo-oligosaccharides (FOS), inulin, isomalt, etc. have been incorporated in various dairy products, especially in yogurts; several of them are discussed in the text and others are given in Table 7.2.

Table 7.2 Recent reports of various dairy products enriched with dietary fibers

Source of DF	Fortified food product	Major observations	Reference
Orange fiber	Yogurt	Fiber pasteurization in the mix enhances its integration in the gel matrix.	Sendra et al., 2010
Wine grape pomace (WGP)	Yogurt, salad dressings	The viscosity and ph of WGP-yogurt increased and decreased, respectively, but syneresis and % lactic acid as well as ph of salads were stable during 3 weeks storage at 4°C.	Tseng and Zhao, 2013
Passion fruit fiber	Yogurt	The apparent viscosity and thixotropy of yogurts were higher at the end of storage; appearance, color and odor of the passion fruit fiber yogurts were "good."	Espírito-Santo et al., 2013
Inulin or inulin combined with a grain mixture or a milled mixture of flakes	Yogurt	Affective acceptance was significantly lower for reduced-sugar yogurt with visible fiber than for reduced-sugar yogurt with inulin; cereal size and cereal taste are important factors in product formulation because of their impact on general acceptance.	Hoppert et al., 2013
Apple, wheat, and bamboo fibers	Yogurt	Bamboo and wheat fiber strained yogurts were acceptable while apple fibers developed ragged structure and had dominant apple taste and strong odor.	Seçkin and Baladura, 2012

(Continued)

Table 7.2 (Continued) Recent reports of various dairy products enriched with dietary fibers

Source of DF	Fortified food product	Major observations	Reference
Dried grape pomace	Yogurt	Yogurt fortified with 3% dried grape pomace had similar appearance, flavor, texture, consistency, and overall acceptance ratings as control yogurt, but increased fiber level to 4%–5% significantly decreased scores and acceptability.	Mohamed et al., 2014
Peach	Yogurt	Peach-flavored yogurts containing the prebiotic did not significantly influence the flavor and so did not much impact consumer acceptance.	Gonzalez et al., 2011
Oligo-fructose	Non-flavored yogurt	Addition of oligofructose showed no influence on the ph, proteolysis or the viability of *Str. Thermophilus* or *Lb. Bulgaricus* during refrigerated storage for 28 days ($p > 0.05$).	Cruz et al., 2013
Inulin (*Jerusalem artichoke*)	Synbiotic yogurt	DF supported the growth of probiotic *Lb. Acidophilus* P106 and high level (5%) led to more reduction of blood glucose, cholesterol levels, and total lipids compared with control in mice.	El-Kholy and Mahrous, 2015
Inulin and isomalt	Frozen yogurt	Sensory properties of the inulin and isomalt containing samples (6.5%) were similar to those of control, LAB counts were 8.12 and 8.49 log values after 3 months of storage period.	Isik et al., 2011
Flaxseed mucilage	Kefir	Flaxseed mucilage demonstrated good prebiotic activity, enhanced LAB growth in kefir model along with high antioxidant beneficiary.	HadiNezhad et al., 2013
Inulin	Kefir	Kefir with inulin had higher firmness, while no significant differences in odor and consistency between kefirs with and without inulin; substitution of SMP by inulin allowed for reducing 15% and 37% of caloric value in comparison with SMP and WMP kefir, respectively.	Glibowski and Kowalska, 2012

(Continued)

Table 7.2 (Continued) Recent reports of various dairy products enriched with dietary fibers

Source of DF	Fortified food product	Major observations	Reference
Inulin (2.5%) and *L. Casei*	Ice cream	Enhanced nutritional and sensory properties.	Di Criscio et al., 2010
Oligo-fructose, inulin with *B. animalis* and *B. longum*	Ice cream	Both prebiotics significantly increased apparent viscosity and developed the melting properties in ice cream during storage; however, the highest increase in firmness and the longest 1st dripping time were obtained with inulin ($P < 0.05$).	Akalin and Eris, 2008
Inulin (2.5%)	Ice cream	Inulin increased viscosity, adhesiveness, cohesiveness, elasticity, gumminess, chewiness, and fat instability in low-fat ice cream.	Ismail et al., 2013
Inulin (2% to 7%)	Caprine milk cheese	Penetrometry parameters were affected by the levels of replacement of fat with inulin; samples containing inulin were characterized by lower values of compressive force, stiffness, viscosity and adhesiveness (except for the sample with 2% fat substitution).	Salvatore et al., 2014
Inulin	Processed cheese spread	As the levels of inulin (0% to 8 %) the firmness and work of shear of cheese spread increased, whereas the stickiness and work of adhesion decreased.	Giri et al., 2014

Several milk-based products occur traditionally in different countries at a glance, which carry cereals, nuts, fruits, and vegetables as a non-dairy ingredient complementing milk with the DFs, such as milk-based porridges, milk shakes, fruit smoothies, and *raita* (fermented milk with pieces of fruits and vegetables) are highly palatable and liked by all age groups.

Yogurt fortified with orange by-product showed increased viscosity and improved water absorption (Sendra et al., 2010). Soukoulis et al., (2009) reported that DFs from oat, wheat, apple, and inulin were able to control the crystallization and re-crystallization of frozen dairy products by elevating the glass transition temperature. The effect of different bulking agents such as maltodextrin, sorbitol, and polydextrose on the physicochemical, sensory, and textural properties of artificially sweetened misti dahi (a sweetened variety of dahi) was studied by Raju and Pal (2011). Misti dahi is analogous to sweetened yogurt, but has a pleasant caramel color and flavor. Authors noticed that maltodextrin increased acidity, water activity and viscosity of dahi while decreased syneresis compared to sorbitol and polydextrose. Maltodextrin also found to increase hardness, adhesiveness and gumminess values of the product.

FOS and inulin were acceptable in ice cream, when substituted for up to 20% of the sugar (Wood, 2011). Ice creams supplemented with probiotic bacterium *Lb. casei* and inulin (2.5%) confirmed good nutritional and sensory properties (Di Criscio et al., 2010). Along with enhancing functional properties, inulin (1.5 %) improved low-fat cheese texture, produced from ultra-filtered milk (Miocinovic et al., 2011). The sensory characteristics were also improved with an increase in the inulin content. Combination of oligofructose and inulin (5% each) improved the technological and sensory acceptability of petit-suisse cheese and further enhanced viable counts of *Lb. acidophilus* and *B. animalis* subsp. *lactis* (Cardarelli et al., 2008).

Addition of inulin in kefir did not influence acidity or viability of LAB (Montanuci et al., 2012). Depending on the type of milk and starter culture used, it influenced the firmness, syneresis, and survival of acetic acid bacteria, *Lactococcus, Leuconostoc,* and yeasts, which either increased or remained unchanged during the storage period. The samples with 9% of the inulin blend or with 0.03% carrageenan displayed identical rheological behavior compared to the full-fat control sample and showed similar creaminess, smoothness, and thickness values; however, it affected the sweetness and flavor sensory values of the low-fat semi-solid dairy desserts (Bayarri et al., 2010).

Apart from improving technological parameters, prebiotic DFs also enhance the viability of health-beneficial bacteria; therefore they are often used in functional dairy foods (Khedkar et al., 2017). Milk supplemented with cellobiose or a combination of cellobiose and FOS enhanced the viability of *B. infantis* during four weeks of storage (Basholli-Salihu et al., 2013). Research findings showed that the synergism between starters (*B. breve* + *B. longum* + *Lb. rhamnosus*) in co-cultures affected the degree of rice fibers fermentation (Fernando et al., 2011). One of the studies demonstrated that flaxseed mucilage acts as a good source of prebiotic, enhancing growth of LAB in kefir model. Pure flaxseed mucilage showed better prebiotic functionality compared to the crude flaxseed mucilage without causing a drastic decline in pH (HadiNezhad et al., 2013). All prebiotics showed similar effect on the viability of probiotics at the end of the 30-day storage period; inulin and polydextrose were preferred over soluble corn fiber with respect to consumer acceptance (Allgeyer et al., 2010). Further, when stressed by low-temperature storage, beta-glucan had shown protective effect on bifidobacteria in yogurt (Rosburg et al., 2010).

Several *in vivo* animal studies also supported the positive role of DFs on the survival of health beneficial bacteria. Mahrous et al., (2014) reported significant decrease in the levels of cholesterol and bile acid in the serum of mice fed with yogurt fermented by *Lb. acidophilus* P106 with 0.75% oats. The yogurt with 0.75% oat had excellent sensory evaluation and satisfactory acceptance by the consumers. In one study, buckwheat flour and oat bran-supplemented samples enhanced stability of *Lb. paracasei* IMC 502®, *Lb. rhamnosus* IMC 501®, and SYNBIO® in probiotic fiber-enriched fermented milks during storage (Coman et al., 2013). Inulin and kiwifruit pectin enhanced the adhesion of *Lb. rhamnosus* and decreased adhesion of *Salmonella typhimurium* to Caco–2 cells. Inulin and citrus pectin significantly enhanced the adhesion of *B. bifidum* to Caco–2 cells (Parkar et al., 2010).

7.2.3 In meat and meat products

Suitability of DF incorporation into meat preparation is due to their water retention, natural pleasant flavor, and decrease in cooking loss and further, their fat-mimetic characteristics offer an interesting concept to meat industry. Incorporation of DFs would help to enhance the desirability of meat products, and further, their sources are generally agricultural by-products that are comparatively cheap and thus, their addition in meat products reduces its overall cost (Mehta et al., 2015). Numerous studies have shown that fiber fortification at nutritionally significant levels (2–3 g/serving) can be accomplished without adverse impact on the organoleptic quality of meat sausages (Yilmaz and Gecgel, 2009; Petersson et al., 2014b).

The DFs obtained from oat (Yang et al., 2010; Akesowan, 2013), wheat (Taludkar and Sharma, 2009; Mahmoud and Badr, 2011), and rye bran (Petersson et al., 2014a, b) in various meat products were more fully investigated as shown in Table 7.3. In one investigation, all three DFs (tomato fiber, beet root fiber, inulin) increased water-retaining capacity in cooked chicken, but only tomato fiber reduced losses from cooking while addition of tomato fiber and beet root fiber reduced lipid oxidation processes (Cava et al., 2012). Apart from this, addition of seaweed *Himanthalia Elongata* (10%–40% w/w) showed reduced cooking losses in beef patties, while the microbiological counts and lipid oxidation were significantly lower ($P < 0.05$) than control samples (Cox and Abu-Ghannam, 2013). Fruit fibers also showed improvement in the cooking properties of pork burger (López-Vargas et al., 2014), and beef burgers (Eldemery, 2009). In sausages, fiber alone or in combination with hydrocolloids shows great suitability. Fibers are added to the tumbler together with brine or separately in a later step in case of restructured hams. In dry sausages, fiber application reduces drying time while insoluble fibers help to overcome organoleptic problems in ground meat products (Bodner and Sieg, 2009; Akesowan, 2013).

Table 7.3 Recent reports of various meat products and sea foods enriched with dietary fibers

Source of DF	Fortified food product	Major observations	Reference
Long-chain powdered cellulose (0-8 g/100 g)	Surimi seafood	Increase in gel elasticity, indicating enhanced thermal gelation of surimi and enhanced water holding capacity.	Debusca et al., 2014
Xanthan, guar, carrageenan, and locust bean gum	Meatballs	Gums decreased moisture content of the products and meatballs with locust bean gum (1%) received higher acceptability.	Demirci et al., 2014
DF extracted from makgeolli lees	Reduced-fat frankfurters	20% fat frankfurters with the addition of 2% makgeolli lees fiber were similar in quality to regular frankfurters with 30% fat.	Choi et al., 2014
Barley β-glucan and resistant starch (RS)	Sausage	RS decreased cooking yield, while BG increased it. Resistant starch increased hardness and RS/BG combination showed antagonistic effect on hardness.	Amini Sarteshnizi et al., 2014
Rye bran	Low-fat sausage	Rye bran treated with hydrolytic enzymes reduced the frying loss to 15.2%–16.4%; improved firmness while the effect of untreated rye bran to sausages was detrimental.	Petersson et al., 2014a
Rye bran, oat bran, and barley fiber	Low-fat sausage	Sausages with oat bran showed low process and frying loss and high firmness and acceptability as compared to other fibers.	Petersson et al., 2014b
Albedo-fiber powder obtained from yellow passion fruit	Pork burger	Improved nutritional values, moisture and fat retention, and cooking yield; decreased microbiological counts.	López-Vargas et al., 2014

(*Continued*)

Table 7.3 (Continued) Recent reports of various meat products and sea foods enriched with dietary fibers

Source of DF	Fortified food product	Major observations	Reference
κ-Carrageenan, polydextrose, oat bran, and corn flour (0.5% and 1%)	Light pork sausages made with konjac flour	Polydextrose and oat bran showed significant decreases ($p < 0.05$) in cooking loss of the sausages with respect to control sausage; all texturizing ingredients (0.5%) significantly increased ($p < 0.05$) the sausage firmness, except oat bran.	Akesowan, 2013
Barley β-glucan, inulin, and their mixture	Low-fat cooked meat batters	β-glucan caused stickiness by itself and inulin powder caused excessive hardness; however, combination of β-glucan and inulin compensated undesirable effect of fat reduction.	Álvarez and Barbut, 2013
Soy flour, split-pea flour, and wheat starch	Low-fat hamburger	Soy flour in combination with starch led to increase in cooking yield and addition of split-pea flour in mixed formula decreased shrinkage while improving texture properties.	Tabarestani, and Tehrani, 2012
Pumpkin (*Cucurbita maxima* Duch) fiber	Chicken frankfurters	Addition of pumpkin fiber produced acceptable chicken frankfurters and improved their quality characteristics.	Choi et al., 2012
Wheat bran	Reduced-fat beef burger	Wheat bran decreased cooking loss in reduced-fat beef burger.	Mahmoud and Badr, 2011
Oat	Pork and chicken sausages	Flavor scores were improved by the addition of hydrated oatmeal in pork and chicken sausages	Yang et al., 2010

(Continued)

Table 7.3 (Continued) Recent reports of various meat products and sea foods enriched with dietary fibers

Source of DF	Fortified food product	Major observations	Reference
Corn starch, wheat semolina, wheat flour, and tapioca starches	Buffalo meat nuggets	Corn starch in buffalo meat nuggets produced more stable emulsion than other binders used; product yield, drip loss, and ph did not vary significantly between the products with different binders.	Devadason et al., 2010
Wheat and oat bran	Chicken meat patties	Both brans significantly increased the water holding capacity (whc) and emulsion stability (es). Oat bran showed better effect on whc and es than wheat bran.	Taludkar and Sharma, 2009
Orange albedo	Beef burgers	The nutritional and cooking properties were improved compared to control treatment.	Eldemery, 2009

Fibers can be applied in premixes depending on such properties as particle size, bulk density, ability to lump, flowability, and dusting. Fibers or fine powders are mixed with a very small amount of food grade oil, which prevents dusting during handling (Bodner and Sieg, 2009).

7.2.4 In miscellaneous foods

Traditionally, DFs have been hard to work with in beverage applications because fiber often negatively affects the flavor, mouthfeel, color, and clarity of a drink (Patel et al., 2017). But ingredient companies have improved the stability and processing capabilities of DFs. Advances in ingredient technology enable beverage scientists to add significant levels of fiber to a range of mainstream beverages, from juices to enhanced waters. Fiber-enriched beverages give consumers another viable option to increase their fiber intake. From 2010 to 2014, there was a 56% increase in drinks launched globally containing fiber, ranging from teas to juices and smoothies (http://tateandlylefibers.com/Content/pdfs/tnl0227-fiberspromoatbevarticles-6.19.15.pdf).

Pectins and pectin extracts are considered as an excellent source of soluble dietary fiber in beverages, particularly due to their fruit origin and stability in low pH. There was no significant difference in sensory scores perceived from almost all evaluated attributes except the turbidity and odor attributes, as compared to guava juice without the addition of crude pectin; however, a deodorization process may be needed for further commercial guava pectin production and use (Thongsombat et al., 2007).

The prebiotic effect of the fermented cashew apple juice, containing oligosaccharides, is evaluated through the growth of probiotic strain *Lb. johnsonii* B-2178 (Vergara et al., 2010). A synbiotic mixture of probiotic *Lb. rhamnosus* GG and prebiotics oligofructose and inulin was applied on fresh cut apple wedges (Roble et al., 2010). Fructan analysis indicated that all prebiotics remained stable over the fourteen days' storage period and an intake of 100 g of apple delivered 2–3 g of prebiotics. Similarly, a combined effect of long-chain and short-chain inulin in different proportions (7.5 g/100 g) to low-fat custards resulted in improved rheological and sensory properties. Further, the use of this blend inulin with carrageenan gave thicker, creamier custard, which had more consumer preference to that of the full-fat custard (Tárrega et al., 2010).

Different prebiotic fibers (oat bran, β–glucan and green banana flour) provided substratum for adherence of *Lb. casei* while trehalose acted as a cell protectant prolonging their viability (Guergoletto et al., 2010). On the other hand, Keenan et al., (2011) indicated that apple purees enriched with two commercial FOS (Beneo GR® [inulin] and HSI®) showed stability for almost a month at 4°C.

Konar et al., (2015) investigated the influence of calcium fortification on physical and rheological properties of sucrose-free prebiotic milk chocolates containing inulin and maltitol. The calcium-containing samples shown to exhibit positive differences in other physical properties (brightness and water activity) that could be noteworthy and significant with respect to visual quality and shelf life. The dark chocolate, DC-1, containing inulin had at least 12 months of shelf life at 18°C, 60% RH with better acceptance than control dark chocolate DC-0 (with high content of sugar); moreover, it did not experience microbiological and inulin content changes (Norhayati et al., 2013). In another investigation also, a functional milk chocolate containing 50 g/kg inulin did not show substantial differences from the control samples (Morris and Morris, 2012).

Some of the DF fortified food products available in the market are compiled in Table 7.4.

7.3 Downfalls, toxicity, and safety of dietary fibers

The majority of the DFs are natural food components present in edible plants; hence, safety is not an issue and the foods are consumed as a part of the traditional diet. Inulin and oligofructose are highly studied prebiotics. Several toxicological studies have shown that chicory

Table 7.4 Commercially available dietary fiber fortified food products fortified with dietary fibers

Product(s)	Dietary fiber type	Country
Yoplait elivaé'—Yogurt	Inulin—natural chicory fiber	Yoplait, New Zealand
Chobani® Greek yogurt	Oat	USA
b-Activ—probiotic dahi	Inulin	Mother dairy, India
Oatgurt, oat spread, fruit oat drink (mango, orange, strawberry), ice cream (chocolate, strawberry)	Oat	Oatly, Sweden
Fiber one—Cottage cheese, chocolate bars, cereals, breads	Oat	General Mills, Inc., USA and Canada
Grape juice	Inulin	Welch Foods Inc., USA
Apple, orange, cranberry	Inulin	Sysco Corporation · Houston, Texas, USA
FIBER BASICS® fiber juice	Acacia gum	Home Care Nutrition, USA
Benefiber®—fiber drink mix	Wheat dextrin	Novartis Consumer Health, Inc., NJ, USA
Elevate Fiber Water and Froose®	Inulin, fruit pectin	FNB Holdings LLC, Pennsylvania, USA
Juice+fiber (apple, orange, grape)	-	Nutrition Express, Ltd., USA
Pasta	Inulin	Dreamfields Foods, USA
Macaroni and cheese pasta, Thinables crackers	Wheat Starch (Resistant Starch)	Fiber Gourmet, Inc., FL, USA
Pasta, cupcakes, brownie	Oat fiber	Linda's Diet Delites, NJ, USA
Potters high fiber biscuits	Wheat, soya bran	Goodness Foods, UK
Horlicks Nutribics	Honey, oat	GlaxoSmithKline (GSK), UK
Digestive biscuit, Nutrichoice hifiber biscuit	Wheat bran	Britannia, Oman, UAE
Cactus Dietary Fiber Biscuit, Cactus red bean bread	Oat	Orgamoon, Korea

fructooligosaccharides do not increase morbidity or mortality or lead to toxicity; these substances are non-mutagenic, -carcinogenic, or -teratogenic (Carabin and Flamm, 1999). Many *in vivo* animal and human studies have been carried out to identify their physiological and potential health benefits and also to evaluate their possible intolerance. The only biological effects observed have been attributed to their action as nondigestible, fermentable carbohydrates causing self-limited gastrointestinal distress. Further, the ensuing gastrointestinal symptoms are dose-dependent as confirmed by various studies. The results indicated that these fructans are well-tolerated at amounts up to 20 g/d; diarrhea can develop with intake of 30 g/d or more (Briet et al., 1995; Den Hond et al., 2000).

The major problem associated with several DFs (such as polydextrose, inilin, and oligofructose) used to fortify food products is gas formation, bloating, and diarrhea in hosts, if used in a large amount. Moreover, a wide variety of nutrients, especially vitamins and minerals found in whole foods, may be missed by choosing fiber-fortified products.

7.4 Legislation and regulatory aspects of dietary fibers

Firm regulations exist regarding incorporation of DFs to specific food products in developed countries such as the United States, Australia, and Europe. However, in major developing countries relevant food regulations are often incomplete or poorly applied. It requires greater transparency and clarity, specifically with respect to maximum amounts permitted in specific foodstuffs, since high amounts of DF can cause side effects as discussed earlier. Such transparency can be achieved by proper labeling on the product and related aspects must be addressed by food control authorities of the respective nations.

7.5 Conclusion and future prospects

Prebiotics DFs have established significant effect on human health and have great possibilities for incorporation into a wide range of common foodstuffs. Their role is played by fermentable carbohydrates, which stimulate, preferentially, the growth of probiotic bacteria (bifidobacteria and lactic acid bacteria), thus enhancing the gastrointestinal and immune systems. In addition, prebiotics have been shown to increase the absorption of calcium and magnesium, influence blood glucose levels, and improve plasma lipids. Long-term clinical trials are required to confirm the health benefits of prebiotics in humans.

References

Abdullah, M. M., Gyles, C. L., Marinangeli, C. P., Carlberg, J. G., and Jones, P. J. 2015. Dietary fiber intakes and reduction in functional constipation rates among Canadian adults: A cost-of-illness analysis. *Food and Nutrition Research 59*. doi:http://dx.doi.org/10.3402/fnr.v59.28646.

Acosta-Estrada, B. A., Lazo-Vélez, M. A., Nava-Valdez, Y., Gutiérrez-Uribe, J.A., and Serna-Saldívar, S. O. 2014. Improvement of DF, ferulic acid and calcium contents in pan bread enriched with nejayote food additive from white maize (Zea mays). *Journal of Cereal Science* 60(1):264–269.

Aggarwal, D., Sabikhi, L., and Kumar, M. S. 2016. Formulation of reduced-calorie biscuits using artificial sweeteners and fat replacer with dairy–multigrain approach. *NFS Journal* 2:1–7.

Akalin, A. S., and Eris D. 2008. Effects of inulin and oligofructose on the rheological characteristics and probiotic culture survival in low-fat probiotic ice cream. *Food Microbiology and Safety M1–M5.*

Akesowan, A. 2013. Quality of light pork sausages containing konjac flour improved by texturizing ingredients. *The Journal of Animal and Plant Sciences* 23(4):1012–1018.

Aldoori, W. H., Giovannucci, E. L., Stampfer, M. J., Rimm, E. B., Wing, A. L., and Willett, W. C. 1997. *Prospective study of diet and the risk of duodenal ulcer in men American Journal of Epidemiology* 145(1):42–50.

Allgeyer, L. C., Miller, M. J., and Lee, S. Y. 2010. Sensory and microbiological quality of yogurt drinks with prebiotics and probiotics. *Journal of Dairy Science* 93:4471–4479.

Almeida, E. L., Chang, Y. K., and Steel, C. J. 2013. Dietary fiber sources in frozen part-baked bread: Influence on technological quality. *LWT-Food Science and Technology* 53(1):262–270.

Álvarez, D., and Barbut, S. 2013. Effect of inulin, β-Glucan and their mixtures on emulsion stability, color and textural parameters of cooked meat batters. *Meat Science* 94 (3):320–327.

Amini Sarteshnizi, R., Hosseini, H., Bondarianzadeh, D., Colmenero, F. J., and Khaksar, R. 2014. Optimization of prebiotic sausage formulation: Effect of using β-glucan and resistant starch by D-optimal mixture design approach. *LWT-Food Science and Technology* 62(1):704–710.

Aryana, K. J., and McGrew, P. 2007. Quality attributes of yogurt with Lactobacillus casei and various probiotics. *LWT Food Science and Technology* 40:1808–1814.

Baba, M. D., Manga, T. A., Daniel, C., and Danrangi, J. 2015. Sensory evaluation of toasted bread fortified with banana flour: a preliminary study. *American Journal of Food Science and Nutrition* 2(2):9–12.

Baek, J. J., Kim, Y., and Lee, S. 2014. Functional characterization of extruded rice noodles with corn bran: Xanthophyll content and rheology. *Journal of Cereal Science* 60(2):311–316.

Bandyopadhyay, K., Chakraborty, C., and Bhattacharyya, S. 2014. Fortification of mango peel and kernel powder in cookies formulation. *Journal of Academia and Industrial Research* 2:661–664.

Basholli-Salihu, M., Mueller, M., Unger, F. M., and Viernstein, H. 2013. The use of cellobiose and fructooligosaccharide on growth and stability of Bifidobacterium infantis in fermented milk. *Food and Nutrition Sciences* 4:1301–1306.

Bayarri, S., Chuliá, I., and Costell, E. 2010. Comparing l-carrageenan and an inulin blend as fat replacers in carboxymethyl cellulose dairy desserts. Rheological and sensory aspects. *Food Hydrocolloids* 24:578–587.

Bchir, B., Rabetafika, H. N., Paquot, M., and Blecker, C. 2014. Effect of pear, apple and date fibers from cooked fruit by-products on dough performance and bread quality. *Food and Bioprocess Technology* 7(4):1114–1127.

Bodner, J. M., and Sieg, J. 2009. Fiber. In: Tarté, R. (Ed.). *Ingredients in Meat Products: Properties, Functionality and Applications*, New York, NY: Springer Science; pp. 83–109. doi: 10.1007/978-0-387-71327-4_4.

Briet, F., Achour, L., Flourie, B., et al., 1995. Symptomatic response to varying levels of fructooligosaccharides consumed occasionally or regularly. *European Journal of Clinical Nutrition* 49: 501–507.

Buriti, F. C., Freitas, S. C., Egito, A. S., and dos Santos, K. M. 2014.Effects of tropical fruit pulps and partially hydrolysed galactomannan from Caesalpinia pulcherrima seeds on the dietary fiber content, probiotic viability, texture and sensory features of goat dairy beverages. *LWT-Food Science and Technology* 59(1):196–203.

Business wire. 2016. *Research and Markets: Global DF Market 2015-2019—It is forecast that the Global DF Market is set to Grow at a CAGR 16.54% in Terms of Revenue During 2014-2019.* Available from http://www.businesswire.com/news/home/20150804006509/en/Research-Markets-Global-Dietary-Fiber-Market-2015-2019 (accessed April 18, 2016).

Capriles, V. D., and Arêas, J. A. 2013. Effects of prebiotic inulin-type fructans on structure, quality, sensory acceptance and glycemic response of gluten-free breads. *Food and function* 4(1):104–110.

Carabin, I. G., and Flamm, W. G. 1999. Evaluation of safety of inulin and oligofructose as dietary fiber. *Regulatory Toxicology and Pharmacology* 30:268–282.

Cardarelli, H. R., Buriti, F. C. A., Castro, I. A., and Saad, S. M. I. 2008. Inulin and oligofructose improve sensory quality and increase the probiotic viable count in potentially synbiotic petit-suisse cheese. *Lebensmittel-Wissenschaft and Technologie* 41:1037–1046.

Cava, R., Ladero, L., Cantero, V., and Ramírez, R. M. 2012. Assessment of different DFs (tomato fiber, beet root fiber, and inulin) for the manufacture of chopped cooked chicken products. *Journal of Food Science* 7(4):C346–C352.

Chauhan, A., Saxena, D. C., and Singh, S., 2015. Total dietary fiber and antioxidant activity of gluten free cookies made from raw and germinated amaranth (Amaranthus spp.) flour. *LWT-Food Science and Technology* 63(2):939–945.

Choi, Y. S., Kim, H. W., Hwang, K. E. et al., 2012. Effects of pumpkin (Cucurbita maxima Duch.) fiber on physicochemical properties and sensory characteristics of chicken frankfurters. *Korean Journal for Food Science of Animal Resources* 32(2):174–183.

Choi, Y. S., Kim, H. W., Hwang, K. E. et al., 2014. Physicochemical properties and sensory characteristics of reduced-fat frankfurters with pork back fat replaced by DF extracted from makgeolli lees. *Meat Science* 96(2):892–900.

Coman, M. M., Verdenelli, M. C., Cecchini, C. et al., 2013. Effect of buckwheat flour and oat bran on growth and cell viability of the probiotic strains Lactobacillus rhamnosus IMC 501®, Lactobacillus paracasei IMC 502® and their combination SYNBIO®, in synbiotic fermented milk. *International Journal of Food Microbiology* 167(2):261–268.

Cox, S., and Abu-Ghannam, N. 2013. Enhancement of the phytochemical and fiber content of beef-patties with Himanthalia Elongata seaweed. *International Journal of Food Science and Technology* 48(11):2239–2249.

Cruz, A. G., Cavalcanti, R. N., Guerreiro, L. M. R. et al., 2013. Developing a prebiotic yogurt: Rheological, physico-chemical and microbiological aspects and adequacy of survival analyses methodology. *Journal of Food Engineering,* 114(3):323–330.

de Camargo, A. C., Vidal, C. M. M., Canniatti-Brazaca, S. G., and Shahidi, F. 2014. Fortification of cookies with peanut skins: Effects on the composition, polyphenols, antioxidant properties, and sensory quality. *Journal of Agricultural and Food Chemistry* 62(46):11228–11235.

Debusca, A., Tahergorabi, R., Beamer, S. K., Matak, K. E., and Jaczynski, J. 2014. Physicochemical properties of surimi gels fortified with dietary fibers. *Food Chemistry* 148:70–76.

Demirci, Z. O., Yılmaz, I., and Demirci, A. Ş. 2014. Effects of xanthan, guar, carrageenan and locust bean gum addition on physical, chemical and sensory properties of meatballs. *Journal of Food Science and Technology* 51(5):936–942.

Den Hond, E., Geypens, B., and Ghoos, Y. 2000. Effect if high performance chicory inulin on constipation. *Nutrition Research* 20:731–736.

Devadason, I. P., Anjaneyulu, A. S.,and Babji, Y. 2010. Effect of different binders on the physico-chemical, textural, histological, and sensory qualities of retort pouched buffalo meat nuggets. *Journal of Food Science* 75(1):S31–S35.

Dhingra, D., Michael, M., Rajput, H., and Patil, R. T. 2012. Dietary fiber in foods: a review. *Journal of Food Science and Technology* 49(3), 255–266.

Di Criscio, T., Frantianni, A., Minogna, R. et al., 2010. Production of functional probiotic, prebiotic and symbiotic ice creams. *Journal of Dairy Science* 93:4555–4563.

Eldemery, M. E. 2009. Effect orange albedo as a new source of dietary fiber on characteristics of beef burger. Recent Trends of Developing Institutional and Academic Performance in Higher Specific Education Institutions in Egypt and Aeab World. *Faculty of Specific Education Mansoura University - Egypt April*, 8–9, 2009.

El-Kholy, W. M., and Mahrous, H. 2015. Biological studies on bio-yogurt fortified with prebiotic obtained from Jerusalem artichoke. *Food and Nutrition Sciences* 6:1552–1564.

Elleuch, M., Bedigian, D., Roiseux, O., Besbes, S., Blecker, C., and Attia, H. 2011. Dietary fiber and fiber-rich by-products of food processing: Characterisation, technological functionality and commercial applications: A review. *Food Chemistry* 124:411–421.

Espírito-Santo, A. P., Lagazzo, A., Sousa, A. L. O. P., Perego, P., Converti, A., and Oliveira, M. N. 2013. Rheology, spontaneous whey separation, microstructure and sensorial characteristics of probiotic yoghurts enriched with passion fruit fiber. *Food Research International* 50(1):224–231.

Fernando, W. M. A. D. B, Flint, S., Zou, M., Brennan, C. S., Ranaweera, K. K., and Bamunuarachchi, A. 2011. The effect of rice fiber fractions on the growth of co-cultures of probiotics. *Journal of Food Science and Technology* 48(1):14–25.

Foschia, M., Peressini, D., Sensidoni, A., and Brennan, C. S. 2013.The effects of dietary fiber addition on the quality of common cereal products. *Journal of Cereal Science* 58(2):216–227.

Giri, A., Kanawjia, S. K., and Khetra, Y. 2014. Textural and melting properties of processed cheese spread as affected by incorporation of different inulin levels. *Food and Bioprocess Technology* 7(5):1533–1540.

Glibowski, P., and Kowalska, A. 2012. Rheological, texture and sensory properties of kefir with high performance and native inulin. *Journal of Food Engineering* 111(2):299–304.

Gonzalez, N. J., Adhikari, K., and Madriz, M. F. S. 2011. Sensory characteristics of peach-flavored yogurt drinks containing prebiotics and synbiotics. *LWT - Food Science and Technology* 44:158–163.

Guergoletto, K. B., Magnani, M., Martin, J. S., Andrade, C. G. T. D., and Garcia, S. 2010. Survival of Lactobacillus casei (LC-1) adhered to prebiotic vegetal fibers. *Innovative Food Science and Emerging Technologies* 11:415–421.

HadiNezhad, M., Duc, C., Han N. F., and Hosseinian, F. 2013. Flaxseed soluble dietary fiber enhances lactic acid bacterial survival and growth in kefir and possesses high antioxidant capacity. *Journal of Food Research* 2(5):152–163.

Heredia-Olea, E., Martínez-Martínez, A., Payan-Tamez, S., Palomera-Santandreu, I., Guajardo-Flores, S. and Pérez-Carrillo, E. 2015. Effect of inulin and oatmeal addition on fat and dietary fiber content in hot press wheat flour tortilla. *Journal of Food Research* 4(2):44.

Ho, L. H., Aziz, N. A. A., and Azahari, B. 2013. Physico-chemical characteristics and sensory evaluation of wheat bread partially substituted with banana (Musa acuminata X balbisiana cv. Awak) pseudo-stem flour. *Food Chemistry,* 139(1):532–539.

Hoppert, K., Zahn, S., Jänecke, L., Mai, R., Hoffmann, S., and Rohm, H. 2013. Consumer acceptance of regular and reduced-sugar yogurt enriched with different types of dietary fiber. *International Dairy Journal* 28(1):1–7.

Hou, G., and Jimenez, V. 2013. Development of Barley-Fortified Instant Noodles. Proceedings Whole Grain Summit 2012. AACC International., pp. 53–54. https://www.aaccnet.org/publications/plexus/cfwplexus/library/books/Documents/WholeGrainsSummit2012/CPLEX-2013-1001-26B.pdf

http://tateandlylefibers.com/Content/pdfs/tnl0227-fiberspromoatbevarticles-6.19.15.pdf.

Huang, T., and Zhang, X. 2015. Dietary fiber intake and mortality from all causes, cardiovascular disease, cancer, infectious diseases and others: A meta-analysis of 42 prospective cohort studies with 1,752,848 participants. *North American Journal of Medicine and Science,* 8(2):59–67.

InterAct Consortium. 2015. Dietary fiber and incidence of type 2 diabetes in eight European countries: The EPIC-InterAct Study and a meta-analysis of prospective studies. *Diabetologia* 58(7):1394–1408.

Isik, U., Boyacioglu, D., Capanoglu, E., and Erdil, D. N. 2011. Frozen yogurt with added inulin and isomalt. *Journal of Dairy Science* 94(4):1647–1656.

Ismail, E. A., Al-Saleh, A. A., and Metwalli, A. A.M. 2013. Effect of inulin supplementation on rheological properties of low-fat ice cream. *Life Science Journal* 10(3):1742–1746.

Ismail, T., Akhtar, S., Riaz, M., and Ismail, A. 2014. Effect of pomegranate peel supplementation on nutritional, organoleptic and stability properties of cookies. *International Journal of Food Sciences and Nutrition* 65(6):661–666.

Jun, Y., Bae, I. Y., Lee, S., and Lee, H. G. 2014. Utilisation of preharvest dropped apple peels as a flour substitute for a lower glycaemic index and higher fiber cake. *International Journal of Food Sciences and Nutrition* 65(1):62–68.

Jung, J., Cavender, G., and Zhao, Y. 2015. Impingement drying for preparing dried apple pomace flour and its fortification in bakery and meat products. *Journal of Food Science and Technology* 52(9):5568–5578.

Kayacier, A., Yüksel, F., and Karaman, S. 2014. Response surface methodology study for optimization of effects of fiber level, frying temperature, and frying time on some physicochemical, textural, and sensory properties of wheat chips enriched with apple fiber. *Food and Bioprocess Technology* 7(1):133–147.

Keenan, D. F., Brunton, N., Butler, F., Wouters, R., and Gormley, R. 2011. Evaluation of thermal and high hydrostatic pressure processed apple purees enriched with prebiotic inclusions. *Innovative Food Science and Emerging Technologies* 12:261–68.

Khedkar, C.D., Kalyankar, S.D., Patel A.R., and Khedkar C.C. 2017. Effect of synbiotic-assisted modulation of gastrointestinal microbiota on human health. In: Nutrients in Dairy and Their Implications for Health and Disease. Watson, R.R., Collier R.J., & Preedy V.R., Academic Press, Elsevier, pp: 223–36

Kip, P., Meyer, D., and Jellema, R. H. 2006. Inulins improve sensoric and textural properties of low-fat yogurts. *International Dairy Journal* 16:1098–1103.

Konar, N., Poyrazoglu, E. S., and Artik, N. 2015. Influence of calcium fortification on physical and rheological properties of sucrose-free prebiotic milk chocolates containing inulin and maltitol. *Journal of Food Science and Technology* 52(4):2033–2042.

Lebesi, D. M., and Tzia, C. 2011. Effect of the addition of different dietary fibers and edible cereal bran sources on the baking and sensory characteristics of cupcakes. *Food and Bioprocess Technology* 4(5):710–722.

Lohsiriwat, V. 2012. Hemorrhoids: from basic pathophysiology to clinical management. *World Journal of Gastroenterology* 18(17):2009–2017.

López-Vargas, J. H., Fernández-López, J., Pérez-Álvarez, J. Á., and Viuda-Martos, M. 2014. Quality characteristics of pork burger added with albedo-fiber powder obtained from yellow passion fruit (Passiflora edulis var. flavicarpa) co-products. *Meat Science* 97(2):270–276.

López-Vargas, J. H., Fernández-López, J., Pérez-Álvarez, J. A., and Viuda-Martos, M. 2013. Chemical, physico-chemical, technological, antibacterial and antioxidant properties of dietary fiber powder obtained from yellow passion fruit (Passiflora edulis var. flavicarpa) co-products. *Food Research International* 51(2):756–763.

Mahmoud, K. A., and Badr, H. M. 2011. Quality characteristics of gamma irradiated beefburger formulated with partial replacemen of beef fat with olive oil and wheat bran fibers. *Food Nutrition and Science* 2:655–666.

Mahrous, H., Kholy, W. M. E., and Elsanhoty, R. M. 2014. Production of new synbiotic yogurt with local probiotic isolate and oat and study its effect on mice. *Journal of Advance Dairy Research* 2:121.

Martinez, C. S., Ribotta, P. D., Añón, M. C., and León, A. E., 2014. Effect of amaranth flour (Amaranthus mantegazzianus) on the technological and sensory quality of bread wheat pasta. *Food Science and Technology International* 20(2):127–135.

Martínez, R., Torres, P., Meneses, M. A., Figueroa, J. G., Pérez-Álvarez, J. A. and Viuda-Martos, M. 2012. Chemical, technological and in vitro antioxidant properties of mango, guava, pineapple and passion fruit dietary fiber concentrate. *Food Chemistry* 135(3):1520–1526.

Mehta, N., Ahlawat, S. S., Sharma, D. P., and Dabur, R. S. 2015. Novel trends in development of DF rich meat products-a critical review. *Journal of Food Science Technology* 52(2):633–647.

Menon, R., Padmaja, G., and Sajeev, M. S. 2015. Cooking behavior and starch digestibility of NUTRIOSE® (resistant starch) enriched noodles from sweet potato flour and starch. *Food Chemistry* 182:217–223.

Miocinovic, J., Puđa, P., Radulovic et al., 2011. Development of low fat UF cheese technology. *Mljekarstvo* 61(1):33–44.

Mir, S. A., Bosco, S. J. D., Shah, M. A., Santhalakshmy, S., and Mir, M. M. 2015. Effect of apple pomace on quality characteristics of brown rice based cracker. *Journal of the Saudi Society of Agricultural Sciences*. doi: 10.1016/j.jssas.2015.01.001.

Mishra, N., and Chandra, R. 2012. Development of functional biscuit from soy flour and rice bran. *International Journal of Agricultural and Food Science* 2(1):14–20.

Mohamed, A. G., Abeer F. Z., and Nadia, M. S. 2014. Physiochemical and sensory evaluation of yogurt fortified with DF and phenolic compound. *Life Science Journal* 11(9):816–822.

Montanuci, F. D., Pimentel, T. C., Garcia, S., and Prudencio, S. H. 2012. Effect of starter culture and inulin addition on microbial viability, texture, and chemical characteristics of whole or skim milk Kefir. *Ciência e Tecnologia de Alimentos Campinas* 32(4):850–61.

Morris, C., and Morris, G. A. 2012. The effect of inulin and fructooligosaccharides supplementation on the textural, rheological and sensory properties of bread and their role in weight management: A review. *Food Chemistry* 133:237–248.

Moyano, G., Sáyago-Ayerdi, S. G., Largo, C., Caz, V., Santamaria, M., and Tabernero, M. 2016. Potential use of dietary fiber from Hibiscus sabdariffa and Agave tequilana in obesity management. *Journal of Functional Foods* 21:1–9.

Msaddak, L., Siala, R., Fakhfakh, N., Ayadi, M. A., Nasri, M., and Zouari, N., 2015. Cladodes from prickly pear as a functional ingredient: effect on fat retention, oxidative stability, nutritional and sensory properties of cookies. *International Journal of Food Sciences and Nutrition*, 66(8):851–857.

Mustafa, U., Naeem, N., Masood, S., and Farooq, Z. 2016. Effect of bamboo powder supplementation on physicochemical and organoleptic characteristics of fortified cookies. *Food Science and Technology* 4(1):7–13.

Nagi, H. P. S., Kaur, J., Dar, B. N., and Sharma, S. 2012. Effect of storage period and packaging on the shelf life of cereal bran incorporated biscuits. *American Journal of Food Technology* 7(5):301–310.

Naknaen, P., Itthisoponkul, T., Sondee, A., and Angsombat, N. 2016. Utilization of watermelon rind waste as a potential source of DF to improve health promoting properties and reduce glycemic index for cookie making. *Food Science and Biotechnology* 25(2):415–424.

Ness-Jensen, E., Hveem, K., El-Serag, H., and Lagergren, J. 2016. Lifestyle Intervention in gastroesophageal reflux disease. *Clinical Gastroenterology and Hepatology* 14(2):175–182.

Norhayati, H., Rasma, S .I., and Mohd, K. A. 2013. Effect of storage conditions on quality of prebiotic dark chocolate. *Malaysian Journal of Nutrition* 19(1):111–119.

O'Shea, N., Arendt, E. K., and Gallagher, E. 2012. Dietary fiber and phytochemical characteristics of fruit and vegetable by-products and their recent applications as novel ingredients in food products. *Innovative Food Science and Emerging Technologies* 16:1–10.

Özbas, Ö. Ö., Seker, I. T., and Gökbulut, I., 2014. Effects of resistant starch and fiber-rich apple and apricot powders on low-fat cookie quality. *International Journal of Arts and Sciences* 7(3):9.

Parkar, S. G., Redgate, E. L., Wibisono, R., Luo, X., Koh, E. T. H., and Schroder, R. 2010. Gut health benefits of kiwifruit pectins: Comparison with commercial functional polysaccharides. *Journal of Functional Foods* 2:210–218.

Patel, A., Shah, D., and Shah N. 2017. Market of functional food products- current scenario and future prospective of fermented milks and fruit juices. *Indian Food Industry Magazine*. 35(3): 34–8.

Petersson, K., Godard, O., Eliasson, A. C., and Tornberg, E. 2014a. The effects of cereal additives in low-fat sausages and meatballs. Part 1: Untreated and enzyme-treated rye bran. *Meat Science* 96(1):423–428.

Petersson, K., Godard, O., Eliasson, A. C., and Tornberg, E. 2014b. The effects of cereal additives in low-fat sausages and meatballs. Part 2: Rye bran, oat bran and barley fiber. *Meat Science* 96(1):503–508.

Piwińska, M., Wyrwisz, J., Kurek, M., and Wierzbicka, A. 2015. Hydration and physical properties of vacuum-dried durum wheat semolina pasta with high-fiber oat powder. *LWT-Food Science and Technology* 63(1):647–653.

Pourfarzad, A., Mahdavian-Mehr, H., and Sedaghat, N. 2013. Coffee silverskin as a source of DF in bread-making: Optimization of chemical treatment using response surface methodology. *LWT-Food Science and Technology* 50(2):599–606.

Previtali, M. A., Mastromatteo, M., Conte, A., De Vita, P., Ficco, D. B. M., and Del Nobile, M. A. 2015. Optimization of durum wheat bread from a selenium-rich cultivar fortified with bran. *Journal of Food Science and Technology* 53(2):1319–1327.

Raju, P. N., and Pal, D. 2011. Effect of bulking agents on the quality of artificially sweetened misti dahi (caramel colored sweetened yogurt) prepared from reduced fat buffalo milk. *Lebensmittel-Wissenschaft und-Technologie* 44(9):1835–1843.

Roble, C., Brunton, N., Gormley, R. T., Ross, P. R., and Butler, F. 2010. Development of potentially synbiotic fresh-cut apple slices. *Journal of Functional Foods* 2:245–254.

Rosburg, V., Boylston, T., White, P. 2010. Viability of bifidobacteria strains in yogurt with added oat beta-glucan and corn starch during cold storage. *Journal of Food Science* 75(5):C439–C444.

Salvatore, E., Pes, M., Mazzarello, V., and Pirisi, A. 2014. Replacement of fat with long-chain inulin in a fresh cheese made from caprine milk. *International Dairy Journal* 34(1):1–5.

Seçkin, A. K, and Baladura, E. 2012. Effect of using some dietary fibers on color, texture and sensory properties of strained yogurt. *GIDA* 37(2):63–69.

Sęczyk, Ł., Świeca, M., and Gawlik-Dziki, U. 2016. Effect of carob (Ceratonia siliqua L.) flour on the antioxidant potential, nutritional quality, and sensory characteristics of fortified durum wheat pasta. *Food Chemistry*, 194:637–642.

Sendra, E., Kuri, V., Fernández-López, J., Sayas-Barberá, E., Navarro, C., and Pérez-Alvarez, J. A. 2010. Viscoelastic properties of orange fiber enriched yogurt as a function of fiber dose, size and thermal treatment. *LWT - Food Science and Technology* 43(4):708–714.

Soukoulis, C., Lebesi, D., and Tzia, C. 2009. Enrichment of ice cream with dietary fiber: Effects on rheological properties, ice crystallisation and glass transition phenomena. *Food Chemistry* 115(2):665–671.

Sudha, M. L., Indumathi, K., Sumanth, M. S., Rajarathnam, S., and Shashirekha, M. N., 2015. Mango pulp fiber waste: Characterization and utilization as a bakery product ingredient. *Journal of Food Measurement and Characterization* 9(3):382–388.

Sun, L., Zhang, Z., Xu, J., Xu, G., and Liu, X. 2015. Dietary fiber Intake Reduces Risk for Barrett's Esophagus and Esophageal Cancer. *Critical Reviews in Food Science and Nutrition* 57(13):2749–2757. doi:10.1080/10408398.2015.1067596

Tabarestani, H. S., and Tehrani, M. M. 2012. Optimization of physicochemical properties of low-fat hamburger formulation using blend of soy flour, split-pea flour and wheat starch as part of fat replacer system. *Journal of Food Process and Preservation* 38(1):278–288.

Taludkar, S., and Sharma, D. P. 2009. Development of dietary fiber rich chicken meat patties using wheat and oat bran. *Journal of Food Science and Technology* 47(2):224–229.

Tárrega, A., Rocafull, A., and Costell, E. 2010. Effect of blends of short and long-chain inulin on the rheological and sensory properties of prebiotic low-fat custards. *LWT-Food Science and Technology* 43(3):556–562.

Thongram, S., Tanwar, B., Chauhan, A., and Kumar, V. 2016. Physicochemical and organoleptic properties of cookies incorporated with legume flours. *Cogent Food and Agriculture*. doi:10.1080/23311932.2016.1172389.

Thongsombat, W., Sirichote, A., and Chanthachum, S. 2007. The production of guava juice fortified with dietary fiber. *Songklanakarin Journal of Science and Technology* 29:187–96.

Threapleton, D. E., Burley, V. J., Greenwood, D. C., and Cade, J. E. 2015. Dietary fiber intake and risk of ischaemic and haemorrhagic stroke in the UK Women's Cohort Study. *European Journal of Clinical Nutrition* 69(4):467–474.

Timmanpyati, S., Mahajan, P., Mehta, S., Pati, P., and Talole, S. 2015. Dietary intake and nutritional status of patients with gall bladder cancer. *Journal of Nutrition Research* 3(1):54–61.

Tiwari, B. K., Brennan, C. S., Jaganmohan, R., Surabi, A., and Alagusundaram, K. 2011. Utilisation of pigeon pea (Cajanus cajan L) by products in biscuit manufacture. *LWT-Food Science and Technology* 44(6):1533–1537.

Tseng, A., and Zhao, Y. 2013. Wine grape pomace as antioxidant dietary fiber for enhancing nutritional value and improving storability of yogurt and salad dressing. *Food Chemistry* 138(1):356–365.

Urushidani, S., and Kuriyama A. 2015.Dietary fiber and blood pressure. *Journal of Hypertension* 33(8):1716. doi:10.1097/HJH.0000000000000643.

Vergara, C.M.D.A.C., Honorato, T.L., Maia, G.A., and Rodrigues, S. 2010. Prebiotic effect of fermented cashew apple (Anacardium occidentale L) juice. *LWT-Food Science and Technology* 43(1):141–145.

Walker, R., Tseng, A., Cavender, G., Ross, A., and Zhao, Y., 2014. Physicochemical, nutritional, and sensory qualities of wine grape pomace fortified baked goods. *Journal of food science* 79(9):S1811–S1822.

Waters, D. M., Jacob, F., Titze, J., Arendt, E. K., and Zannini, E. 2012. Fiber, protein and mineral fortification of wheat bread through milled and fermented brewer's spent grain enrichment. *European Food Research and Technology* 235(5):767–778.

Witwer R. S. 2008. Natural resistant starch in glycemic management: From physiological mechanisms to consumer communications. In: Pasupuleti, V. K, and Anderson, J. W. (Eds.). *Nutraceuticals, Glycemic Health and Type 2 Diabetes.* Ames, IA: Blackwell Publishing Professional; pp. 401–438.

Wood, J. M. 2011. Sensory evaluation of ice cream made with prebiotic ingredients substituted for sugar. *Master thesis submitted to the Nutrition and Health Sciences, Department of at DigitalCommons@University of Nebraska - Lincoln.*

Yang, H. S., Kim, G. D.,Choi, S. G.,and Joo, S. T. 2010. Physical and sensory properties of low fat sausage amended with hydrated oatmeal and various meats. *Korean Journal for Food Science of Animal Resources* 30:365–372.
Yilmaz, I., and Gecgel U. 2009. Effect of inulin addition on physico-chemical and sensory characteristics of meatballs. *Journal of Food Science and Technology-Mysore* 46(5):473–476.
Zha, X. Q., Wang, J. H., Yang, X. F. et al., 2009. Antioxidant properties of polysaccharide fractions with different molecular mass extracted with hot-water from rice bran. *Carbohydrate Polymers* 78(3):570–575.

chapter eight

Fortification of animal foodstuffs

Mariusz Korczyński, Robert Kupczyński, Marita Świniarska, Damian Konkol, and Sebastian Opaliński

Contents

The productivity and health of farm animals, as well as quality of products obtained from them, are affected by two main factors. The first is the genotype of the animal, that is, its functional characteristics, while the second, equally important, is the habitat. Two basic components, which are the conditions of maintenance (welfare) and nutritional factors, must be distinguished defining the breeding environment. Optimal nutrition of farm animals directly determines their growth and development, reproduction, as well as health status. These elements also affect the economics of livestock production and the quality of products obtained from them.

A continuous increase in the demand for animal origin protein has been observed in the world in recent years. This is particularly evident in developing countries and regions, mainly in Asia and South America (FAO, 2012). These tendencies cause the market for food of animal origin and the feed industry to be financially stable. According to IFIF (International Feed Industry Federation, 2015) the value of the global feed market in 2015 amounted to $400 billion and the estimates of that organization for 2016 showed that the market has reached the level of feed production of more than 1 billion Mg. According to FEFAC (The European Feed Manufacturers' Federation, 2017), the biggest markets for feed production in the world are the United States (176 million Mg), China (180 million Mg), and the European Union—28 (161 million Mg). The major feed markets in South America are Brazil and Mexico with production levels of 69 and 31 million Mg, respectively. A significant but dispersed market of feed production is Asia, with the exception of the aforementioned China, this market produced 149 million Mg in 2015. The structure of the global feed market is focused on five main directions. Importantly, it is dominated by the production of feed for pigs, poultry, and cattle, 31.8, 33.7, and 26.8% of global production, respectively. Production of feed, depending on the region of the world, is primarily based on feed materials of plant origin, which results from the physiology of farm animals' digestive tracts. The main feed materials of strategic significance are cereals (including corn), soybeans, fats, meat, and bone meals, as well as waste of food industry.

In addition to feed materials, feed additives are also an important component of complete feeds. At the beginning of the twenty-first century, the European Union decided to regulate and standardize the issues related to the Community feed market. In 2003, attention was mainly focused on feed additives, which resulted in the EU Regulation 1831/2003. The main premise of legislative action was the need to regulate such issues as the definition of feed additives, their labeling, rules, and supervision of their turnover, and, above all, the conditions for their launching on the market with particular emphasis on safety in the food chain guaranteeing the highest level of human health, animal health and welfare, and environment protection. By definition, food additives are chemical substances, their mixtures or microorganisms other than feed material and premixes, which have the features of a particular functionality. They are added to the feed in order to supplement the deficiency of nutrients in a feed ration (vitamins, macro and microelements, feed amino acids), to improve the palatability of feed and its hygienization (raising, flavoring agents, antifungal preparations), to increase the use of feed and stabilize gastrointestinal tract flora (e.g., fermentative bacteria). Another group of feed additives, which raises a lot of controversy in the world, are medical feed additives such as antibiotics or growth hormones. This group of feed additives has been limited in recent years in the 27 EU member states. Only antibiotics with coccidiostatic and histomonostatic activity are allowed, and since 2006, they can be used if necessary as a therapeutic agent (Korczyński and Opaliński, 2012). Due to the progressive phenomenon of multiple drug-resistances of many pathogenic strains that farm animals are exposed to, some attempts are made to use substances of natural origin with antibiotic activity (Kupczyński et al., 2013).

The last direction of feed additives use is to obtain a product of animal origin with improved taste and nutrition value enriching the meat, milk, or eggs with scarce micronutrients or polyunsaturated fatty acids (Chojnacka et al., 2009; Lelis et al., 2009; Dolińska et al., 2011; Słupczyńska et al., 2014). Hence, the function of dietary substances allowing to talk about animal origin food enrichment at the primary level of its production is reserved for feed additives themselves.

8.1 *Functional food*

The concept of functional food is derived from the traditions of the East under the assumptions that there is no clear difference between drugs and food. Starting from the 1980s, the assumptions of functional foods have been promoted in the United States and Europe. The research program FUFOSE (Functional Food Science in Europe) funded by the European Commission started in 1996. A number of criteria that should be met by such foods were identified in the final FUFOSE document of 1999 (Scientific Concepts of Functional Foods in Europe):

- Food can be considered functional when its beneficial, more than nutritional, effect on one or more functions of an organism is proved, and this effect involves an improved health and well-being and/or reduced risk of diseases.
- Functional foods must resemble the form of conventional food and exhibit beneficial effect in amounts that are expected to be normal when consumed with the diet—these are not tablets or capsules, but part of a normal diet.
- Increased health quality of such food is mainly due to the presence of bioactive substances in its composition that stimulate the desired course of metabolic processes, and due to physiologically optimal proportions of particular components.
- Beneficial health effect of this food should be documented with clinical trials conducted on humans, whose diet includes the examined food product.
- Functional food is intended for general consumption as a part of the daily diet.

Functional food is also referred to as food designed for the specific needs of an organism (designer foods, tailored foods). It may also be of nutraceutical nature. Functional features of the products can be achieved by their composition modification, elimination of the component of harmful activity, increase in the concentration of the compound naturally occurring in food (health-promoting), addition of another component, replacement, or improvement of the bioavailability of components essential for one or more functions of an organism (Roberfroid, 2000). Concurrently, functional food, like any other type of food, must ensure consumer's safety, efficiency, and participation in the total diet.

Due to its composition, functional food is divided into the following: enriched food, low-energy, high-fiber, probiotic, low-sodium, low-cholesterol, energizing food, and others. There is also another division due to its effect on the human organism: food for reducing the risk of cardiovascular disease, cancers, and osteoporosis; food for individuals coping with stress; diet for the elderly, people with impaired metabolism and digestion, and sportspeople; diet for pregnant women, nursing mothers, babies, and youth in the phase of intensive growth; and diet for affecting mood and psychomotor performance (Grajeta et al., 2004).

The global market for functional foods is experiencing dynamic and rapid development. The reasons for an increased interest in functional foods are as follows:

- Development of knowledge concerning biologically active substances
- Increased purchasing power of consumers in developed/developing countries
- Populations aging, an increase in health and socialcare costs
- Increased incidence of chronic diseases related to nutrition
- Development of biotechnology and technology of food raw materials processing
- Fashion and promotion of new types of foods that could contribute to an increase in the assortment and quantity of products on the market and help to increase producers' income
- Widely understood healthy lifestyle

8.2 Eggs

As a result of changes in the feed law involving the prohibition of feed antibiotics and hormonal growth regulators use in the EU, the new materials with high digestibility of nutrients are of particular importance in poultry nutrition, and their use is more frequent over time (Shapira, 2010; Świątkiewicz et al., 2014). These are usually natural origin substances with properties that make it possible to keep an animal organism in good condition, and concurrently enriching the products in bioactive components. It is important that humans could affect certain quality features of the product due to rational balanced feed ration, and especially their use in poultry nutrition. In recent years, in an era of diseases of civilization, it is very important and economically justified to obtain the functional product, since the processing industry, including the consumers, are looking for products with certain utility characteristics. This is mainly health-promoting food. An egg is such a product in the case of poultry production, in addition to the meat. Therefore, the consumers pay close attention to the size of the egg, its freshness and above all the content of cholesterol, as well as omega 3 and 6 polyunsaturated fatty acids in the egg. Numerous studies have shown that hens feeding on feed with a high content of these fatty acids is directly reflected in n-3/n-6 ratio in egg yolk. Marine algae, fish oil, or selected plant oils were successfully used in the diet of laying hens in order to enrich eggs with long-chain omega-3 fatty acids (Kralik et al., 2008; Chojnacka et al., 2009; Lelis et al., 2009; Oliveira et al., 2010; Ceylan et al., 2011).

In the case of raw egg material, except nutritional value, features related to the technological quality of raw material are also an important issue. From the point of view of production profitability, the important indices include egg weight, feed consumption per egg, shell strength, and egg yolk color. These are the features that also indirectly affect the economic result of laying hens farms. The birds lay bigger eggs with age, while calcium absorption decreases, resulting in a decrease in the strength of the shell and an increased number of breaks. According to Narváez-Solarte et al. (2006), calcium absorption from the feed ration in the initial period of laying is 50%–60%, and by the end of this period it decreases to a level of 35%–25%. However, this is not the only factor affecting the availability of this element. Other factors important for calcium availability throughout the layer's life include: Ca form administered in the feed; its pH; the content of vitamin D_3; chemical form; and amount of phosphorus, zinc, and magnesium; as well as an activity of certain hormones in the animal organism (Boorman and Guarante, 2001; Jamroz, 2004; de Matos, 2008).

Micro- and macroelements deficit observed for many years in the human diet also resulted in an increased demand for food with a high content of mineral components. This problem concerns about 2 billion people (Chojnacka, 2011). One of the methods of production of animal origin food characterized by a high content of mineral substances is its enrichment at the level of animal breeding by the application of various forms of materials and feed additives containing micro- and macroelements of high bioavailability. The effectiveness of this type of solution is usually expressed by the level of incorporation of an element into animal origin product (Dolińska et al., 2011; Słupczyńska et al., 2014). Therefore, an increasing interest in new materials such as, for example, algae enriched with microelements (Chojnacka et al., 2009; Michalak et al., 2011), fossil materials (Kucukersan et al., 2005; Dobrzański et al., 2009), waste of the food industry as yeast (Dolińska et al., 2006; Dobrzański et al., 2006; Dozier et al., 2008), or other organic waste (Słupczyńska et al., 2014) is observed in the feed industry and among farmers. Appropriate balance of feed mixture in terms of minerals content is also an important issue from the point of view of herd production profitability. The presence of adequate amounts of microelements in farm animals feed is necessary not only to obtain a product with their increased content, but also for the proper growth of the animal and its health (Brisibe et al., 2009; Haenlein and Anke, 2011). A deficiency or excess of a particular nutrient can cause toxic or metabolic disorders in animal organism. The amount of microelements supplied with feed mixture is often insufficient. This is due to their different bioavailability (Fuquay et al., 2011), as well as the presence of antinutritional factors, such reducing the risk of cardiovascular in the gastrointestinal tract, resulting in the formation of insoluble complexes of these elements (Siddhuraju et al., 2002). It should also be noted that the organic forms of some microelements used in poultry nutrition are characterized by an increased bioavailability compared to the standard inorganic forms. The most common form of minerals supplemented in the feed are inorganic salts. Their bioavailability is very low, and in many cases is only a few percent (Fairweather-Tait, 1999). The only advantage of microelements administration in the form of inorganic salts over their organic forms is the low price of their production.

Considering the growing market for functional foods, as well as the ban on the use of growth stimulants and feed antibiotics in farm animals feeding and rather restrictive policy in the range of feed law (mainly in the EU), there is a search for new forms of feed preparations, which can optimize the process of animal origin food production at the primary level.

8.2.1 Cu, Fe, Mn, Zn, I

As nutrients, microelements play an important role in the proper functioning of any living organism. Each of them has quite different, but equally important, functions in the metabolic processes or plays a constructive role in human and animal organisms. Recently, attention is also paid to the deficit of most micronutrients in foods of animal origin, with concurrent attempts to develop the new feed forms of some microelements, which use incorporation in the egg, meat, or milk would be higher. The aim of such procedures is an attempt to obtain the food enriched with these micronutrients (Chojnacka, 2011). One example is seen in the study conducted by Dobrzański et al. (2009) on the use of new forms of organic copper, manganese, and iron in the diet of laying hens. Replacement of Cu, Fe, Mn in the feed ration for laying hens, in an amounts of 47%, 20%, and 58%, respectively, of the daily requirement, with an organic form as enriched yeast, resulted in a higher level of Cu in eggs, feathers, and blood. This proves a better availability of copper from the organic form from copper sulfate. The authors did not report higher content of Fe and Mn in the egg, feathers, and blood after an introduction of organic forms of micronutrients into the mixture, with the exception of the feathers, where higher bioaccumulation of manganese was observed. Also no antagonistic interactions were found between zinc content in eggs, feathers, and blood and microelements introduced into a mixture.

Another study concerning the use of yeasts enriched with iodine in laying hens feeding demonstrated their significant effect on the production parameters and iodine content in the egg (Opaliński et al., 2012). Iodine in an inorganic form was supplemented to the complete mixture of the control birds (1 mg/kg mixture), while the experimental groups I and II were supplemented with iodine-enriched yeast in an amount of 1 and 2 mg/kg of the mixture, respectively. No effect of iodine form on body weight of hens and their egg laying was noted, but based on the results, however, there was a negative effect, especially in case of higher dose, on feed consumption and its use. Chickens receiving 2 mg of iodine in an organic form in the feed were characterized by higher feed consumption and its worse use compared to the control group. Feed consumption for the production of 1 kg egg was the highest in the group receiving organic iodine at a dose of 2 mg/kg of the mixture. It should be emphasized that analysis of the qualitative results of the eggs showed that the use of iodine in an organic form resulted in improved coloring of the yolk and increased egg weight, mainly due to increased weight of albumen. The reduced value is in a quite significant technological parameter of the egg, which is the strength of its shell, was considered the negative effect of the examined iodine form. This weakness was observed in both groups of laying hens supplemented with yeast enriched with iodine, although there were no differences in the level of Ca and P in blood serum of all examined birds. In addition to qualitative evaluation of the eggs, the level of iodine in the egg content was also determined. The results indicated higher iodine content in the egg yolk of hens supplemented with organic iodine form (I and II), by 80% and 90%, respectively, compared to the control group.

The feed market accepted the yeasts enriched with microelements as a valuable carrier of these minerals, the carrier with high availability and biofortification in meat and egg. However, there is still a search for alternative biological forms of these elements. One idea is to use the biosorption process of selected microelement ions on feed material as a natural and obvious source of nutrients in the feeding ration for farm animals. This idea was applied in the study on the use of enriched soybean meal in the process of biosorption in feeding laying hens (Witkowska et al., 2014a). Replacement of inorganic salts of Cu, Zn, Fe (control group) in the feed mixture for laying hens with enriched soybean meal in these microelements (experimental groups: Sm-Cu, -Zn, -Fe, a group which was also given the meal enriched with chromium Sm-Cr) resulted in an improvement in some production results and quality parameters of the eggs.

The detailed analysis of the results demonstrated higher shell strength of the eggs obtained from hens receiving the experimental form of Cu and Cr, as well as better coloring of egg yolks in groups Sm-Cu and Sm-Zn. Production results of the hens from experimental groups showed a lower feed intake in birds treated with chromium and copper. Higher consumption of feed to produce 1 kg of egg was reported in hens receiving Fe in the form of enriched soybean meal compared to other groups. In the further part of the experiment, the share of microelements in the feed ration for the hens was increased by 50% (series II), and 100% (series III) compared to the recommended feeding standards. No significant differences in the quality features of eggs were found based on the results obtained in this part of the experiment, but there was a lower feed intake in the hens treated with Cu, Fe, and Cr in the form of enriched soybean meal compared to the other groups. Also statistically lower feed consumption per egg was noted in all groups of birds fed with organic microelements.

8.2.2 *Fatty acids*

The eggs enriched with n-3 fatty acids are characterized by higher nutritional and health-promoting value. For this reason, they can be successfully classified as functional foods. The fatty acids profile in egg yolk may be significantly altered by the use of suitably modified feed mixtures. Numerous studies demonstrated the possibility of the use of fish meals, fish, linseed, rapeseed oils, marine algae, and some seeds in feeding in order to produce so-called designer eggs (Shapira et al. 2008, Souza et al. 2008, Yi et al. 2014, Coorey et al. 2015).

Yi et al. (2014) demonstrated that the use of linseed oil and dried whitebait in feeding laying hens contributed to changes in the egg yolk fatty acids profile. The addition of 1.5% of linseed oil and a combination of linseed oil (1.5%) and dried whitebait (1.5%) caused an increase in the content of ALA from 0.6% to 4.3% and 3.8%, respectively. Both additives also caused an increase in the percentages of EPA and DHA. Souza et al. (2008) also observed an increase in the concentration of polyunsaturated fatty acids in eggs derived from hens fed with linseed oil.

Fredriksson et al. (2006) compared in their study an effect of rapeseed oil, corn oil, and the combination of these oils with microalgae *Nannochloropsis oculata*. They proved that the supplementation of laying hens' feed mixture with microalgae resulted in an increased concentration of LC PUFA. The change in the content of 18:2n–6, 18:3n–3, 20:4n–6, 20:5n–3, and 22:6n–3 fatty acids was observed in the phospholipid fraction of the yolk. The highest content of EPA and DHA was found in the eggs from groups fed with algae at of 20%.

Cachaldora et al. (2005) compared the use of two oils: microalgae and fish (both in an amount of 1.7%) as laying hens' feed supplements.

The results of the experiment show that the addition of algae oil causes a nearly 46% increase in EPA content, and a 17% increase in DHA content in egg yolk compared to the group receiving fish oil.

The change in omega-3 fatty acids content in egg yolks after microalgae use as a feed additive for laying hens was also noted by Lemahieu et al. (2014). The results of the experiment demonstrated that an increased algae supplementation led to a linear increase in omega-3 acids content in the yolk, and the addition of 2.4% of algal biomass to the feed mixture was found to be optimal.

Bruneel et al. (2013) demonstrated that the use of *Nannochloropsis gaditana* algae (in an amount of 5% of d.m.) resulted in 7% and 53% increases in ALA and DHA content, respectively, in the egg after 2 weeks of experiment carried out on laying hens. EPA content increased from 0 to 2.1 mg/egg. Also Kostik et al. (2015) found that the addition of *Schizochytrium* spp. microalgae as a source of n–3 acids, in amounts of 1.27 and 1.77%, improved the DHA content in hen's egg yolk. Park et al. (2015) also confirmed in their study that the addition of *Schizochytrium* algae to the feed for laying hens results in an improved fatty acid profile in the egg. The possibility of producing DHA-enriched eggs by appropriate dietary supplementation with microalgae was also presented by Rizzi et al. (2009).

Michalak et al. (2016) demonstrated the possibility of using marine algae and supercritical extract from *Spirulina* sp. algae in feeding laying hens. The results of this study show that the use of marine algae extract as an additive to drinking water (0.2%) resulted in a slight increase in both omega-3 and omega-6 fatty acids in the yolk. An increase in the content of GLA (12%), ETE (13%) and DPA (11%) in egg yolk compared to the control group was noted after 120 days of the experiment. An increase of about 12% in EPA content, and of about 20% DPA with respect to the control, was noted in the case of *Spirulina* microalgae application to the feed (in an amount of 15 g·kg-1).

The addition of products such as fish oil or flax seed to the mixture, aside from the modification in the fatty acids profile and improvement in n–6/n–3 ratio in the enriched eggs, also causes some side effects in the form of fishy taste and smell in the eggs. This undesirable effect depends, inter alia, on the additive concentration, and on the degree of lipids peroxidation (Jiang et al. 1992; Van Elswyk et al. 1995; Scheideler et al. 1997; Lewis et al. 2000).

Chia seeds used as a component of health-promoting diet have become a popular product in recent years. Coorey et al. (2015) demonstrated that their use in feeding laying hens creates the possibility of eggs' enrichment in omega-3 acids. Moreover, no negative effect on the sensory properties of egg product was observed. The absence of the so-called fishy flavor in eggs derived from hens fed with the feed containing chia seeds was also observed by Ayerza and Coates (2000, 2002) and Ayerza et al. (2002).

An attempt to use fish oil, linseed oil, alfalfa, and mineral-organic preparations (Humokarbowit and Humobentofet) in order to improve production results and egg raw material quality in laying hens was undertaken in the study conducted by Dobrzański et al. (2012). The study did not demonstrate any effect of the applied preparations on body weight of birds and their production results. Qualitative analysis showed that eggs obtained from hens receiving oils, alfalfa, and mineral-organic preparations were characterized by greater thickness and strength of shells and worse coloration of egg yolks. Sensory analysis of the eggs obtained during the experiment showed a deterioration in their taste value. This was especially observed in eggs obtained from experimental groups hens whose feed mixture was supplemented with linseed oil and fish oil. Concurrently, a more favorable fatty acid profile, mainly ALA and DHA, was noted in the same eggs, but the observations were not confirmed statistically. There is still a need for studies of fish and linseed oils used to improve the quality of egg raw material.

To conclude this section, the proposed new generation of mineral-organic preparations can be considered useful in improving the efficiency of breeding laying hens as a result of optimization of production results and quality features of the eggs, as well as maintenance of birds in good condition.

8.3 Meat

Meat is one of the basic raw materials of animal origin used in food production. This raw material provides many valuable nutrients so it should be a regular part of the human diet. Meat protein is characterized by the presence of all essential amino acids and is about 94% (Litwińczuk et al., 2012). The fat contained in the muscles is a source of long-chain polyunsaturated fatty acids, whose share in meat is from 11% to 29% of total fatty acids (Williams, 2007). Meat is also a source of cholesterol, of which a suitable level is essential in the diet for the proper functioning of an organism. Meat is an important source of vitamins B, and is concurrently characterized by the lower share of fat-soluble vitamins (A, D, E, K). Muscle tissue is also a source of macro- and microelements such as potassium, phosphorus, sodium, magnesium, zinc, iron, and copper (Jensen et al., 2004). An increase in consumer awareness has had the result that today's raw material should be characterized not only by good organoleptic, but also by primarily health-promoting features. Health-promoting features are determined, inter alia, by the fatty acids profile, mineral components, and content of other biologically active compounds. Consumers' demands can be met thanks to so-called functional foods. Aside from the nutritional aspect, functional foods also exhibit a beneficial psychological or physiological effect on the human organism (Litwińczuk, 2012). Meat is classified in such a food group due to the possibility of its enrichment with mineral components.

Mineral components, especially microelements, play an extremely important role in human nutrition since they are responsible for maintaining homeostasis. The group of microelements includes elements such as manganese, iron, zinc, copper, selenium, or iodine. Manganese is a component of many important enzymes, it is an agent stabilizing blood sugar level, is involved in the synthesis and metabolism of carbohydrates, fats and cholesterol, and plays an important role in the normal formation of bones and cartilage, as well as participating in the synthesis of DNA and RNA (Jędrzejczak, 2004). As a component of hemoglobin, iron is involved in the transport and storage of oxygen, is responsible for the maintenance of humoral and cellular immunity, and plays an important role in the normal development of the brain, muscles, and other tissues. Iron deficiencies cause anemia; they may also impair mental development and be responsible for physical fitness decline (Jędrzejczak, 2004). Zinc is a component or activator of about 80 enzymes, is essential for the proper functioning of respiratory and reproductive systems, and is also involved in the elimination of free radicals. Its deficiency in an organism causes a number of diseases of the muscular, nervous, digestive, reproductive, humoral, and immune systems (Puzanowska-Tarasiewicz et al., 2009). Copper is an integral component of many proteins, and as a component of enzymes it is involved in oxidation-reduction processes (Kurzępa, 2014). Selenium determines the correct course of many physiological and biochemical processes. It is a component of enzymes and proteins. It demonstrates a synergistic effect with vitamin E, protecting an organism from the harmful effect of free radicals and demonstrating an immunostimulating activity (Nakane, 1992). It reduces the toxic effect of xenobiotics, including heavy metals (Grosicki, 1999). It delays the aging of tissues and alleviates menopausal symptoms (Wiąckowski, 1995). Iodine is involved in the biosynthesis of the thyroid hormones thyroxine and triiodothyronine (Gołkowski, 2010).

The content of microelements in meat is variable and depends on factors such as the species of animal from which the meat was obtained, part of the carcass, kind of feed, or season of the year. However, it may be modified, e.g., through the use of various feed additives. Meat, which is a subject of the studies concerning its composition modification, mainly includes pork, beef and poultry, because they are consumed in the greatest quantities.

Pork is a source of human protein of high biological value. Gawęcki et al. (2003) demonstrated that the biological value of protein in pork is higher than in poultry and beef. There is general opinion recommending limiting pork consumption due to its high fat content. This opinion is false, because many years of breeding work have significantly reduced the caloric content of pork. Also the balance of fatty acids has changed. Intramuscular fat is the most desirable pork fat, and its value is considered an indicator of good quality meat. According to Ellis (2006), it is in the range of 1.8%–2.6%, and according to Fernandez et al. (1999) it may be as high as 3.5%. Pork is a rich source of B vitamins, especially vitamin B_1 and B_{12}, and fat-soluble vitamins, especially vitamin E. Considering its mineral components content, it can be concluded that pork is characterized by lower sodium content compared to meat of other animal species, and a relatively high content of iron, which is absorbed at the level of 20%–50% (Blicharski et al., 2013). These data indicate that pork should be enriched with micronutrients as a functional food. The use of feed additives in order to enrich the meat with microelements is increasingly common, but the factor determining the success of the process is the form of an element which we want to introduce into certain product. It should be borne in mind that the animals make better use of the elements present in organic form than these, which are in the form of inorganic salts. Mahan and Parrett (1996) demonstrated a higher share of selenium in the muscles of pigs fed with an organic Sel-Plex® additive compared to animals fed with sodium selenite. Animals receiving additives of sodium selenite, excreted most selenium in the urine. Sel-Plex® aroused an interest of the entrepreneurs from South Korea, who through the use of this additive created the so-called SelenPork characterized by almost twenty-fold higher selenium content compared to normal pork (D'Souza et al., 2005). Other studies proved that selenium concentration in the muscles of pigs fed with an addition of yeast enriched in this element was about two-fold higher compared to animals treated with sodium selenite (EFSA, 2008). Olivera et al. (2005) demonstrated that muscle tissue and liver of pigs supplemented with selenium-enriched yeast was characterized by higher selenium concentration compared to animals treated with sodium selenite or without any additive. Vernerová et al. (2008) also found higher levels of selenium in the meat of pigs fed with organic selenium. The study conducted by Witkowska et al. (2014b) demonstrated that the meat of pigs fed with soybean seeds enriched with copper, manganese, iron, and zinc in the biosorption process contained a level from 4.3% to 20.3% higher of these microelements compared to meat of animals supplemented with these microelements in an inorganic form. In addition, meat from the experimental groups was classified as high quality meat, and animals increased daily growth and carcass weight. The study by Saeid et al. (2013a,b) showed no statistically significant differences relating to the production, metabolic, and physiological parameters of pigs. An addition of copper-enriched *Spirulina maxima* algae to the feed for fattening pigs not only caused a significant decrease in serum total cholesterol and LDL, but also did not cause a significant increase in the level of copper, zinc, and iron. Another study by Saeid et al. (2013 a,b) concerning the use of *Spirulina maxima* algae enriched with copper as a feed additive also showed no effect on the production parameters of pigs. However, it demonstrated an increase in the content of copper, manganese, and selenium to a level of 18%, 25%, and 23%, respectively in meat of pigs examined. A 16 and 95% decrease in the content of zinc and selenium, respectively, was observed in the liver of the examined pigs. Banoch et al. (2010) proved that the meat of pigs supplemented with *Laminaria spp.* algae enriched with iodine was richer in this element than the meat of pigs fed with an additive of inorganic iodine. It was also demonstrated that iodine content in the muscles of animals fed with the additives of *Laminaria digitata* and *Ascophyllum nodosum* algae was higher compared to the animals treated with the addition of iodine in an inorganic form (Smet, 2012).

Poultry meat is characterized by a high nutritional value and its culinary treatment is easy. It is a low-energy and low-fat meat, which provides substantial quantities of high-quality protein and other nutrients. Protein content in poultry meat ranges between 18% and 25%. Poultry meat proteins contain all exogenous and endogenous amino acids constituting an excellent source of nitrogen (Insel et al., 2001). It is assumed that the ratio of essential amino acids for poultry is 80% to 84%. Poultry meat is the source of vitamins B, especially vitamins B_1, B_2, B_3, B_6, and B_{12}, and also fat-soluble vitamins (A, D, E). Water poultry meat and meat from chickens and turkeys legs is a good source of iron. Other mineral substances contained in poultry meat include zinc, selenium, copper, sodium, potassium, calcium, magnesium, and chlorine (Smolińska and Kopeć, 2009). The study on poultry meat enrichment with microelements was, inter alia, conducted by Ševčíková et al. (2006) using yeast and *Chlorella* algae enriched with selenium as a feed additive. The study demonstrated higher concentration of selenium in the muscles of broilers treated with enriched additives compared to the control group. Olivera et al. (2005) showed that the meat of chickens fed with the addition of yeast enriched with selenium contains higher level of this element than meat from animals treated with the addition of sodium selenite. Similar conclusions were reached by Kinal et al. (2012), who demonstrated that thigh muscles, kidneys, and bones of broilers fed the diet supplemented with selenium-enriched yeast contained higher amounts of this element compared to the animals treated with sodium selenite addition. Potapenko et al. (2015) demonstrated that broilers' enrichment of diet with the drug "Ekstraselen + Vit" manufactured on a basis of selenium nanoparticles and vitamins increases the concentration of this element in the meat of the animals examined. Another study was conducted by Čepulienë et al. (2008). They found that the meat of chickens that were supplied with drinking water containing a stable concentrate of iodine formulation (Lithuanian Patent) was enriched in iodine by 16% to 76% compared to the meat of chickens treated with potassium iodide as an additive. Herkel et al. (2016) found that the use of phytogenic mixture of essential oils increased the concentration of zinc in the pectoral muscles, magnesium and copper in the thigh muscles, and manganese in the liver of turkeys. Brooks et al. (2012) demonstrated that the broilers supplemented with manganese propionate were characterized by higher manganese content in the bones, compared to the broilers fed with manganese sulphate addition. Salim et al. (2012) proved that supplementation of organic forms of zinc increases the content of this element in the thigh muscles of female and male fattening chickens.

Beef is characterized by protein content of 18%–23% and intramuscular fat level below 5%. Intramuscular fat of beef meat contains about 44% saturated fatty acids, 46% monounsaturated fatty acids, and 10% polyunsaturated fatty acids. Beef contains about 1% mineral components and higher level of assimilable iron compared to meat of other farm animals species (Kołczak, 2008). Enrichment of beef in microelements through the use of feed additives is more difficult than in the case of other two kinds of meat, since there is no direct transfer of nutrients from the feed to animal tissues in ruminants. Pehrson et al. (1999) found that the ruminants absorb lower amounts of selenium supplemented with the feed compared to monogastric animals, since part of this element may be used by rumen microflora. Dannenberg et al. (2013) did not demonstrate an effect of silage supplemented with n–3 and n–6 fatty acids on the content of iron, copper, zinc, and selenium in bovine meat and products of its processing.

Although many attempts have been made to enrich the meat in microelements and other biologically active components, studies in this field should be continued. In a time of diseases of civilization and global nutritional deficiencies, functional foods should not only be promoted but also widely available. Modern livestock production provides such a possibility.

8.4 Milk

Milk and dairy products are commonly consumed by humans. They supply the human diet with 15% to 25% fat, where 25%–35% of the acids are saturated. Chemical composition of milk is affected by many factors, such as breed, age, individual variation, nutrition, or mammary gland health status. Increasingly often, milk is perceived not only as a source of nutrients covering the demands of the organism, but also as a factor in human health and well-being.

Bioactive substances present in milk include immunoglobulins, hormones, cytokines, growth factors, polyamides, nucleotides, peptides, fatty acids (mono- and polyunsaturated), fat soluble vitamins, carotenoids, and phospholipids (Séverin and Wenshui, 2005). The rapid development of functional dairy products enriched with n–3 fatty acids, conjugated linoleic acid (CLA), phytosterols, isoflavones, vitamins, and minerals has been observed in recent years. Commercial products are commonly enriched with pro- and prebiotics. An interest is also focused on preparations

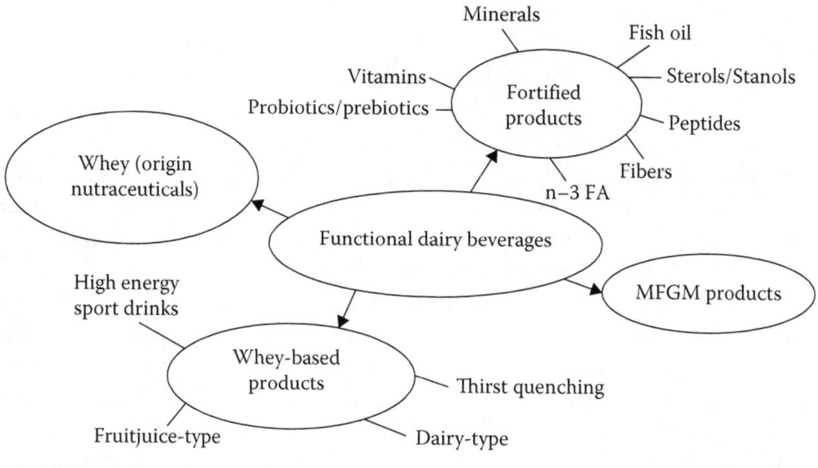

Figure 8.1 Category of functional dairy beverages (Hözer, B. and Kirmaci, H. A., *Int. J. Dairy Technol.*, 63, 1–15, 2010).

enriched with n–3 fatty acids, mainly γ-linolenic acid (C18:3 n-3, ALA), eicosapentaenoic acid (C20:5 n–3, EPA), and docosahexaenoic acid (C22:6 n–3, DHA) (Figure 8.1). Their positive effects on human health result from the reduction of the risk of cardiovascular diseases and their impact on nervous system development in children (especially DHA). In Europe, the first milk enriched with n–3 fatty acids appeared in the late 1980s in Ireland (Omega-3 product) (Hözer and Kirmaci, 2010).

Milk and its products are also an important source of minerals in the human diet. Milk is an important source of calcium, phosphorus, sodium, potassium, iodine, and magnesium. Milk is the main source of calcium in the European diet, and its content and bioavailability are closely correlated with the concentration of casein (Gaucheron, 2005). Macro- and microelements present in milk are involved in maintenance of metabolic processes in the organism and affect the chemical and functional properties of milk proteins. The content of elements in milk may directly indicate the quality of raw material and dairy products, and indirectly the degree of contamination of animals and the human environment, since milk production is closely related to the state of the environment, that is, air, soil, and water as well as the feed consumed by cows (Malbe et al., 2010; Kołacz et al., 2017).

8.4.1 Fatty acids

Fat is a very important component of milk, determining its nutritional value and technological usefulness. Lipids are the basic and the best compounds that provide energy for the organism. They are also building material for biochemically active substances and hormones (cholesterol, phospholipids, glycolipids) and affect the dynamic properties of cell membrane. Fat allows the absorption of fat-soluble vitamins and the other hydrophobic, biologically active compounds, including carotenoids. Among the 588 fatty acids identified in milk fat, about 94% of them are bound to the simple lipids, that is, triacylglycerols (Glasser et al., 2007). The predominant group are saturated fatty acids—SFA (about 68%); mono- and polyunsaturated ones constitute about 29% and 3% of milk fat, respectively (Jensen, 2002). Fatty acid content of intramuscular fat in cattle is about 44% SFA, 46% MUFA, and 10% PUFA. The ratio of n–6/n–3 acids in beef is slightly less than 3, with a tendency to SFA decrease with an increasing meatiness of the cattle (Kołczak, 2008). The content of saturated and *trans* fatty acids is sometimes associated with an increased risk of many metabolic disorders and related diseases, such as obesity, atherosclerosis, cardiovascular diseases, and others (Barłowska and Litwińczuk, 2009). However, the effect of *trans* fatty acids derived from ruminants is not clear (Mensink, 2005). The content of *trans* acids in the milk of ruminants is mainly determined by the content of vaccenic acid *trans*–11 C18:1 (TVA). Its average concentration in milk fat is almost 78% (Moate et al., 2007). Some studies have demonstrated a negative relationship between the incidence of coronary diseases in humans and the consumption of animal origin *trans* fatty acids (Pietinen et al., 1997). An anti-atherosclerotic effect was also confirmed in laboratory animals (Lock et al. 2005). In addition, TVA can inhibit the growth of cancer cells (McGuire and McGuire, 2000).

In recent years, a great interest is also noted in the case of CLA isomers (conjugated linoleic acid). This term defines the group of positional and geometric isomers of linoleic acid–octadecadienoic (C18: 2). Conjugated linoleic acid is also called rumenic acid. The double bonds in CLA molecules present in the animal fats are most common at carbons 9 and 11 and 10 and 12, although there are other CLA isomers (Fritsche et al., 2000). These isomers may have spatial configurations of *cis* and *trans*, that is, they may occur in the *cis-cis, trans-trans, cis-trans,* and *trans-cis* form. A number of advantageous properties of different CLA isomers were confirmed *in vitro,* as well as on animal models and in clinical studies (McGuire and McGuire, 1999; Kritchevsky et al., 2000; Belury, 2002; Burdge et al., 2004; Brownbill et al., 2005):

- Inhibition (*in vitro* and *in vivo*) of cancer cells development (*cis*–9, *trans*–11 CLA)
- Delayed atherosclerosis development
- Adipose tissue reduction (*trans*–10, *cis*–12 CLA)
- Delayed type II diabetes development
- Immunomodulatory and anti-inflammatory activity, improved bone mineralization
- Bacteriostatic and antioxidant activity

In the human organism, the long-chain n–3 acids are included in phospholipids of cell membranes, with particularly high levels observed in the tissues of the central nervous system, retina, and testes. The proportion of these acids in tissues is largely dependent on their dietary ratio (Sanders, 2000). These acids are also precursors of intrasystemic synthesis of eicosanoids (compounds of the status of hormone), mainly prostaglandins series 3, prostacyclins, leukotrienes, lipoxins, and thromboxanes (Tavani et al., 2005). Deficiency of EPA and DHA are important causes of the development of a number of diseases of civilization, which include cardiovascular diseases. These acids inhibit the stimulation of inflammatory, thrombotic processes, allergic response, carcinogenesis, and atherosclerosis (Simopoulos, 2008). Eicosanoids affect, inter alia, the regulation of cardiovascular system, blood pressure, thrombosis, triglycerides content, inflammatory processes, immune system function, cell proliferation and tumor growth, regulation of hormones and neurotransmitters, gene expression, pain perception, and reduced therapeutic dose and toxicity of certain drugs. Eicosanoids produced from EPA exhibit an antithrombotic, anti-inflammatory activity, inhibiting an excessive shrinkage of the vessels and carcinogenesis. Different activity in low concentrations was found for eicosanoids formed from arachidonic acid (n–6) (Sanders, 2000; Stillwell et al., 2005).

8.4.2 Modification of fatty acids profile

The fatty acid content in the milk of cows is determined chiefly by nutritional factors. Fats are a commonly used component of the feed rations for high-yielding dairy cows, which results from difficulties to cover their energy needs in the first period of lactation. Milk fat of cows fed on pasture is characterized by more beneficial fatty acid profile and contains more health-promoting components (TVA, CLA, EPA, DHA, vitamins A and E, β–carotene) compared to the milk fat of cows fed with the TMR system or bulky feed and concentrates (Nałęcz-Tarwacka et al., 2009). Due to the fact that the ratio of n–6 to n–3 in grassland vegetation is low, that is, about 0.3%, the feeding with pasture green forage may cause even a two- to threefold increase in linolenic acid content in milk. In the case of high-yielding cows, the TMR system is standard, therefore any method of fatty acid profile change arouses interest.

The source of fatty acids in the milk fat of ruminants are the acids formed in the rumen processes, lipids derived from the feed ration and mobilized reserve fat in an organism (Barłowska and Litwińczuk, 2009). Short-chain saturated fatty acids (C:4 to C:14) are synthesized *de novo* in mammary gland from acetic acid formed in the rumen, and β-hydroxybutyric acid formed in prestomachs. About 50% palmitic acid (C16:0) is also synthesized *de novo,* the rest is derived from blood lipids.

Higher fatty acids (> C:18) generally originate from the circulatory system, including the direct absorption from the gastrointestinal tract of reserve fat (Szumacher-Strabel, 2005). The main source of *cis*-9, *trans*-11 CLA isomer in milk fat of cows is endogenous synthesis of vaccenic acid *trans*-11 C18:1 (TVA), derived from rumen fluid under the influence of enzyme Δ^9-desaturase (stearoyl-CoA desaturase). About 80% (64–78%) of *cis*-9, *trans*-11 CLA present in the milk fat is synthesized by Δ^9-desaturase from TVA in the mammary gland (McGuire and McGuire, 2000; Kay et al., 2004; Bodkowski et al., 2016). Hydrogenation of polyunsaturated fatty acids is performed by bacteria from the group A (mainly *Butyrivibriofibrisolvens*, *Eubacterium* spp., *Micrococcus* spp., *Ruminococcusalbus*) and group B (*Fucocillu* spp.). The role of bacteria and protozoa in linoleic acid biohydrogenation is presented in Figure 8.2. The study conducted by Boeckaert et al. (2009) indicates that bacteria adhering to the particles of the feed (SAB, solid adhering bacteria) perform complete biohydrogenation of *cis*-9, *cis*-12 C18:2 to C18:0, while the bacteria suspended in the rumen liquid (LAB, liquid adhering bacteria) carry out a partial biohydrogenation to *trans*-10 C18:1/*trans* 11 C18:1. Bacteria *Butyrivibrio* spp. tolerate increased amounts of unsaturated fatty acids introduced into the rumen, and their population significantly increases after the combined use of fish oil and sunflower oil in cows feeding (Palmquist and Griinari, 2006). The easiest dietary way to increase the amount of *cis*-9, *trans*-11 CLA in milk fat is stimulation of an increase in vaccenic acid production by rumen bacteria.

Fat effect on ruminal transformations, metabolism and FA content in milk fat depends on its amount in the feed ration, its kind, physical form and fatty acid profile (Castañeda-Gutieérrez et al., 2009). Lipid

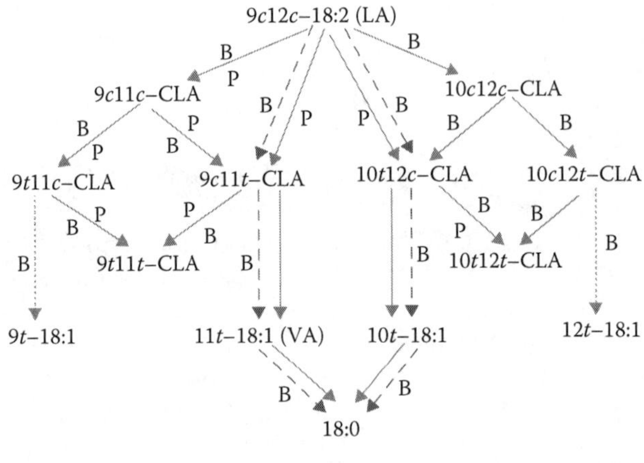

Figure 8.2 Metabolic pathways for the biosynthesis of CLA and related compounds from linoleic acid by rumen bacteria (B) and protozoa (P). (From Or-Rashid, M. M. *Appl. Microbiol. Biotechnol.*, 84, 1033–1043, 2009.)

supplementation may affect various metabolic processes that determine the fatty acid profile of milk. Dietary factors affecting CLA concentration in milk fat are presented in Table 8.1. The concentration of CLA and n-3 can be increased in cow milk by the application of plant oils (Kelly et al., 1998), raw (Donovan et al., 2000; Osborne et al., 2008) and protected fish oil (Castañeda-Gutiérrez et al., 2007; Kupczyński et al., 2012), fish and plant oils used concomitantly (AbuGhazaleh and Holmes, 2007), lipid complex enriched in EPA and DHA (Bodkowski et al., 2016), fish oil with algae (AbuGhazaleh et al., 2009), and encapsulated fish oil or microalgae (Vahmani et al., 2013). It was found evaluating an effect of plant oils (peanut, sunflower, and linseed oil) that the highest increase ($p \leq 0.001$) in CLA content in milk followed sunflower oil administration (Kelly et al., 1998).

One of the methods of CLA and n-3 fatty acids content increasing in the milk is fish oil introduction into cows' feed rations. An increase in CLA concentration after fish oil application may be from 100% to 400% (Donovan et al., 2000; Osborne et al., 2008; Bodkowski et al., 2016). In the

Table 8.1 Influence of Dietary Factors that Affect Concentrations of Conjugated Linoleic Acid (Cla) in Milk Fat

Dietary factor	CLA content in milk fat
1. Fats	
Unsaturated vs. saturated	Increase by addition of unsaturated fat
Type of plant oil	Increase with oils high in unsaturated fatty acids
Level of plant oil	Dose-dependent increase
Ca salts of plant oils	Increase
Processed seeds	Increase
Fish oil	Increase
Marine algae	Increase
2. Feeding system	
Pasture vs. TMR	Pasture–increase
Plants growth stage	Increase with less mature plants
Forage concentration ratio	Variable effect
Ratio of forage to concentrate	Increased CLA in forage predominance
Nonstructural carbohydrate level	Minor effect
3. Rumen environment	
Acidosis	Decrease
DCAD	Minimal effect
Buffers	Little effect with sufficient fiber
4. CLA supplement	Increase dependent on a dose and isomers used

Source: Adapted from Jensen, R. G., *J. Dairy Sci.*, 85: 295–350, 2002.

study conducted by Castañeda-Gutieérrez et al. (2007), high doses of fish oil in the form of calcium soaps did not cause as significant increase in CLA in milk fat (1.04 g/100 g fatty acids) as intraruminal infusion (6.05 g/100 g fatty acids). It is a kind of fish oil phenomenon, since used in an unprotected form it causes an increase in vaccenic acid content in rumen fluid, which is then a substrate for CLA synthesis in enzymatic reactions in the mammary gland (Loor, 2005).

The dynamics of the changes in CLA content during the application of fish oil is differentiated, but even its long-term use leads to a higher CLA content than in the case of standard feed. A clear increase in CLA content is observed after 5 days of supplementation (Shingfield et al., 2006). Also, the combined use of fish oil and plant oils with a high share of linoleic acid is an effective method (Shingfield et al., 2006; Whitlock et al., 2006; AbuGhazaleh and Holmes, 2007; AbuGhazaleh et al., 2009). Having in mind an increase in the content of PUFAs (including EPA and DHA) in milk fat, with a concurrent decrease in short-chain acid content (C4:0–C12:0), oil applying oil to the mineral carrier (Kupczyński et al., 2012) or the use of lipid complexes with high EPA and DHA content, which can be added TMR ration (Bodkowski et al., 2016), can be used in practice.

After an introduction of > 2% DM of fish oil to the diet of cows, the product (such as butter or cream) is characterized by a softer consistency, salty taste, with an unchanged color (Kupczyński et al., 2014). Supplementation of cows' diet with low amounts (45 g/kg DM) of fish oil and sunflower oil caused no differences in the organoleptic evaluation, including flavor (Jones et al., 2005).

Supplementation of feed rations with algae or fish oil with algae also led to an increase of CLA content in milk fat (Table 8.2). Franklin et al. (1999) compared the effect of *Schizochytrium sp.* algae given to cows in unprotected and protected form. CLA content of control cows' milk fat was 0.37 g/100 g

Table 8.2 An Effect of Feeding on The Content of Selected Fatty Acids in Cows' Milk, G/100 G of Fatty Acids

	Group				
Fatty acids	FO	2/3 FO	1/3 FO	ALG	SEM
C18:1 t11	11.80	12.83	13.87	13.53	0.779
CLA c9t11	3.41	3.69	4.47	4.21	0.08
C20:5 n–3 (EPA)	0.04	0.03	0.04	0.04	0.58
C22:6 n–3 (DHA)	0.03	0.04	0.06	0.05	0.18

Source: AbuGhazaleh, A. A. et al., *J. Dairy Sci.*, 92, 6156–6159, 2009.

FO = 150 g fish oil (FO) per day; 2/3FO = 100 g of FO + 50 g of algae per day; 1/3FO = 50 g of FO + 100 g of algae per day; ALG = 150 g of algae per day

fatty acids, and after 6 weeks of algae supplementation it was as high as 2.31 (protected algae) and 2.62 g/100 g fatty acids (unprotected algae). An increase in DHA content in milk fat to 0.76 g/100 g (protected algae) was also observed, while DHA content in the milk of control cows was below the detection limit. Neither form of algae affected milk yield, and its flavor was acceptable to the consumer. Total content of n–3 isomers in milk fat may increase about threefold after marine algae application (Boeckaert et al., 2008). As in the case of fish oil, milk fat content was reduced, with a higher content of PUFAs (Boeckaert et al., 2008; AbuGhazaleh et al., 2009).

The possibilities of increasing the content of n–3 fatty acids in milk are limited, since the transfer of EPA and DHA from the feed ration to milk and other tissues is low (HeraviMoussavi et al., 2007). Protection against biohydrogenation in rumen affects the increase of the content of these fatty acids in milk fat only to a small degree (Castañeda-Gutieérrez et al., 2007). EPA and DHA transfer to milk fat is 21.27% and 18.9%, respectively, for fish oil infusion to abomasum, 3.08% and 4.36% for fish oil Ca salt administration (high doses), and 1.86% and 3.30% for ruminal infusion of fish oil (Castañeda-Gutieérrez et al., 2007). Loor et al. (2005) found that with high doses of fish oil the value of the DHA transfer to milk coefficient may be as high as 13%. However, studies showing such great potential of these acids transfer to milk fat are sparse. Dietary addition of rumen-protected microalgae in cows feeding increased DHA content in milk fat to a higher degree than protected fish oil, 0.20 and 0.14 g/100 g of fatty acids, respectively (Vahmani et al., 2013).

The importance of odd- and branched-chain fatty acids (OBCFA) has also been emphasized in recent years. The main OBCFA in cow milk fat are isomers of tridecanoic acid (*iso* C13:0), tetradecanoic acid (*iso* C14:0), pentadecanoic acid (C15:0, *iso* C15:0, *anteiso*C15:0), hexadecanoic acid (*iso* C16:0), and heptadecanoic acid (C17:0, *iso* C17:0, *anteiso* C17:0) (Fievez et al., 2012; Baumann et al., 2016). These acids demonstrate many interesting features, including that they can be a diagnostic tool in ruminal fermentation evaluation, have anti-cancer properties, and may also be markers of milk fat intake and feed quality (Wongtangtintharn et al., 2005; Lin et al., 2012; Fievez et al., 2012). However, Baumann et al. (2016) suggest that lipid supplementation (PUFA) can affect the profile of milk OBCFA.

Yogurt is the most consumed healthy and nutritious food around the world. Technological methods are used by many food companies. Yogurt and other dairy products are rich in calcium. Generally, the sensory properties should not be modified using large amounts of minerals. A good method of Ca fortification of yogurt is the use of micronized tricalcium citrate. Also, organic forms of Zn and Mg are used in yogurt enrichment (Gahruie et al., 2015). Due to the fact that dairy products are poor in Fe, fortification with this element is taken into account. However, fortification with compounds such as ferrous sulfate and ferric ammonium leads to the processes of fat oxidation.

8.4.3 Minerals and vitamins

The main mineral components include macroelements (Ca, P, Na, K, Cl, Mg, Si), microelements (Cu, Fe, Mn, Mo, J, Se), and trace elements (Table 8.3). Their content usually dooes not exceed 1% (0.65%–0.8% on average). The presence of trace amounts of heavy metals (e.g., Pb, Cd, As, Cd) is also possible, and the allowable limits for them are specified in particular countries. Mineral concentration in milk is related to physical-chemical equilibria, which are important in processing, nutritive value, and shelf life of dairy products. Mineral components together with lactose form the osmotic pressure of milk. A considerable part of calcium is bond in the casein-calcium complex. Mineral components are also involved in many biochemical reactions, since these elements are part of enzymes and coenzymes or catalyze

Table 8.3 Nutritional Composition of Milk and Yogurts (100 g)

Components	Unit	Full-fat milk	Full-fat yogurt
Energy	Kcal	68	70
Protein	G	3.3	3.8
Fat	G	3.8	3.8
Lactic acid	G	0	0.8
Potassium	mg	157	157
Calcium	mg	120	120
Phosphorus	mg	92	92
Magnesium	mg	12	12
Sodium	mg	48	48
Iodine	mg	0.46	0.46
Chlorine	mg	102	102
Retinol	µg	52	28
Carotene	µg	21	21
Vitamin B_1	µg	30	60
Vitamin B_2	µg	170	270
Vitamin B_6	µg	60	100
Vitamin B_{12}	µg	0.4	0.2
Vitamin C	mg	1	1
Vitamin D	µg	0.03	0.04
Vitamin E	µg	90	50
Folic acid	µg	6	18
Nicotinic acid	µg	100	200
Pantothenic acid	µg	350	500
Biotin	µg	1.9	2.6
Choline	mg	12.1	–

Source: Adapted from Gahruie, H. H. et al., *Food Sci. Human Well.*, 4, 1–8, 2015.

chemical reactions. They also affect the nutritional value of milk, e.g., one liter of milk covers 100% of the daily requirement of an adult man for Ca, 75% for K and 40% for Mg. On average, 250 mL of milk covers 56% human demand for vitamin B_{12}, but only 4% for folates (Graulet, 2014).

Scientific studies in recent years have been focused on an optimization of animals' supply of the most important microelements, both in terms of form and bioavailability. Thus, inorganic forms of microelements were compared with organic ones (Yasui et al., 2014; Osorio et al., 2016). Recent advances in mineral research indicate that absorption and utilization of trace elements is higher when they are supplemented in organic forms. Metalloproteins, metal polysaccharide, hydroxyanalogue chelates, metals hydroxychlorides, metal amino acid chelates (e.g., Zn, Cu, Fe, Mn, and Co), and metal amino acid complex were developed in order to increase the possibility of absorption and improve the bioavailability of elements (Mohanta and Garg, 2014). The ligand may be hydrolyzed protein (e.g., soy), glycine, or amino acids.

Responding to the demand for mineral components is significant in terms of production, since the deficiency of certain elements may cause a 20%–30% decrease in productivity (Mohanta and Garg, 2014), as well as in terms of health and immune (Yasui et al., 2014; Osorio et al., 2016). Zinc deficiency in the feed rations of cows is clearly associated with a higher risk of metritis, mastitis, and retained placenta occurrence at the beginning of lactation (Enjalbert et al., 2006; Siciliano-Jones et al., 2008). Similar results occur in the case of Cu and Se deficit. In the practical feeding of ruminants, attention should be paid to the fact that chelating and sequestering agents which occur as natural compounds in feedstuffs may increase or decrease mineral absorption and utilization.

Meta analysis by Rabiee et al. (2010) demonstrated that supplementation of organic forms of trace elements increases milk yield with a negligible increase in fat and protein content (Table 8.4). This analysis also indicates a potentially positive effect of organic forms of supplementation on reproduction. However, Formigoni et al. (2011) demonstrated that partial substitution of Zn, Cu, and Mn sulfates with organic trace minerals during the dry phase and lactation resulted in higher colostrum immunoglobulins and milk fat, as well as lower calf mortality at calving. No unambiguous results of the studies on trace elements supplementation may be due to the coverage of the demand for these elements, the age of the animals, as well as the share of fiber in the feed ration (NRC, 2001).

The use of trace elements supplementation is of primary importance especially during the transition period and at the beginning of cows' lactation, because at that time they play a special role in the antioxidant processes (Osorio et al., 2016). The deficit of these elements may affect immunity and increase the risk of a variety of diseases (e.g., endometrial inflammation, mastitis). Most often, the positive effect of trace elements

Table 8.4 Effect of Trace Mineral Supplementation in Ruminants

Animal	Organic mineral	Results of research	Reference
Dairy cows	Organic trace minerals	Meta-analysis (20 research papers) -Milk yield increase (by 0.93 kg) -Minimum increase in fat and protein content -Except milk solids concentrations - No effect on SCC	Rabiee et al., 2010
Dairy cows	Organic or inorganic Zn, Mn, Cu, and Co	Both forms improved reproduction and productivity Organic complexes -Milk yield increase (especially in 2nd lactation) -Fat content increase -Fewer cases of hooveswhite line separation	Nocek et al., 2006
Dairy cows	Organic or inorganic Zn, Mn, Cu, and Co	Replacing sulfate minerals with CTM resulted in improved lactation and claw integrity Organic -More milk and energy-corrected milk -Produced more fat and protein -Decreased incidence of sole ulcers	Siciliano-Jones et al., 2008
Dairy cows	Organic or inorganic Zn, Cu, and Mn	Hydroxy trace minerals -Higher body weight after birth -No effect on performance or uterine health -Total antioxidant capacity lower in cows fed hydroxy trace minerals than inorganic sulfate forms	Yasui et al., 2014

(*Continued*)

Table 8.4 (Continued) Effect of Trace Mineral Supplementation in Ruminants

Animal	Organic mineral	Results of research	Reference
Dairy cows	Organic (AA complexes) or inorganic Zn, Cu, and Mn	AA complex	Osorio et al., 2016
		-Higher feed intake (2 kg DM)	
		-3.3 kg/d more milk and 0.14 kg/d more protein during the first 30 DIM	
		-Lower content of ketones and GGT in blood	
		-Improved antioxidant status	
		-Increased concentration of liver tissue Co and Cu	
Bulls	Zn, Mn, Cu, and Co	Increase in motile sperm—Increase in progressive sperm	Rowe et al., 2014
		Increase in sperm with rapid motility	
Goats	Inorganic Cu, Fe, Zn, and Mn	In milk was higher than in the control: Cu(II) – 8.2%, Mn(II) – 29.2%, Zn(II) –14.6	Witkowska et al., 2015
		Higher Zn content in cheese	

supplementation in this period concerned productivity, reduced lameness, and improved health of the hoof (Nocek et al., 2006; Siciliano-Jones et al., 2008; Rabiee et al., 2010). An increased efficiency after application of amino acid complexes of trace elements results from an increase in dry matter intake from the feed ration (Osorio et al., 2016). Higher digestibility of organic forms noted in the studies mostly affects the yield of fat and protein, but not the percentage of these components (Kincaid and Socha 2004; Siciliano-Jones et al., 2008; Yasui et al., 2014). Any effect of supplementation on trace elements' content in the blood and other physiological parameters is usually minimal.

Organic forms of trace elements have a beneficial effect on oxidative status and inflammation, with moderate impact on changes in concentration of glucose and fatty acids (Nayeri et al., 2014). An improvement in antioxidant status affects the secretory functions of the liver and immune status (Osorio et al., 2016). Increase in overall health status and epithelial tissue integrity while reducing the energy required can affect the reduction of negative energy balance in early lactation. Supplementation of hydroxy sources of Zn, Cu, and Mn during the transition period and early lactation modulated plasma markers related to oxidative metabolism, resulting in trends for decreased thiobarbituric acid-reactive substances (TBARS) concentration and decreased total antioxidant capacity (TAC) compared to the supplementation of these minerals as sulfates (Yasui et al., 2014).

The use of targeted supplementation before the birth of cows has a beneficial effect on colostrum quality. An application of complexed trace minerals (Zn, Cu, and Mn) resulted in a significant increase in Zn and IgG in colostrum, which undoubtedly positively affects the transfer of calves' passive immunity. The presented possibilities of changing milk composition can have a broader meaning. The modern dairy industry is looking for not only technological solutions of biofortification, but also uses biotechnological achievements in applying nutritional methods to reach specific consumer tastes or to produce foods with targeted composition. Targeted supplementation of cows' feed rations allows increase of the concentration of Ca, Se, I, Fe, vitamin B_{12}, and folates (Knowles et al., 2006). The challenge remains to create supplement formulations that deliver maximum active ingredient to whole milk, milk fractions, or subsequent dairy products. Currently, these are the supplements added to feed, water or intraruminal boluses.

Copper is mainly involved in immune processes. Since Cu is a component of ceruloplasmin and SOD and is involved in the metabolism of vitamin A and E, it clearly affects the state of oxidative equilibrium in an organism. Experimental studies demonstrated an improvement in clinical condition of the mammary gland after supplementation with Cu sulfate and Cu proteinate after intramammary infusion of *E. coli* (Scaletti and Harmon, 2012). Among ruminants, sheep are the most sensitive to deficit or excess Cu (Rooke et al., 2010). In terms of physiological transformations, Cu supplementation is fully justified, but it is not very important for the consumer of the products derived from ruminants (milk and meat).

Selenium is an important trace element in the diet of humans and animals. This results from the fact that it is involved as an antioxidant in the elimination of reactive oxygen species, beneficially affects immune system functioning, and reduces the risk of cancer. Two forms, that is, inorganic (such as selenite and selenate) or organic (Se yeast, Se-Cys, Se-Met), were used in ruminants. The organic form is actively transported through and absorbed in the intestine and nonspecifically incorporated into body proteins in place of Met during protein synthesis, providing a means of reversible Se storage in organs and tissues. The inorganic form is absorbed via passive diffusion, and little is retained in tissue reserves (Liu et al., 2015). An increased biotransformation of Se to milk and cheese can be achieved in an effective manner using the organic forms (Moschini et al., 2010; Liu et al., 2015). This allows an almost sevenfold increase in the content of Se in whole milk, from 5.5 to 35.8 mg/L (Liu et al., 2015). Comparing Se transfer from the ration to the milk of goats, it was found that a similar increase in Se content in milk can be obtained using selenium in the form of lactate and proteinate, but that higher increase is observed after the use of selenium yeast due to high content of selenomethionine (Pechova et al., 2008).

Iodine deficit is observed in many countries, and therefore, supplementation with this element is included in the prevention programs of food modification rrelated to the consumer's health. Such programs include, for example, the use of iodized salt. The content of iodine in milk of cows shows seasonal variation, depending on the phase of lactation or the use of iodophor preparations for teat dipping or parlor installation cleaning. Fluctuations in iodine concentration in milk can range from 30 to 300 mg/l (Underwood and Suttle, 1999). Supplementation of cows' diet with iodine compounds effectively increases iodine content in milk (Moschini et al., 2010). However, such actions are justified only in areas deficient in iodine, since rapid increase in iodine intake in humans increases the risk of iodine toxicity in susceptible individuals and young children. For these reasons, in Europe, EFSA suggested that the maximum iodine content in dairy cattle rations be set at 4000 μg/kg of feed (EFSA, 2005). Standard iodine content in rations is usually exceeded, thus supplementation should be careful. Iodine concentrations in milk must be monitored closely.

Iron content in the feed rations fully cover the cows' needs, mainly due to the Fe content in plants, pasture, as well as some Fe content in premixes. Iron is associated with hematopoietic processes, but also with the changes of oxygen, energy, and Fe-dependent enzymes. Iron sulfate is the form used most often, and it is added to some premixes. Few studies used iron-amino acid complex (Weiss et al., 2010). However, these studies did not demonstrate any significant effect on the milk yield, with the observed decrease in SCC.

Zinc (Zn) is trace element essential for animals, and it is involved in many physiological functions in the body through numerous metalloenzyme systems. The immune system has a large turnover of cells, which necessitates a high rate of proliferation, differentiation, and apoptosis (Haase et al., 2006). This element also plays a protective role against the harmful effect of free radicals. Administration of Zn in an organic form has higher effect on rumen microflora compared to zinc oxide (Spears and Kegley, 2002). Zn proteinate is more soluble in rumen. An application of organic or inorganic Zn in feeding cows usually leads to increased milk yield and a decreased SCC level in the milk (Cope et al., 2009). This was also confirmed by the study of Wang et al. (2013), who compared the use of Zn-proteinate chelate with the use of zinc sulfate and found that the organic form improves milk yield, which results from increased fermentation in the rumen and immune system stimulation. Regardless of the form (organic vs. inorganic), supplementation is associated with a similar increase in Zn content in milk (Sobhanirad et al., 2010). Zinc concentrations in milk from the ZnM were higher ($P<0.05$) than the control group (9.82 vs. 6.13 mg/L, respectively). It was also demonstrated that supplementation of Zn in an organic form can improve the hoof state (Noori et al., 2013), since Zn participates in the formation of horn tissue keratin. Another possible effect of Zn is the formation of teat canal keratin and other mechanisms of the mammary gland defense against pathogens.

The possibility of milk enrichment with I, Se, Co is also provided by the use of intraruminal boluses or the combined use of boluses with dietary supplementation with marine algae (López-Alonso et al., 2016). The effect of using a bolus is not maintained over time, so manufacturer's instructions should be followed. The use of intraruminal boluses containing, in addition to trace elements, as well as vitamins (A, D_3, E) can have a positive effect on the mammary gland, improving its health status and production results (Khorsandi et al., 2016). Such supplementation is also justified during heat stress.

Milk is an important source of fat-soluble vitamins for humans, especially vitamin A, D, and E. The contents of these vitamins and β-carotene in milk depends mainly on factors related to the diet of cows and to a lesser degree on genetic and physiological factors (Calderón et al., 2007). β-carotene is the main precursor of vitamin A in ruminants. Higher concentration of terpenoids, vitamin E, and β-carotene was found in the milk and cheese of ruminants grazing on mountain pastures compared to conventional farms (Valdivielso et al., 2016). Comparative studies indicate that cows kept on organic farms had a similar level of vitamins A and E in blood serum and milk as did cows receiving the addition of synthetic vitamins (Johansson et al. 2014). This demonstrates the clear homeorhetic mechanisms regulating the transfer of vitamins A and E to milk. However, worse supply with these vitamins was associated with an increased number of cases of mastitis, which justifies the additional supplementation.

Dietary supplementation of ruminants with water-soluble vitamins is rarely used in practice. Formerly, there were opinions that cows' need for B vitamins is covered by the synthesis of rumen microorganisms. More recent studies indicate that B9 + B12 injections promote liver regeneration and reduced catabolism of lipids in early lactation (Ouattara et al., 2016). Additional supplementation may also provide reproductive benefits. The possibility of affecting their content in milk is considerably reduced, since oral administration leads to their significant degradation by rumen microflora (Graulet et al., 2007). The transfer of folic acid from diet to milk is also moderate. The methods of milk biofortification with vitamin B_{12} are important, since it is better absorbed from milk than from synthetic supplements.

References

AbuGhazaleh, A. A., and Holmes, L. D. 2007. Diet supplementation with fish oil and sunflower oil to increase conjugated linoleic acid levels in milk fat of partially grazing dairy cows. *Journal of Dairy Science* 90: 2897–2904.

AbuGhazaleh, A. A., Potu, R. B., and Ibrahim, S. A. 2009. The effect of substituting fish oil in dairy cow diets with docosahexaenoic acid-micro algae on milk composition and fatty acids profile. *Journal of Dairy Science* 92: 6156–6159.

Ayerza, R., and Coates, W. 2000. Dietary levels of chia: Influence on yolk cholesterol, lipid content and fatty acid composition for two strains of hens. *Poultry Science* 79: 724–739.

Ayerza, R., and Coates, W. 2002. Dietary levels of chia: Influence on hen weight, egg production and sensory quality for two strains of hens. *Br. Poult. Sci. Poultry Science* 43(2): 283–290.

Ayerza, R., Coates, W., and Lauria, M. 2002. Chia seed (Salvia hispanica L.) as an ω-3 fatty acid source for boilers: Influence on fatty acid composition, cholesterol and fat content of white and dark meats, growth performance and sensory characteristics. *Poultry Science* 81(6): 826–837.

Banoch, T., Fajt, Z., Drabek, J., and Svoboda, M. 2010. Iodine and its importance in human and pigs. *Veterinarstvi* 60(12): 690–694.

Barłowska, J., and Litwińczuk, Z. 2009. Właściwości odżywcze i prozdrowotne tłuszczu mleka. *Medycyna Wet* 65: 171–174.

Baumann, E., Chouinard, P. Y., Lebeuf, Y., Rico, D. E., and Gervais, R. 2016. Effect of lipid supplementation on milk odd-and branched-chain fatty acids in dairy cows. *Journal of Dairy Science* 99: 6311–6323.

Belury, M. A. 2002. Dietary conjugated linoleic acid in health: Physiological effects and mechanisms of action. *Annual Review of Nutrition* 22: 505–531.

Blicharski, T. (red.) 2013. Aktualna wartość dietetyczna wieprzowiny, jej znaczenie w diecie i wpływ na zdrowie konsumentów. *Warszawa. Wyd. POLSUS.*

Bodkowski, R., Czyż, K., Kupczyński, R., Patkowska-Sokoła, B., Nowakowski, P., and Wiliczkiewicz, A. 2016. Lipid complex effect on fatty acid profile and chemical composition of cow milk and cheese. *Journal of Dairy Science* 99(1): 57–67.

Boeckaert, C., Vlaeminck, B., Dijkstra, J. et al. 2008. Effect of dietary starch or micro alga supplementation on rumen fermentation and milk fatty acid composition of dairy cows. *Journal of Dairy Science* 91: 4714–4727.

Boeckaert, K., Morgavi, D. P., Jouany, J. P., Maignien, L., Boon, N., and Fievez, V. 2009. Role of the protozoan Isotrichaprostoma, liquid-, and solid associated bacteria in rumen biohydrogenation of linoleic acid. *Animal* 3: 961–971.

Boorman, K. N., and Gunaratne, S. P. 2001. Dietary phosphorus supply, egg-shell deposition and inorganic phosphorus in laying hens. *British Poultry Science* 42: 81–91.

Brisibe, E. A., Umoren, U. E., Brisibe, F. et al. 2009. Nutritional characterization and antioxidant capacity of different tissues of Artemisia annua L. *Food Chemistry* 115: 1240–1246.

Brooks, M. A., Grimes, J. L., Lloyd, K. E., Valdez, F., and Spears, J. W. 2012. Relative biovailability in chicks of manganese from manganese propionate. *J. Journal Appl. Poult. Res. Applied Poultry Research* 21(1): 126–130.

Brownbill, R. A., Petrosian, M., and Ilich, J. Z. 2005. Association between dietary conjugated linoleic acid and bone mineral density in Postmenopausal Women. *J. Am. Coll. Nutr.* 24: 177–181.

Bruneel, C., Lemahieu, C., Fraeye, I. et al. 2013. Impact of microalgal feed supplementation on omega-3 fatty acid enrichment of hen eggs. *J. Journal Funct. Foods* 5(2): 897–904.

Burdge, G. C., Lupoli, B., Russell, J. J. et al. 2004. Incorporation of cis-9, trans-11 or trans-10, cis-12 conjugated linoleic acid into plasma and cellular lipids in healthy men. *Journal of Lipid Research* 45: 736–741.

Cachaldora, P., De Blas, J. C., Garia-Rebollar, P., Alvarez, C., and Mendez, J. 2005. Short communication. Effects of type and level of supplementation with dietary n−3 fatty acids on yolk fat composition and n−3 fatty acid retention in hen eggs. *Sp. J. Ag. Res.* 3: 209–212.

Calderón, F., Chauveau-Duriot, B., Martin, B., Graulet, B., Doreau, M., and Noziére, P. 2007. Variations in carotenoids, vitamins A and E and color in cow's plasma and milk during late pregnancy and the first three months of lactation. *Journal of Dairy Science* 90: 2335–2346.

Castañeda-Gutieérrez, E., de Veth, M. J., Lock, A. L., Dwyer, D. A., Murphy, K. D., and Bauman, D. E. 2007. Effect of supplementation with calcium salts of fish oil on n-3 fatty acids in milk fat. *Journal of Dairy Science* 90: 4149–4156.

Castañeda-Gutieérrez, E., Pelton, S. H., Gilbert, R. O., and Butler, W. R. 2009. Effect of peripartum dietary energy supplementation of dairy cows on metabolites, liver function and reproductive variables. *Animal Reproduction Science.* 112: 301–315.

Čepulienë, R., Bobinienë, R., Sirvydis, V., Gudavičiūtë, D., Miđkinienë, M., and Kepalienë, I. 2008. Effect of stable iodine preparation on the quality of poultry products. *Veterinarija ir zootechnika* 42(64): 38–43.

Ceylan, N., Ciftci, I., Mizrak, C., Kahraman, Z., and Efil, H. 2011. Influence of different dietary oil sources on performance and fatty acid profile of egg yolk in laying hens. *Journal of Animal Feed Sciences* 20: 71–83.

Chojnacka, K. 2011. Zastosowanie metody biosorpcji w wytwarzaniu żywności biofortyfikowanej w mikroelementy. *Przemysł. Chemiczny* 90(5): 707–710.

Chojnacka, K., Górecki, H., Zielińska, A., and Michalak, I. 2009. Technologia wytwarzania biologicznych dodatków paszowych na bazie alg. *Przemysł Chemiczny* 88(6): 634–639.

Coorey, R., Novinda, A., Williams, H., and Jayasena, V. 2015. Omega-3 fatty acid profile of eggs from laying hens fed diets supplemented with chia, fish oil, and flaxseed. *J. Food Sci.* 80(1): 180–187.

Cope, C. M., Mackenzie, A. M., Wilde, D., and Sinclair, L. A. 2009. Effect of level and form of dietary zinc on dairy cow performance and health. *Journal of Dairy Science.* 92: 2128–2135.

D'Souza, D. N., Mullan, B. P., and Dunshea, F. R. 2005. Pork as a functional food. *Energy (kj)* 440(660): 529.

Dannenberg, D., Nuernberg, K., Herdmann, A., Nuernberg, G., Hagemann, E., and Kienast, W. 2013. Dietary PUFA intervention affects fatty acid and micronutrient profiles of beef and related beef products. *Foods* 2(3): 295–309.

de Matos, R. 2008. Calcium metabolism in birds. *Veterinary Clinics of North Am.—America–Exotic Animal Practice* 11(1): 59–82.

Dobrzański, Z., Dolińska, B., Chojnacka, K., Opaliński, S., and Ryszka, F. 2006. Znaczenie drożdży w żywieniu zwierząt gospodarskich. *Acta Sco. Pol. Med. Vet. Scientiarum Polonorum, Seria Medicina Veterinara* 5(2): 49–6666.

Dobrzański, Z., Korczyński, M., Opaliński, S., Kosmalski, B., and Trziszka, T. 2012. Wpływ różnych tłuszczów i dodatków paszowych na cechy fizyczno-chemiczne jaj kur Lohman Brown. *Acta Scientiarum Polonorum Medicina Veterinaria* 11: 11–23.

Dobrzański, Z., Trziszka, T., Herbut, E., Krawczyk, J., and Tronina, P. 2009. Effect of humic preparations on productivity and quality traits of eggs from greenleg partridge hens. *Annals of Animal Science* 9(2): 165–174.

Dolińska, B., Opaliński, S., Zieliński, M., Chojnacka, K., Dobrzański, Z., and Ryszka, F. 2011. Iodine concentration in fodder influence the dynamics of iodine levels in hen's egg components. *Bio. Trace Element Res.* 144: 747–752.

Dolińska, B., Ryszka, F., and Dobrzański, Z. 2006. Optimization of processes of incubation of yeasts *Saccharomyces cerevisiae* enriched with microelements. *Chemistry Agricultural* 7: 175–180.

Donovan, D. C., Schingoethe, D. J., Baer, R. J., Ryali, J., Hippen, A. R., and Franklin, S. T. 2000. Influence of dietary fish oil on conjugated linoleic acid and other fatty acids in milk fat from lactating dairy cows. *Journal of Dairy Science* 83: 2620–2628.

Dozier, W. A., Kerr, B. J., Corzo, A., Kidd, M. T., and Weber, T. E., Bregendal, K. 2008. Apparent metabolizable energy of glycerin for broiler chickens. *Poultry Science* 87: 317–322.

EFSA. 2008. Selenium-enriched yeast as source for selenium added for nutritional purposes in foods for particular nutritional uses and foods (including food supplements) for the general population. *EFSA Journal* 766: 1–42.

Ellis, M. 2006. High quality pork production system. *Meat Science* 1: 99–100.

Enjalbert, F., Lebreton, P., and Salat O. 2006. Effects of copper, zinc and selenium status on performance and health in commercial dairy and beef herds: Retrospective study. *Journal of Animal Physiology and Animal Nutrition (Berl.)* 90: 459–466.

European Food Safety Authority. 2005. *Opinion of the Scientific Panel on Additives and Products or Substances used in Animal Feed on the use of iodine in feedingstuffs*. Accessed April 2010.

Fairweather-Tait, S. J. 1999. The importance of trace element speciation innutritional sciences. *Fresenius J. Anal. Chem.* 363: 536–540.

FAO Statistical YearBook. 2012. http://www.fao.org/docrep/015/i2490e/i2490e00.htm.

Fernandez, X., Monin, G., Talmant, A., Mourot, J., and Lebret, B. 1999. Influence of intramuscular fat content on the quality of pig meat 2, Consumer acceptability of m. longissimus lumborum. *Meat Science* 53: 67–72.

Fievez, V., Colman, E., Castro-Montoya, J. M., Stefanov, I., and Vlaeminck, B. 2012. Milk odd- and branched-chain fatty acids as biomarkers of rumen function. *Animal Feed Science Technology* 172: 51–65

Formigoni, A., Fustini, M., Archetti, L., Emanuele, S., Sniffen, C., and Biagi, G. 2011. Effects of an organic source of copper, manganese and zinc on dairy cattle productive performance, health status and fertility. *Animal Feed Science Technology*. 164: 191–198.

Franklin, S. T., Martin, K. R., Baer, R. J., Schingoethe, D. J., and Hippen, A. R. 1999. Dietary marine algae (*Schizochytriumsp.*) increases concentrations of conjugated linoleic, docosahexaenoic and transvaccenic acids in milk of dairy cows. *Journal of Nutrition* 129: 2048–2054.

Fredriksson, S., Elwinger, K., and Pickova, J. 2006. Fatty acid and carotenoid composition of egg yolk as an effect of microalgae addition to feed formula for laying hens. *Food Chemistry* 99: 530–537.

Fritsche, J., Fritsche, S., Solomon, M. B. et al. 2000. Quantitative determination of conjugated linoleic acid isomers in beef fat. *European Journal of Lipid Science Technology* 102: 667–672.

Fuquay, J. W., Fox, P. F., and McSweeney, P. L. H. (Eds.). 2011. *Encyclopedia of Dairy Sciences*. 2nd ed. London: Elsevier.

Gahruie, H. H., Eskandari, M. H., Mesbahi, G., and Hanifpour, M. A. 2015. Scientific and technical aspects of yogurt fortification: A review. *Food Science and Human Wellness* 4: 1–8.

Gaucheron, F. 2005. The minerals of milk. *Reprod. Nutr. Dev* 45: 473–483.

Gawęcki, J. (red.) 2003. Białka w żywności i żywieniu, Wyd. II poprawione i uzupełnione. Poznań. Wydawnictwo Akademii Rolniczej im. *A. Cieszkowskiego w Poznaniu*. 22–41.

Glasser, F., Doreau, M., Ferlay, A., and Chilliard, Y. 2007. Estimation of milk fatty acid yield from milk fat data. *Journal of Dairy Science* 90: 2302–2304.

Gołkowski, F. 2010. Jod-pierwiastek istotny w profilaktyce, diagnostyce i leczeniu. *Interdyscyplinarne aspekty nauk o zdrowiu* 81.

Grajeta, H. 2004. Żywność funkcjonalna w profilaktyce chorób układu krążenia. *Advances in Clinical Experimental Medecine* 13, 503–510.

Graulet, B. 2014. Ruminant milk: A source of vitamins in human nutrition. *Animal Frontiers* 4:, 24–30.

Graulet, B., Matte, J. J., Desrochers, A., Doepel, L., Palin, M. F., and Girard C. L. 2007. Effects of dietary supplements of folic acid and vitamin B-12 on metabolizm of dairy cows in early lactation. *Journal of Dairy Science*. 90: 3442–3455.

Grosicki, A. 1999. Interakcje selenu z wybranymi metalami ciężkimi. Materiały Konferencyjne: Skażenie środowiska a zdrowie. *Augustów*. 92.

Haase, H., Mocchegiani, E., and Rink, L. 2006. Correlation between zinc status and immune function in the elderly. *Biogerontology* 7: 421–428.

Haenlein, G. F. W., and Anke, M. 2011. Mineral and trace element research in goats: A review. *Small Ruminant Research* 95: 2–19.

HeraviMoussavi, A. R., Gilbert, R. O., Overton, T. R., Bauman, D. E., and Butler, W. R. 2007. Effects of feeding fish meal and n-3 fatty acids on milk yield and metabolic responses in early lactating dairy cows. *Journal of Dairy Science* 90, 136–44.

Herkel, R., Gálik, B., Bíro, D. et al. 2016. The effect of a phytogenic additive on nutritional composition of turkey meat. *J. Cent. ECentralur. Ag.* 17(1).

Hözer, B., and Kirmaci, H. A. 2010. Functional milks and dairy beverages. *International Journal of Dairy Technology* 63: 1–15.

Insel, P., Turner, R. E., and Ross, D. 2001. *Nutrition*, Boston, Toronto: Jones & Bartlett Publication.

International Feed Industry Federation. 2015. http://www.ifif.org/pages/t/Global+feed+production.

Jamroz D., Podkówka W., Chachułowa J. 2004. Animal feeding and fodder science, PWN, Warszawa.

Jędrzejczak, R. Iron and manganese in food. *PZH* 55: 13–20.

Jensen, R.G. 2002. The composition of bovine milk lipids. *Journal of Dairy Science*. 85: 295–350.

Jensen, W. K., Devine, C., and Dikeman, M. 2004. *Encyclopedia of Meat Sciences*. Amsterdam, London. Elsevier Academic Press.

Jiang, Z., Ahn, D. U., Ladner, L., and Sim, J. S. 1992. Influence of feeding full-fat flax and sunflower seeds on internal and sensory qualities of egg. *Poultry Science* 71(2): 378–382.

Johansson, B., Persson Waller, K., Jensen, S. K., Lindqvist, H., and Nadeau, E. 2014. Status of vitamins E and A and β-carotene and health in organic dairy cows fed a diet without synthetic vitamins. *Journal of Dairy Science* 97: 1682–1692.

Jones, E. L., Shingfield, K. J., Kohen, C. et. al. 2005. Chemical, physical, and sensory properties of dairy products enriched with conjugated linoleic acid. *Journal of Dairy Science* 88: 2923–2937.

Kay, J. K., Mackle, T. R., Auldist, M. J., Thomsan, N. A., and Bauman, D. E. 2004. Endogenoussynthesis of cis-9, trans-11 conjugatedlinoleicacid in dairycowsfedfreshpasture. *Journal of Dairy Science* 87: 369–378.

Kelly, M. L., Berry, J. R., Dwyer, D. A. et al. 1998. Dietary fatty acid sources affect conjugated linoleic acid concentrations in milk from lactating dairy cows. *Journal of Nutrition* 128: 881–885.

Khorsandi, S., Riasi, A., Khorvash, M., Mahyari, S. A., Mohammadpanah, F., and Ahmadi, F. 2016. Lactation and reproductive performance of high producing dairy cows given sustained-release multi-trace element/vitamin ruminal bolus under heat stress condition. *Livestock Science* 187: 146–150.

Kinal, S., Król, B., and Tronina, W. 2012. Effect of various selenium sources on selenium biovailability, chicken growth performance, carcass characteristic and meat composition od broiler chickens. *Vet. med.* 15(1): 07.

Kincaid, R. L., and Socha, M. T. 2004. Inorganic versus complexed trace mineral supplements on performance of dairy cows. *Professional Animal Scientist* 20: 66–73.

Knowles, S. O., Grace, N. D., Knight, T. W., McNabb, W. C., and Lee, J. 2006. Reasons and means for manipulating the micronutrient composition of milk from grazing dairy cattle. *Animal Feed Science and Technology* 131: 154–167.

Kołacz, R., Dobrzański, Z., Kupczyński, R., Cwynar, P., Opaliński, S., and Pogoda-Sewerniak, K. 2017. Impact of the copper industry on the content of selected heavy metals and biochemical indicators in the blood of dairy cows. *Medycyna Weterynaryjna*. 73: 171–175.

Kołczak, T. 2008. Jakość wołowiny. *Żywność, Nauka, Technologia, Jakość* 1 (56): 5–22.

Korczyński M., and Opaliński S. 2012. Dodatki paszowe jako potencjalna perspektywa dla przemysłu chemicznego. *Przemysł Chemiczny* 5: 792–795.

Kostik, V., Gjorgjeska, B., Bauer, B., and Filev, K. 2015. Production of shell eggs enriched with n-3 fatty acids. *J. ofPharm.* 5(8): 48–51.

Kralik, G., Skrtić, Z., Suchy, P., Strakova, E., and Gajcević, Z. 2008. Feeding Fish oil and linsed oil to laying hens to increase the n-3 PUFA in egg yolk. *Acta Veterinaria Brno* 77: 561–568.

Kritchevsky, D., Tepper, S. A., Wright, S., Tso, P., and Czarnecki, S. K. 2000. Influence of conjugated linoleic acid (CLA) on establishment and progression of atherosclerosis in rabbits. *Journal American College Nutrition* 19: 472–477.

Kucukersan, S., Kucukersan, K., Colpan, I., Goncuoglu, E., Reisli, Z., and Yesilbag, D. 2005. The effects of humic acid on egg production and egg traits of laying hen. *Veterinary Medicine Czech* 50(9): 406–410.

Kupczyński. R., Kuczaj. M., Szołtysik. M., and Stefaniak. T. 2012. Influence of fish oil, palm oil and glycerol on milk fatty acid composition and metabolism in cows during early lactation. *Archiv. Tierzucht* 55: 540–551.

Kupczyński, R., Piasecki, T., and Bednarski, M. 2013. Zioła i propolis jako dodatki funkcjonalne dla przemysłu paszowego. *Przemysł Chemiczny* 92(8): 1549–1553.

Kupczyński, R., Szołtysik, M., Janeczek, W., Zachwieja, A., and Budzińska, K. 2014. Wpływ preparatu mineralno-tłuszczowego na zawartość kwasów tłuszczowych w mleku krów i produktach mleczarskich. *Przemysl Chemiczny* 93: 1467–1471.

Kurzępa J. (red.) 2014. Chemia organizmów żywych. *Radom. Radomskie Towarzystwo Naukowe* 13.

Lelis, G. R., Silva, M. D., Tavernari, F., Albino, L. F. T., and Rostagno, H. S. 2009. Performance of layers fed diets containg different oils. *Revista Brasileira Ciencia de Ciência Avícola* 11(4): 235–240.

Lemahieu, C., Bruneel, C., Termote-Verhalle, R., Muylaert, K., Buyse, J., and Foubart, I. 2014. Effect of different microalgal n–3 PUFA supplementation doses on yolk color and n–3 LC-PUFA enrichment in the egg. *Algal Research* 6: 119–123.

Lewis, N. M., Seburg, S., and Flanagan, N. L. 2000. Enriched eggs as a source of n-3 polyunsaturated fatty acids for humans. *Poult. Sci.* 79: 971–974.

Lin, T., Yin, X., Cai, Q. et al. 2012. 13-Methyltetradecanoic acid induces mitochondrial-mediated apoptosis in human bladder cancer cells. *Urologic Oncology* 30: 339–345.

Litwińczuk, Z. (red.) 2012. Towaroznawstwo surowców i produktów zwierzęcych, Warszawa. *Powszechne Wydawnictwo Rolnicze i Leśne*. 287–305.

Liu, H. Y., Zhu, W. Z., Lu, B. Y., Wei, Z. H., and Ren, D. X. 2015. Effect of feed selenium supplementation on milk selenium distribution and mozzarella quality. *Journal of Dairy Science* 98: 8359–8367.

Lock, A. L., Horne, A. A. M., Bauman, D. E., and Salter, A. M. 2005. Butter naturally enriched in conjugated linoleic acid alters tissue fatty acids and improves the plasma lipoprotein profile in cholesterol-fed hamsters. *Journal Nutrition* 135: 1934–1939.

Loor, J. J., Ferlay, A., Ollier, A., Ueda, K., Doreau, M., and Chilliard, Y. 2005. High-concentrate diets and polyunsaturated oils alter trans and conjugated isomers in bovine rumen, blood and milk. *Journal of Dairy Science* 88: 3986–3999.

López-Alonso, M., Rey-Crespo, F., Orjales, I., Rodríguez-Bermúdez, R., and Miranda, M. 2016. Effects of different strategies of mineral supplementation (marine algae alone or combined with rumen boluses) in organic dairy systems. *Journal of Animal Physiology and Animal Nutrition (Berl.)* 100: 836–843.

Mahan, D. C., and Parrett, N. A. 1996. Evaluating the efficacy of selenium-enriched yeast and sodium selenite on tissue selenium retention and serum glutathione peroxidase activity in grover and finisher swine. *J.Journal Anim. Animal Sci.* 74: 2967–2974.

Malbe, M., Otstavel, T., Kodis, I., and Viitak, A. 2010. Content of selected micro and macro elements in dairy cows' milk in Estonia. *Agron. Res.* 8: 323–326.

McGuire M. A., and McGuire M. K. 2000. Conjugated linoleic acid (CLA): A ruminant fatty acid with beneficial effects on human health. *Proceedings of American Society of Animal Science 1999.* http://www.asas.org/jas/symposia/proceedings/0938.pdf.

Mensink, R. P. 2005. Metabolic and health effects of isomeric fatty acids. *Current Opinion Lipidology* 16: 27–30.

Michalak, I., Chojnacka, K., Dobrzański, Z. Górecki, H., Zielińska A., Korczyński, M., Opaliński, S., 2011. Effect of macroalgae enriched with microelements on egg quality parameters and mineral content of eggs, eggshell, blood, feathers and droppings. *J.Journal Anim. Phys. Anim. Nutr.* 95: 374–387.

Michalak, I., Świniarska, M., Korczyński, M., Opaliński, S., Rój, E., and Chojnacka, K. 2016. Supercritical Algal Extracts as the Component of Pro-Health Preparations for Animals. *BIT's 9th Annual World Congress of Industrial Biotechnology*. Seoul. Seul, Korea Południowa.

Moate, P. J., Chalupa, W., Boston, R. C., and Lean, I. J. 2007. Milk fatty acids. I. Variation in the concentration of individual fatty acids in bovine milk. *Journal of Dairy Science*. 90: 4730–4739.

Mohanta, R. K., and Garg, A. K. 2014. Organic trace minerals: Immunity, health, production and reproduction in farm animals. *Indian Journal of Animal Nutrition* 31: 203–212.

Moschini, M., Battaglia, M., Beone, G. M., Piva, G., and Masoero, F. 2010. Iodine and selenium carry over in milk and cheese in dairy cows: Effect of diet supplementation and milk yield. *Animal* 4: 147–155.

Nakane, A. 1992. TNS in Listeriosis, w: Bentler B. (red.): *Tumor Necrosis Factors-The Molecules and Their Emerging Role in Medicine*. New York, NY: Raven Press.

Nałęcz-Tarwacka, T., Grodzki, H., Kuczyńska, B., and Zdziarski, K. 2009. Wpływ dawki pokarmowej na zawartość składników frakcji tłuszczowej mleka krów. *Medycyna Wet* 65: 487–491.

Narváez-Solarte, W., Rostagno, H. S., Soares, P. S., Uribe-Velasquez, F. S., and Silva, M. A. 2006. Nutritional requirement of calcium in white laying hens from 46 to 62 week of age. *International Journal Poultry Science* 5(2): 181–184.

National Research Council. 2001. *Nutrient Requirements of Dairy Cattle*. 7th rev. ed. Washington, DC: National Academy of Science.

Nayeri, A., Upah, N. C., Sucu, E. et al. 2014. Effect of the ratio of zinc amino acid complex to zinc sulfate on the performance of Holstein cows. *Journal of Dairy Science* 97: 4392–4404.

Nocek, J. E., Socha, M. T., and Tomlinson, D. J. 2006. The effect of trace mineral fortification level and source on performance of dairy cattle. *Journal of Dairy Science* 89: 2679–2693.

Noori, G. R., Amanlou, H., Mahjoubi, E., Zahmatkesh, D., Mousavi, S. S., and Shahrami, E. 2013. Top-dressing of the different feed additives is effective to prevent lameness and to increase feedlot cattle performance during a short-term period. *Journal of Applied Animal Research* 41: 263–268.

Oliveira, D. D., Baiao, N. C., Cancadao, S. V. et al. 2010. Effect of lipid sources in the diet of laying hens on the fatty acids profile of egg yolk. *Poult. SciScience* 89(11): 2484–2490.

Olivera, P., Backović, D., and Slađana, Š. 2005. Dietary selenium supplementation of pigs and broilers as a way of producing selenium enriched meat. *Acta Veterinaria* 55(5–6): 483–492.

Opaliński S., Dolińska B., Korczyński M., Chojnacka K., Dobrzański Z., Ryszka F.:2012. Effect of iodine-enriched yeast supplementation of diet on performance of laying hens, egg traits, and egg iodine content. *Poult. Sci.*91: 1627–1632.

Or-Rashid, M. M., Wright, T. C., and McBride, B. W. 2009. Microbial fatty acid conversion within the rumen and the subsequent utilization of these fatty acids to improve the healthfulness of ruminant food products. *Applied Microbiology Biotechnology* 84: 1033–1043.

Osborne, V. R., Radhakrishnan, S., Odongo, N. E., Hill, A. R., and McBride, B. W. 2008. Effects of supplementing fish oil in the drinking water of dairy cows on production performance and milk fatty acid composition. *Journal Animal Science* 86: 720–729.

Osorio, J. S., Trevisi, E., Li, C., Drackley, J. K., Socha, M. T., and Loor, J. J. 2016. Supplementing Zn, Mn, and Cu from amino acid complexes and Co from cobalt glucoheptonate during the peripartal period benefits postpartal cow performance and blood neutrophil function. *Journal of Dairy Science*. 99: 1868–1883.

Ouattara, B., Bissonnette, N., Duplessis, M., and Girard, C. L. 2016. Supplements of vitamins B9 and B12 effectaffect hepatic and mammary gland gene expression profiles in lactating dairy cows. *BMC Genomics* 17: 640.

Palmquist, D. L., and Griinari, J. M. 2006. Milk fatty acid composition in response to reciprocal combinations of sunflower and fish oils in the diet. *Animal Feed Science Technology* 131: 358–369.

Park, J. H., Upadhaya, S. D., and Kim, I. H. 2015. Effect of dietary marine microalgae (Schizochytrium) powder on egg production, blood lipid profiles, egg quality, and fatty acid composition of egg yolk in layers. *Asian-Australasian J. Animal Sci.* 28: 391–397.

Pechova, A., Misurova, L., Pavlata, L., Dvorak, R. 2008. Monitoring of changes in selenium concentration in goat milk during short-term supplementation of various forms of selenium. *Biological Trace Element Research* 121: 180–191.

Pehrson, B., Ortman, K., Madjid, N., and Trafikowska, U. 1999. The influence of diet ary selenium as selenium yeast or sodium selenite on the concentration of selenium in the milk of suckler cows and on the selenium status of their calves. *J.Anim. Sci.* 77: 3371–3376.

Pietinen, P., Ascherio, A., Korhonen, P., Hartman, A. M., Willett, W. C., Albanes, D., and Virtamo, J. 1997. Intake of fatty acids and risk of coronary heart disease in a cohort of Finnish men. *American Journal of Epidemiology* 145: 876–887.

Potapenko, E. V., Evdokimow, I. A., Oboturova, N. P., and Serov, A. V. 2015. Efficiency of adding Essentials micronutiens to the diet od broiler chickens. *Foods and Raw Materials* 3(2): 82–88.

Puzanowska-Tarasiewicz, H., Kuźmicka, L., and Tarasiewicz, M. 2009. Biological function of some elements and their compounds. III. Zinc – component and activator of enzymes, Polish Medical Journal 27(161): 419.

Rabiee, A. R., Lean, I. J., Stevenson, M. A., and Socha, M. T. 2010. Effects of feeding organic trace minerals on milk production and reproductive performance in lactating dairy cows: A meta-analysis. *Journal of Dairy Science*. 93: 4239–4251.

Rizzi, L., Bochocchio, D., Bargellini, A., Parazza, P., and Simiolo, M. 2009. Effects of dietary microalgae, other lipid sources, inorganic selenium and iodine on yolk n-3 fatty acid composition, selenium content and quality of eggs in laying hens. *J. Sci, Food Ag.* 89: 1775–1781.

Roberfroid, M. B. 2000. Concepts and strategy of functional food science: The European perspective. *American Journal of Clinical Nutrition* 71, 1660–1664.

Rooke, J. A., Flockhart, J. F., and Sparks, N. H. 2010. The potential for increasing the concentrations of micro-nutrients relevant to human nutrition in meat, milk and eggs. *Journal of Agricultural Science*. 148: 603–614.

Rowe, M. P., Powell, J. G., Kegley, E. B., Lester, T. D., and Rorie, R. W. 2014. Effect of supplemental trace-mineral Skurce on bull semen quality. *Professional Animal Science* 30: 68–73.

Rozporządzenie (WE) Nr 1831/2003

Saeid, A., Chojnacka, K., Korczyński, M., Korniewicz, D., and Dobrzański, Z. 2013a. Biomass of Spirulina Maxima enriched by biosorption process as a New feed supplement for swine. *J. Appl. Phyc. Applied Phycology* 25(2): 667–675.

Saeid. A., Chojnacka. K., Korczyński. M., Korniewicz. D., and Dobrzański. Z. 2013b. Effect on supplementation of Spirulina maxima enriched with Cu on production performance, metabolical and physiological parameters in fattening pigs. *J. Appl. phyc.y Phycology* 25(5): 1607–1617.

Salim, H. M., Lee, H. R., Jo, C., Lee, S. K., and Lee, B. D. 2012. Effect of sex and diet ary organic zinc on growth performance, carcass traits, tissue mineral kontent and blood parameters of broiler chickens. *Biol.l Trace Elem. Res. Trace Element Research* 147(1–3): 120–129.

Sanders, T. A. B. 2000. Polyunsaturated fatty acids in the food chain in Europe. *American Journal of Clinical Nutrition* 71: 176–178.

Scaletti, R. W., Harmon, R. J. 2012. Effect of dietary copper source on response to coliform mastitis in dairy cows. *Journal of Dairy Science* 95: 654–662.

Scheideler, S. E., Froning, G., Cuppett, S. 1997. Studies of consumer acceptance of high omega-3 fatty acid-enriched eggs. *J. Appl. Poult. Res.* 6: 137–146.

Ševčíková, S., Skřivan, M., Dlouhá, G., and Koucký, M. 2006. The effect of selenium Skurce on the performance and meat quality od broiler chickens. *Czech Journal of Animal Science* 51(10): 449–457.

Séverin, S., and Wenshui, X. 2005. Milk biologically active components as nutraceuticals: Review. *Critical Reviews in Food Science and Nutrition* 45: 645–656.

Shapira, N. 2010. Every egg may have a targeted purpose: Toward a differential approach to egg according to composition and functional effect. *World Poult. Sci. J.* 66(3): 66(3): 271–284.

Shapira, N., Weill, P., and Loewenbach, R. 2008. Egg fortification with n-3 polyunsaturated fatty acids (PUFA): Nutritional be nefits versus high n-6 PUFA western diets, and consumer acceptance. *Israel Med. Assoc.J.* 10: 262–265.

Shingfield, K. J., Reynolds, C. K., Hervas, G., Griinari, J. M., Grandison, A. S., and Beever, D. E. 2006. Examination of the persistency of milk fatty acid composition responses to fish oil and sunflower oil in the diet of dairy cows. *Journal of Dairy Science* 89: 714–732.

Siciliano-Jones, J. L., Socha, M. T., Tomlinson, D. J., and De-Frain, J. M. 2008. Effect of trace mineral source on lactation performance, claw integrity, and fertility of dairy cattle. *Journal of Dairy Science* 91: 1985–1995.

Siddhuraju, P., Makkar, H. P. S., and Becker, K. 2002. The effect of ionising radiation on antinutritional factors and the nutritional value of plant materials with reference to human and animal food. *Food Chemistry* 78: 187–205.

Simopoulos, A. P. 2008. The Importance of the omega-6/omega-3 fatty acid ratio in cardiovascular disease and other chronic diseases. *Experimental Biology Medicine* 233: 674–688.

Słupczyńska, M., Jamroz, D., Orda, J., and Wiliczkiewicz, A. 2014. Effect of various sources and levels of iodine, as well as the kind of diet, on the performance of young laying hens, iodine accumulation in eggs, egg characteristics, and morphotic and biochemical indices in blood. *Poultry Science* 93: 2536–2547.

Smet, S. De. 2012. Meat, poultry and fish composition: Strategies for optimizing human intake of Essentials nutriens. *Animal Frontiers* 2(4): 10–16.

Smolińska, T., and Kopeć, W. (red.) 2009. Processing of poultry meat - biological and technological bases.Wrocław. Wydawnictwo Uniwersytetu Przyrodniczego we Wrocławiu. 179–193.

Sobhanirad, S., Carlson, D., and Kashani, R. B. 2010. Effect of zinc methionine or zinc sulfate supplementation on milk production and composition of milk in lactating dairy cows. *Biological Trace Element Research* 136: 48–54.

Souza, J. G., Costa, F. G. P., Queiroga, R. C. R. E., Silva, J. H. V., Schuler, A. R. P., and Goulart, C. C. 2008. Fatty acid profile of eggs of semi-heavy layers fed feeds containing linseed oil. *Brazil. J. Poult. Sci.* 10: 37–44.

Spears, J. W., and Kegley, E. B. 2002. Effect of zinc source (zinc oxide vs. proteinate) and level performance, carcass characteristics, and immune response of growing and finishing steers. *Journal of Animal Science* 80: 2747–2752.

Stillwell, W., Shaikh, S.R., Zerouga, M., Siddiqui, R., and Wassall, S. R. 2005. Docosahexaenoic acid affects cell signaling by altering lipid rafts. *Reprod. Nutrition Development* 45: 559–579.

Świątkiewicz, S., Arczewska-Włosek, A., and Józefiak, D. 2014. The efficacy of organic minerals in poultry nutrition: Review and implicationsof recent studies. *WorldWorld's Poult. Sci. J.*70(3): 475–486.

Szumacher-Strabel, M. 2005. Wpływ dodatku tłuszczów do dawek pokarmowych dla owiec kóz na zawartość nienasyconych kwasów tłuszczowych w płynie żwaczowym i mleku, ze szczególnym uwzględnieniem izomerów sprzężonego kwasu linolowego. *Roczn. AR w Poznaniu. Rozprawy Nauk.* 365.

Tavani, A., Franceschi, S., Levi, F., and La Vecchia, C. 2005. Fish, omega-3 polyunsaturated fat intake and cancer at selected sites. *World Review Nutrition Diet* 94: 166–175.

The European Feed Manufacturers' Federation. 2017. http://www.fefac.eu/files/69455.pdf

Underwood, E. J., and Suttle, N. 1999. *Mineral Nutrition of Livestock,* 3rd ed. CABI publishing Wallingford, UK.

Vahmani, P., Fredeen, A. H., Glover, K. E. 2013. Effect of supplementation with fish oil or microalgae on fatty acid composition of milk from cows managed in confinement or pasture systems. *Journal of Dairy Science* 96: 6660–6670.

Valdivielso, I., Bustamante, M. A., Aldezabal, A. et al. 2016. Case study of a commercial sheep flock under extensive mountain grazing: Pasture derived lipid compounds in milk and cheese. *Food Chem,* 197: 622–633.

Van Elswyk, M. E., Dawson, P. L., and Sams, A. R. 1995. Dietary menhadenoil influences sensory characteristics and head space volatile soft shell eggs. *J. Food Sci.* 60: 85–89.

Vernerová, J., Pipek, P., and Sklenářová, M. 2008. Kvalita vepřového masa obohaceného selénem. *Věda a výskum.* In Maso 1: 86–89

Wang, R. L., Liang, J. G., Lu, L., Zhang, L. Y., Li, S. F., and Luo, X. G. 2013. Effect of zinc source on performance, zinc status, immune response, and rumen fermentation of lactating cows. *Biological Trace Element Research* 152: 16–24.

Weiss, W. P., Pinos-Rodriguez, J. M., and Socha, M. T. 2010. Effects of feeding supplemental organic iron to late gestation and Elary lactation dairy cows. *Journal of Dairy Science.* 93: 2153–2160.

Whitlock, L. A., Schingoethe, D. L., AbuGhazaleh, A. A., Hippen, A. R., and Kalscheur, K. F. 2006. Milk production and composition from cows fed small amounts of fish oil with extruded soybeans. *Journal of Dairy Science*. 89: 3972–3980.

Wiąckowski, S. K. 1995. *Próba ekologicznej oceny żywienia, żywności i składników pokarmowych*. Warszawa. PWN.

Williams, P. G. 2007. Nutritional composition of red meat. *Nutrition & Dietetics* 64(4): 113–119.

Witkowska Z., Chojnacka K., Korczyński M. et al. 2014a. Soybean meal enriched with microelements by biosorption—A new biological feed supplement for laying hens. Part I. Performance and egg traits. *Food Chemistry* 151, 86–92, IF: 3,259.

Witkowska Z., Michalak I., Korczyński M., et al. 2015. Biofortification of milk and cheese with microelements by dietary feed bio-preparations. *Journal of Food Science and Technology*. DOI 10.1007/s13197-014-1696-9, IF: 2,024.

Witkowska, Z., Saeid, A., Korczyński, M., Dobrzański, Z., and Chojnacka, K. 2014b. Biofortification of meat with microelements by biological dietary feed supplements. *J.Nutr. Food Sci.* 4(6): 1.

Wongtangtintharn, S., Oku, H., Iwasaki, H., Inafuku, M., Toda, T., and Yanagita, T. 2005. Incorporation of branched-chain fatty acid into cellular lipids and caspase-independent apoptosis in human breast cancer cell line SKBR-3. *Lipids Health Disease* 4(1): 29.

Yasui, T., Ryan, C. M., Gilbert, R. O., Perryman, K. R., and Overton, T. R. 2014. Effects of hydroxy trace minerals on oxidative metabolism, cytological endometritis, and performance of transition dairy cows. *Journal of Dairy Science*. 97: 3728–3738.

Yi, H., Hwang, K. T., Regenstein, J. M., and Shin, S. W. 2014. Fatty acid composition and sensory characteristics of eggs obtained from hens fed flaxseed oil, dried whitebait and/or fructo-oligosaccharide. *Asian-Australasian J.Anim. Sci.* 27(7): 1026–1034.

chapter nine

Fortification of plant foodstuffs

Łukasz Tuhy, Mateusz Samoraj, and Katarzyna Chojnacka

Contents

9.1 Introduction

Fortification of food is one of the methods leading to the obtainment of so-called enriched products. The term *fortification* was not strictly defined and there are some discrepancies in scientific literature dealing with food fortification. The most widespread definition of fortification includes the changes in nutrient composition of food not affecting its energy value. It is used to increase the nutritional value of paramount foodstuff and leads to its use as a tool for overcoming nutrient deficiency and malnutrition (Tarabella and Burchi, 2012). According to Cannella et al., (2007), fortification should not be confused with food enrichment nor supplementation. First, it can be defined as increasing of nutrients existing in food but often lost in food processing while supplementation concerns nutrients that are not naturally found in the foodstuff.

Because nutrient malnutrition is a global problem and investigation of tools for its reduction are of particular interest, fortification of plant foodstuff becomes a more and more popular subject of research (Hotz, 2009). Due to the high importance of crops in human nutrition, vegetables, fruits, and cereals were shown to be commonly fortified with different nutrients.

9.2 Vegetables

In Africa, cassava was reported as one of most important staple foods after maize. It is used for the production of cassava mahewu—a fermented beverage, the consumption of which is high. Fermentation makes it possible to obtain products characterized by higher content of amino acids, vitamins, and improved mineral bioavailability. In the study conducted by Salvador (2015), the possibility of cassava mahewu fortification with iron was investigated. Analysis of results suggests that fortified bitter cassava can deliver more bioavailable iron and contribute to increased iron consumption and reduced iron deficiency in vulnerable populations.

Other studies confirmed the positive influence of various plant extracts (grape seeds, green tea, thyme, parsley, oregano extracts) and butylated hydroxytoluene on the fortification of tomato chips with phenolic compounds. During experiments, reduced peroxide value development and astringency development were observed. Preparations examined revealed high potential as a tool useful in the fortification with antioxidants resulting in increased preservation of tomato chips (Rababah et al., 2012).

Fortification of tomato, aubergine, and chili with different nutrients was a subject of interest conducted by Ponnuswamy and Vijayalakshmi (2011). Soaking of vegetable seeds with gelatin, potassium phosphate, and potassium nitrate lead to plant fortification significantly improving seed germination and plant vigour.

Besides organic compounds, fortification of foodstuffs with trace elements is also of particular interest. Rahman and co-workers (2015) proved the possibility of plant fortification with selenium via foliar application of K_2SeO_4. Furthermore, experiments carried out on lentil confirmed possible fortification of vegetables with the use of genetic biofortification. Kápolna et al., (2012) in their work described fortification of onion and carrots with selenium by foliar application of nutrient. The analysis of bulbs and leaves showed 50–200 times increased content of selenium in vegetables, depending on the part of plant.

Fortification of plants with inorganic compounds can be an effective way for biochemical modifications and hence biochemical profile of vegetables. Tomato fertilization with selenium by seed soaking, soil, and foliar application of preparations was examined. It was reported that foliar application of selenium fertilizer was the most efficient method for plant fortification with this nutrient. Simultaneously, increased total protein, phenolic content, and antioxidant activity was observed (Nancy and Arulselvi, 2014).

Great attention was also paid on the fortification of sprouts due to high nutritional value and bioavailability of essential elements. In the study conducted by Przybysz et al., (2016), sprouts from *Brassica oleracea, Raphanus sativus, Medicago sativa* L., *and Vigna radiate* L the presence of higher iron concentration led to increased micronutrient concentration in sprouts, promoted ROS, and increased antioxidative activity through enzyme activation or phenolic compounds synthesis.

In other studies, the role of folate fortification of food was emphasized and potatoes were shown to be appropriate organism for this purpose.

Solanum species were screened for the identification of high folate content organisms and *Solanum tuberosum, Solanum vernei,* and *Solanum boliviense* were chosen for further processing. Genetic diversity was shown to be a promising approach for folate fortification of paramount crops (Robinson et al., 2015). Vacuum impregnation of whole potatoes was used for the fortification of vegetables with ascorbic acid the concentration of which was increased with increasing duration of the process. It was proved that fortified potatoes provided recommended allowance of ascorbic acid (Hironaka et al., 2011). Fortification of lettuce with selenium and iodine was observed when they were applied foliarly in the form of KIO_3 and Na_2SeO_4, respectively. Lettuce fertilization improved nutrients absorption by leaves. The results suggest that transfer of iodine and selenium to plants occurs through phloem (Smoleń et al., 2014).

Biofortification of onion and broccoli with selenium was carried out to examine its possible effect on plant growth parameters as well as ascorbic acid, phenolic compounds, and antioxidant content in plants. Increased content of nutrient in soil resulted in its higher content in plants without negative effects on the health-related compounds for both tested vegetables (Adhikari, 2012).

9.3 Fruits

Another effective tool for controlling nutrients deficiency is fortification of fruits. Kumar and coworkers (2011) obtained 6.32- and 4.58-fold increase in iron and zinc content, respectively, via genetic transformation of genome.

Shikov and coworkers (2012) carried out the fortification of strawberries with polyphenols. The application of rose petal extracts allowed enhanced antioxidant capacity and significant pigment retention. Hence, it seems to be a promising tool for development of functional foodstuff.

Due to the low content of iodine in plant foodstuff, an attempt was made to fortify tomatoes using potassium iodide and potassium iodate. Tomatoes were shown to constitute a perfect target for iodine fortification and the resulting content of element exceeded recommended dietary allowance (RDA) for adults (Caffagni et al., 2011).

Tomato fruits also constitute a subject of fortification with vitamin E. Currently, there are a lot of molecular techniques to increase vitamin E content of tomatoes (Raiola et al., 2015).

In the study conducted by Chakraborty and Samanta (2015), Alphonso mango was fortified with aloe vera and the nutritional quality of new product was investigated. Fortified food exhibited over 110% increase of ascorbic acid content, sixfold increase in the polyphenol content, and improved radical scavenging activity.

Younas and coworkers examined apricots coated with chitosan/alginate and fortified with zinc for their physicochemical properties. Edible coating and zinc fortification significantly affected food stability. Apricots fortified with zinc were shown to be characterized by minimum weight and moisture losses during storage (Younas et al., 2014). Direct feeding of banana bunches with iron and manganese combined with urea increased crop yield and led to biofortification of plants with these nutrients. The author put forward a hypothesis that described a technique of banana fortification with iron and manganese that was useful for combating anemia (Kotur, 2015).

Fortification of tomato fruits with iodine was also carried out in pot trials where iodine was delivered as root treatment. It was confirmed that iodine fertilization significantly increased nutrient content in fruits not affecting plant growth and development (Kiferle et al., 2013).

Transgenic tomatoes characterized by overexpression of cDNA encoding selenocysteine methyltransferase were shown to be able to convert inorganic selenium to methylselenocysteine. Genetic modification made it possible to obtain plants with a higher accumulation of selenium than when provided with selenite or selenate (Brummell et al., 2011).

Higher potassium content and improved antioxidant capacity parameters were observed for cherry tomatoes subjected to biofortification program with K. It was postulated that consumption of these tomatoes would be beneficial for health due to high nutritional value (Constn-Aguilar et al., 2015).

Increased food processing combined with reduced consumption of fruits and vegetables led to reduction in potassium intake by humans. Experiments carried out by Montoya et al., 2013 showed agronomic fortification to be beneficial method for K content increase in cucumbers. Fortification was obtained through fertilization with the use of potassium sulfate.

Zinc fertilization of "Fugi" apple trees enhanced fruit fortification with this nutrient simultaneously activating carbohydrate metabolism and sugar accumulation in apples (Zhang et al., 2013).

9.4 Cereals

Minimizing the negative results of nutrients deficiency can also be achieved via fortification of cereals with inorganic and organic compounds necessary for human nutrition.

The attempt to fortify sunflower with selenium was made through foliar application of sodium selenite. Incorporation of selenium into plant system resulted in higher crop field and increased content of crucial fatty acids (i.e., linoleic, palmitoleic, palmitic, and oleic) (Skarpa, 2013).

Mictonutrient content of bioavailable zinc and iron in maize may be improved in several approaches. In the work of Moretti and coworkers two ways to reach the goal were presented. The first one is maize fortification with sodium iron ethylenediaminetetraacetate (NaFeEDTA), ferrous fumarate, or ferrous sulfate with the use of mechanical or enzymatic methods. Ferrous sulfate led to degradation of phytic acid, which is the main inhibitor of iron and zinc adsorption. Experiments confirmed higher bioavailability of micronutrients from maize, which contain lower phytic acid level (Moretti et al., 2014). In the second approach, maize was fortified with copper, manganese, and zinc in field conditions. In the experiment, new fertilizers were produced via biosorption conducted on the biomass of *Spirulina platensis*. Fertilization with biomass-based fertilizers lead to agronomic fortification (micronutrient content was significantly higher) and yield increase (Tuhy et al., 2015). In field trials on maize potential of blackcurrant seed post-extraction residues enriched with micronutrients as organic fertilizer was investigated. A biological form of micronutrient source was compared with commercial mineral micronutrient fertilizer. About 10% higher content of micronutrient was achieved in comparison with plants fertilized with commercial reference micronutrient fertilizer (Samoraj et al., 2015).

In other studies, supplementation with iron and nitrogen was tested and verified to affect iron content in grains and shoots of durum wheat, under greenhouse conditions. Iron and nitrogen were applied to soil—as FeEDTA or $FeSO_4$ and $Na(NO_3)_2$—and foliarly as FeEDTA, FeEDDHA, Fe-$C_5H_4O_5COOH$ and $FeSO_4$, and $CO(NH_2)_2$. Iron foliar spraying alone was also tested. The experiment showed that neither inorganic nor chelated forms of iron affected its accumulation in plants. Simultanously both treatments with nitrogen provided higher concentration of Fe in wheat grains; similarly, the application of calcium nitrate led to higher content of Fe in shoots and increase Zn amount in grains. It confirms that nitrogen fertilizing plays a key role in crop biofortification with iron (Aciksoz et al., 2011).

In another study, fertilizing durum wheat with zinc increased its accumulation in grains. The treatment increased productivity and is recommended during Zn-deficiency conditions (Cakmak et al., 2010).

Another way of enhancement of Zn and Fe content in grains is exploring genetic diversity of durum wheat. This approach was introduced by HarvestPlus biofortification program. Promising solutions for selenium deficiency are genetic variations between wheat varieties, based on seed banks (Carvalho and Vasconelos, 2013).

In the work of Kumar and coworkers on the genome in hexaploid wheat, wheat (*Aegilops kotschyi* substitution lines, wild species of *Triticum*, and *Aegilops* species) was investigated to determine sequences enabling grain to efficiently accumulate zinc and iron. Wild species have two promising donors for biofortification with either Zn or Fe, *Aegilops speltoides* and *Triticum monococcum*, respectively. Transfer of appropriate genes from *Ae. kotschyi* substitution lines of wheat show high tissue content of Zn and Fe (Kumar et al., 2016).

Borril and coworkers presented a biofortification strategy that relied on genome sequencing and mutant cultivation for identification of genes that participate in zinc and iron uptake and their cellular transport (Borrill et al., 2014).

Iron malnutrition was overcome by mineral enrichment of wheat flour. That will improve nutrition value of staple foods such as bread (Gómez-Galera et al., 2010, Akhtar et al., 2011). Obligatory wheat flour fortification in the majority of developing countries in Latin America causes decrease of anemia (Shrimpton et al. 2005). New strategy of using fortified wheat flour as a tool in Fe hunger prevention was introduced by the Flour Fortification Initiative and the Micronutrient Initiative. It is preventing 540 million people against Fe deficiency (CDCP 2008, Gómez-Galera et al., 2010).

In studies conducted by Velu and coworkers acculation of iron and zinc in grains of a number of pearl millet variations, including hybrid parents and germplasm accessions, for under two-season field trials were tested. Micronutrient content varied within the population by 24.5–64.8 mg/kg and 30.1–75.7 mg/kg for Zn and Fe, respectively. The highest biofortification effect was achieved for commercial varieties, their progenies, and the parental lines of hybrids based on *iniari* germplasm. A strong positive correlation between the results showed Fe–Zn synergistic effect. Simultaneous fertilization with Fe and Zn provide plant supplementation with both micronutrients at the same time (Velu et al., 2007).

Cassava biofortification was successfully performed during the BioCassava Plus program which involves genetic engineering for stress prevention to supply African countries' diet with essential micronutrients such as iron and zinc. The effectiveness of this strategy was proved in field conditions in Nigeria (Sayre et al., 2011).

In the research carried out by Rodrigo and coworkers (2014), barley was fortified with selenium as a result of plant fertilizing with sodium selenate and sodium selenite. In the next step, fortified cereals constituted a base for beer production. The application of selenium-fortified barley made it possible to obtain a beverage characterized by six-fold higher content of examined micronutrient compared with traditional beer (Rodrigo et al., 2014). In other research, oat seeds coating with the use of zinc sulfate led to biofortification of cereals' seeds with zinc (Shivay et al., 2013).

High levels of rice fertilizing that can be observed is due to its sensitiveness to micronutrients shortage. The crops are often subjected to biofortification because of high contribution of rice in human consumption and possible impact on human health. Various strategies for rice fortification were considered and agronomic fortification was found to be the most efficient method not interfering with genome in comparison with genetic fortification tools (Sperotto et al., 2012). Zinc is a micronutrient, the shortage of which was shown to constitute a major problem. Results obtained by Ram and coworkers (2015) showed agronomic fortification to be an effective instrument for crop quality improvement. Moreover, there was no difference in the fertilizer efficiency between soil and foliar application, while the second method worked independently on soil zinc status (Ram et al., 2015). Fortification of rice with zinc during parboiling led to the increase of zinc content (from 1.3 to 4.5 times) in grain. The resulting product was characterized by high bioavailability of delivered nutrient (over 50%) that was confirmed by extraction experiments in a dilute acid (Rerkasem et al., 2010). In other work, rice grains were subjected to transgenic fortification with zinc. Modifications resulted in six-fold higher micronutrient content in comparison with nontransgenic seeds (Masuda et al., 2012). The efficiency of foliar fertilization in micronutrient fortification of Italian rice was confirmed by Giacosa and coworkers (2014). The results also showed a positive effect of selenium fortification on serum selenium and glutathione peroxidase activity after 20 days of supplementation (Giacosa et al., 2014). The need for iron fortification of rice was postulated mainly due to combat micronutrient malnutrition in developing countries. Low availability results from the conversion of iron into unavailable forms in calcareous soils (Ramzani et al., 2016). Plants are not able to produce iron and soil constitutes the sole source of this nutrient. While plants are able to take up Fe^{2+} ions and it is present in soils mainly as Fe^{3+}, rice fortification was indicated as the most promising tool for combating iron shortage in plants and humans (Sautter et al., 2006). Treatment of rice grains with Fe-EDTA during parboiling caused a10- to 50-fold increase in micronutrient concentration and its availability was correlated with increasing iron content (Longbin et al., 2011).

Cassava is a plant foodstuff being consumed by people in the poorest regions of the world. Cassava reveals high resistance to Al, an element commonly present in tropical soils, while it often suffers from micronutrient deficiency. Due to that fact, fortification of cassava in micronutrients constitutes a subject of interest. Local authorities decided to implement the BioCassava Plus program for sub-Saharan regions of Africa. The idea of the program is to use biotechnological approaches for cassava fortification because consumption of non-modified cassava provides less than 20% of required micronutrients. In parallel, genetic modifications increase plant resistance to diseases, reduce cyanogenic glycosides content, and prolong shelf-life (Sayre et al., 2011).

Also maize, which is one of the most widespread crops all over the world, suffers from deficiency of major nutrients, especially zinc. Due to high maize consumption, a zinc deficiency was also revealed in the human diet. This situation means that zinc deficiency in the human diet is one of the main causes of hidden hunger. Within one of the projects, the fortification of maize using agronomic tools was carried out. During tests, foliar fertilization of maize with $ZnSO_4{\cdot}7H_2O$ was applied after sowing.

The treatment significantly improved plant growth and increased zinc content of maize (Imran and Rehim, 2016).

Rice was shown to be a significant staple food for over half the global population and also a source of zinc, although the bioavailability of this nutrient is not satisfactorily high. Wei et al., (2012) showed that fortification of germinated brown rice with zinc (as zinc sulfate) was an efficient method to obtain increased content of the nutrient in grains and improve zinc bioavailability.

In other studies, researchers examined the possibility of rice fortification with zinc and iron, the deficiency of which constitute one of the most serious nutritional problems. Foliar application of zinc and iron sulfates increased nutrients content in rice of over 30% and over 20%, respectively (Dhaliwal et al., 2010).

Soil and foliar application of zinc and iron made it possible to significantly increase the content of available nutrients in wheat. Simultaneously, improvement of plant growth parameters was observed (Naz et al., 2015).

Bacterial and cyanobacterial strains were investigated for their potential in biofortification of wheat in terms of micronutrients and protein content. It was observed that the application of biofertilizers as a complementary fertilization led to protein and micronutrient content increase in wheat grain (Rana et al., 2012).

Agricultural fortification of rice with zinc and iron as well as edible oil with vitamin A was postulated to be recommended to overcome malnutrition and hidden hunger in Asian countries (Leyvraz et al., 2015).

Hotz et al., (2015) proved that addition of zinc and iron sulfates to soaking water during parboiling causes rice fortification with these micronutrients. Furthermore, micronutrients were found to be in bioavailable forms.

References

Aciksoz, S. B., Yazici, A., Ozturk, L., and Cakmak, I. 2011. Biofortification of wheat with iron through soil and foliar application of nitrogen and iron fertilizers. *Plant Soil,* 349(1-2): 215–225

Adhikari, P. (2012). Biofortification of Selenium in broccoli (Brassica oleracea L. var. italica) and onion (Allium cepa L.) (Master's thesis, Norwegian University of Life Sciences, Ås)

Akhtar, S., Anjum, F. M., and Anjum, M. A. 2011. Micronutrient fortification of wheat flour: Recent development and strategies. *Food Res Int,* 44(3): 652–659

Borrill, P., Connorton, J. M., Balk, J., Miller, A. J., Sanders, D., and Uauy, C. 2014. Biofortification of wheat grain with iron and zinc: integrating novel genomic resources and knowledge from model crops. *Frontieres in Plant Science* 5: 53, 98

Brummell, D. A., Watson, L. M., Pathirana, R., Joyce, N. I., West, P. J., Hunter, D. A., and McKenzie, M. J. 2011. Biofortification of tomato (Solanum lycopersicum) fruit with the anticancer compound methylselenocysteine using a selenocysteine methyltransferase from a selenium hyperaccumulator. *Journal of agricultural and food chemistry,* 59(20): 10987–10994

Caffagni, A., Arru, L., Meriggi, P., Milc, J., Perata, P., and Pecchioni, N. 2011. Iodine fortification plant screening process and accumulation in tomato fruits and potato tubers. *Communications in soil science and plant analysis,* 42(6): 706–718

Cakmak, I., Pfeiffer, W. H., and McClafferty, B. 2010. Review: biofortification of durum wheat with zinc and iron. *Cereal Chemistry,* 87(1): 10–20

Cannella, C., Giusti, A. M., and Pinto, A. 2007. Dal cibo per tutti agli alimenti personalizzati. *Pensiero Scientifico Editore,*1: 1–2

Carvalho, S. M., and Vasconcelos, M. W. 2013. Producing more with less: strategies and novel technologies for plant-based food biofortification. *Food Res Int,* 54(1): 961–971

CDCP (Centers for Disease Control and Prevention). 2008. Trends in wheat-flour fortification with folic acid, iron. Worldwide, 2004 and 2007. MMWR 57:8–10

Chakraborty, R., and Samanta, R. 2015. Alphonso Mango Enrichment with Aloe Vera (Aloe barbadensis) by Sequential Drying: Optimization, Kinetics and Quality Evaluation. *Journal of Food Processing and Preservation,* 39(6): 2698–2709

Constn-Aguilar, C., Leyva, R., Romero, L., Soriano, T., Blasco, B., and Ruiz, J. M. (2015). The effect of potassium biofortification over yield and nutritional quality of cherry tomato fruits. *American Journal of Advanced Food Science and Technology, 3(2):* 67–93

Dhaliwal, S. S., Sadana, U. S., Khurana, M. P. S., Dhadli, H. S., and Manchanda, J. S. 2010. Enrichment of rice grains with zinc and iron through ferti-fortification. *Indian Journal of Fertilisers,* 6(7): 28–35

Giacosa, A., Faliva, M. A., Perna, S., Minoia, C., Ronchi, A., and Rondanelli, M. 2014. Selenium fortification of an Italian rice cultivar via foliar fertilization with sodium selenate and its effects on human serum selenium levels and on erythrocyte glutathione peroxidase activity. *Nutrients,* 6(3): 1251–1261

Gómez-Galera, S., Rojas, E., Sudhakar, D., Zhu, C., Pelacho, A. M., Capell, T., and Christou, P. 2010. Critical evaluation of strategies for mineral fortification of staple food crops. *Transgenic Res,* 19(2): 165–180

Hironaka, K., Kikuchi, M., Koaze, H., Sato, T., Kojima, M., Yamamoto, K., and Tsuda, S. 2011. Ascorbic acid enrichment of whole potato tuber by vacuum-impregnation. *Food chemistry,* 127(3): 1114–1118

Hotz, C. 2009. The potential to improve zinc status through biofortification of staple food crops with zinc. *Food Nutr Bull,* 30: 172–78

Hotz, C., Kabir, K. A., Dipti, S. S., Arsenault, J. E., and Bipul, M. 2015. Rice fortification with zinc during parboiling may improve the adequacy of zinc intakes in Bangladesh. *Journal of the Science of Food and Agriculture,* 95(2): 379–385

Imran, M., and Rehim, A. 2016. Zinc Fertilization Approaches for Agronomic Biofortification and Estimated Human Bioavailability of Zinc in Maize Grain. *Archives of Agron Soil Sci,* 63(1): 106–116

Kápolna, E., Laursen, K. H., Husted, S., and Larsen, E. H. 2012. Bio-fortification and isotopic labelling of Se metabolites in onions and carrots following foliar application of Se and 77 Se. *Food Chem,* 133: 650–57

Kiferle, C., Gonzali, S., Holwerda, H. T., Real Ibaceta, R., and Perata, P. 2013. Tomato fruits: a good target for iodine biofortification. *Frontiers in plant science,* 4: 205

Kotur, S. C. 2015. Bio-fortification with iron and manganese for enhanced bunch yield in 'Robusta' banana through direct nutrient-feeding. *Journal of horticultural sciences,* 2015(1): 44–48

Kumar, U., Mathpal, P., Malik, S., Kumar, N., Kumar, S., Chugh, V., and Kumar, S. 2016. Evaluation of iron and zinc in grain and grain fractions of hexaploid wheat and its related species for possible utilization in wheat biofortification. *Plant Genet Resour, 14*(02): 101–111 Leyvraz, M., Laillou, A., Rahman, S., Ahmed, T., Rahman, A. S., Alam, N., Panagides, D. 2015. An Assessment of the Potential Impact of Fortification of Staples and Condiments on Micronutrient Intake of Young Children and Women of Reproductive Age in Bangladesh. *Nutrients, 7*(12): 9960–9971

Longbin, H., Shu, F., and Benjavan, R. 2011. Iron fortification in parboiled rice - A rapid and effective tool for delivering iron nutrition to rice consumers. *Food Nutr Sci 2:* 323–328

Masuda, H., Ishimaru, Y., Aung, M. S., Kobayashi, T., Kakei, Y., Takahashi, M., and Nishizawa, N. K. 2012. Iron biofortification in rice by the introduction of multiple genes involved in iron nutrition. *Sci Rep,* 2: 543

Montoya, S., Ortega, E., Navarro, E., and Lorenzo, M. L. 2013. Cucumber biofortification with potassium. *European Scientific Journal, 9*(33): 101–108

Moretti, D., Biebinger, R., Bruins, M. J., Hoeft, B., and Kraemer, K. 2014. Bioavailability of iron, zinc, folic acid, and vitamin A from fortified maize. *Ann N Y Acad Sci, 1312*(1): 54–65

Nancy, D., and Arulselvi, P. I. 2014. Effect of Selenium Fortification on Biochemical Activities of Tomato (Solanum lycopersicum) Plants. *Indo Am J Pharm Res,* 4: 3997–4005

Naz, S., Yousaf, B., Tahir, M. A., Qadir, A., and Yousaf, A. 2015. Iron and Zinc biofortification strategies in wheat crop by exogenous application of micronutrients. *Food Sci. and Quality Management, 35:* 49–54

Ponnuswamy, A. S., and Vijayalakshmi, V. 2011. Effect of Seed Fortification with Bio-inoculants, Nutrients and Growth Regulators on Seed Germination and Seedling vigour of Tomato (Lycopersicon esculentum), Brinjal (Solanum melongena) and Chilli (Capsicum annum). *Madras Agric J,* 98: 251–52

Przybysz, A., Wrochna, M., Małecka-Przybysz, M., Gawrońska, H., and Gawroński, S. W. 2016. Vegetable sprouts enriched with iron: Effects on yield, ROS generation and antioxidative system. *Sci Hortic,* 203: 110–17

Rababah, T. M., Feng, H., Yang, W., and Yücel, S. 2012. Fortification of potato chips with natural plant extracts to enhance their sensory properties and storage stability. *J Am Oil Chem Soc,* 89(8): 1419–25

Rahman, M. M., Erskine, W., Materne, M. A., McMurray, L. M., Thavarajah, P., Thavarajah, D., and Siddique, K. H. M. 2015. Enhancing selenium concentration in lentil (Lens culinaris subsp. culinaris) through foliar application. *The J Agric Sci,* 153: 656–665

Raiola, A., Tenore, G. C., Barone, A., Frusciante, L., and Rigano, M. M. 2015. Vitamin E Content and Composition in Tomato Fruits: Beneficial Roles and Bio-Fortification. *International journal of molecular sciences, 16*(12): 29250–29264

Ram, H., Sohu, V. S., Cakmak, I., Singh, K., Buttar, G. S., Sodhi, G. P. S., and Mavi, G. S. 2015. Agronomic fortification of rice and wheat grains with zinc for nutritional security. *Current Sci,* 109(6): 1171–1176

Ramzani, P. M. A., Khalid, M., Naveed, M., Irum, A., and Kausar, S. 2016. Iron Biofortification of Cereals Grown Under Calcareous Soils: Problems and Solutions. *Soil Sci, 1:* 231–258

Rana, A., Joshi, M., Prasanna, R., Shivay, Y. S., and Nain, L. 2012. Biofortification of wheat through inoculation of plant growth promoting rhizobacteria and cyanobacteria. *European Journal of Soil Biology, 50:* 18–126

Rerkasem, B., Cakmak, I., and Huang, L. 2010. Zinc fortification of whole rice grain through parboiling process. *Food Chem,* 120(3): 858–863

Robinson, B. R., Sathuvalli, V., Bamberg, J., and Goyer, A. 2015. Exploring Folate Diversity in Wild and Primitive Potatoes for Modern Crop Improvement. *Genes,* 6: 1300–1314

Rodrigo, S., Santamaria, O., Chen, Y., McGrath, S. P., and Poblaciones, M. J. 2014. Selenium speciation in malt, wort, and beer made from selenium-biofortified two-rowed barley grain. *J Agric Food Chem,* 62: 5948–5953

Salvador, E. M. 2015. Development of iron fortified cassava mahewu. Doctoral dissertation, University of Pretoria. South Africa

Samoraj, M., Tuhy, Ł., Baśladyńska, S., and Chojnacka, K. 2015. Biofortification of maize grains with micronutrients by enriched biomass of blackcurrant seeds. *Open Chem, 13*(1): 1236–1244

Sautter, C., Poletti, S., Zhang, P., and Gruissem, W. 2006. Biofortification of essential nutritional compounds and trace elements in rice and cassava. *Proc Nutr Soc,* 65: 153–159

Sayre, R., Beeching, J. R., Cahoon, E. B., Egesi, C., Fauquet, C., Fellman, J., and Maziya-Dixon, B. 2011. The BioCassava plus program: biofortification of cassava for sub-Saharan Africa. *Ann Rev Plant Biol, 62*: 251–272

Shikov, V., Kammerer, D. R., Mihalev, K., Mollov, P., and Carle, R. 2012. Antioxidant capacity and colour stability of texture-improved canned strawberries as affected by the addition of rose (Rosa damascena Mill.) petal extracts. *Food Research International, 46*(2): 552–556

Shivay, Y. S., Prasad, R., and Pal, M. 2013. Zinc fortification of oat grains through zinc fertilisation. *Agric Res,* 2(4): 375–381

Shrimpton, R., Gross, R., Darnton-Hill, I., and Young, M. 2005. Zinc deficiency: what are the most appropriate interventions? *BMJ,* 330:347–349

Skarpa, P. 2013. Fortification of sunflower plants (helianthus annuus l.) With selenium. The Journal of Microbiology, *Biotechnology and Food Sciences,* 2(1): 1569–1579

Smoleń, S., Kowalska, I., and Sady, W. 2014. Assessment of biofortification with iodine and selenium of lettuce cultivated in the NFT hydroponic system. *Scientia Horticulturae, 166*: 9–16

Sperotto, R. A., Ricachenevsky, F. K., de Abreu Waldow, V., and Fett, J. P. 2012. Iron biofortification in rice: it's a long way to the top. *Plant Sci,* 190: 24–39

Tarabella, A., and Burchi, B. 2012. Enriched foodstuff on basis of European regulations N. 1924 and N. 1925 Introduced in 2006: An analysis of consumer protection. *Int J Econ Pract Theor,* 2(1): 28–35

Tuhy, Ł., Samoraj, M., Witkowska, Z., and Chojnacka, K. 2015. Biofortification of maize with micronutrients by Spirulina. *Open Chem, 13*(1): 1119–1126

Velu, G., Rai, K. N., Muralidharan, V., Kulkarni, V. N., Longvah, T., and Raveendran, T. S. 2007. Prospects of breeding biofortified pearl millet with high grain iron and zinc content. *Plant Breed, 126*(2): 182–185

Wei, Y., Shohag, M. J. I., Wang, Y., Lu, L., Wu, C., and Yang, X. 2012. Effect of zinc sulfate fortification in germinated brown rice on seed zinc concentration, bioavailability, and seed germination. *Journal of agricultural and food chemistry, 60*(7): 1871–1879

Younas, M. S., Butt, M. S., Pasha, I., and Shahid, M. 2014. Development of zinc fortified chitosan and alginate based coatings for apricot. *Pak J Agri Sci, 51*(4): 1033–1039

Zhang, Y., Fu, C. X., Liu, F., Fan, X. D., Yan, Y. J., Wang, Y. A., and Zhang, Y. P. 2013. Effects of Aerial Zinc Application on Carbohydrate Metabolism-related Enzymes Activities in Apple Fruit. *Acta Horticulturae Sinica, 8*: 3

Index

C

F

G

H

I

L